NUTRACEUTICALS IN CARDIAC HEALTH MANAGEMENT

AAP Advances in Nutraceuticals

NUTRACEUTICALS IN CARDIAC HEALTH MANAGEMENT

Raj K. Keservani, PhD
Rajesh K. Kesharwani, PhD
Praveen Kumar Jain, PhD
Bhushan R. Rane, PhD
Nayan A. Gujarathi, PhD
Editors

AAP APPLE ACADEMIC PRESS

First edition published 2025

Apple Academic Press Inc.
1265 Goldenrod Circle, NE,
Palm Bay, FL 32905 USA

760 Laurentian Drive, Unit 19,
Burlington, ON L7N 0A4, CANADA

CRC Press
2385 NW Executive Center Drive,
Suite 320, Boca Raton FL 33431

4 Park Square, Milton Park,
Abingdon, Oxon, OX14 4RN UK

Library and Archives Canada Cataloguing in Publication

Title: Nutraceuticals in cardiac health management / Raj K. Keservani, PhD, Rajesh K. Kesharwani, PhD, Praveen Kumar Jain, PhD, Bhushan R. Rane, PhD, Nayan A. Gujarathi, PhD, editors.
Names: Keservani, Raj K., 1981- editor | Kesharwani, Rajesh Kumar, 1978- editor | Jain, Praveen Kumar, editor. | Rane, Bhushan R., editor. | Gujarathi, Nayan A., 1980- editor.
Series: AAP advances in nutraceuticals.
Description: First edition. | Series statement: AAP advances in nutraceuticals | Includes bibliographical references and index.
Identifiers: Canadiana (print) 20240460189 | Canadiana (ebook) 20240460219 | ISBN 9781774917565 (hardcover) | ISBN 9781774917572 (softcover) | ISBN 9781003545644 (ebook)
Subjects: LCSH: Heart—Diseases—Diet therapy. | LCSH: Heart—Diseases—Prevention. | LCSH: Functional foods—Therapeutic use. | LCSH: Medicine, Preventive.
Classification: LCC RC684.D5 N88 2025 | DDC 616.1/20654—dc23

Library of Congress Cataloging-in-Publication Data

CIP data on file with US Library of Congress

ISBN: 978-1-77491-756-5 (hbk)
ISBN: 978-1-77491-757-2 (pbk)
ISBN: 978-1-00354-564-4 (ebk)

ABOUT THE BOOK SERIES: AAP ADVANCES IN NUTRACEUTICALS

Series Editor:
Raj K. Keservani, PhD, MPharm
Faculty of B. Pharmacy, CSM Group of Institutions, Allahabad, India

Rajesh K. Kesharwani, PhD
Nehru Gram Bharati (Deemed to be University), Prayagraj, India

Anil K. Sharma, PhD, MPharm
Department of Pharmacy, School of Medical and Allied Sciences,
GD Goenka University, Gurugram, India

In the modern era, mankind has witnessed a paradigm shift with respect to fundamental eating behavior. The lack of physical workouts and busy schedules at offices and in households have promoted the consumption of junk foods, which eventually results in numerous diseases and disorders since the nutritional content from fast food is inadequate. Plumpness and obesity have become a global health threat. The leading causes of death from most developing nations are noncommunicable diseases such as cardiovascular diseases, cancer, arthritis, osteoporosis, and liver toxicity. Patients suffering from such lifestyle ailments are a bit apprehensive towards prolonged use of costly modern therapeutics, which encourages instead the use of alternative approaches for management of such diseases and disorders.

The emerging sector of the nutraceutical industry encompasses products derived from nature, dietary supplements, and functional foods. Nutraceuticals are used for treatment and prevention of a broad range of diseases, such as the common cold, arthritis, sleep-related disorders, cancers, cardiovascular complications, metabolic disorders, and others.

The research on nutraceuticals is increasing day by day, considering the beneficial effects of food or food supplements in the management of diverse diseases. The issue of paramount concern is standardization and establishment of clinical efficacy of nutraceuticals, which is in fact a challenge for researchers around the globe.

This book series aims at realizing the significance of the variety of nutraceuticals for human well-being. The books in the series also emphasize the role of dieticians and nutritionists for the prescription of judicious eating habits. The key food components such as carbohydrates, proteins, and lipids as well as micronutrients (vitamins, minerals) are demonstrated to maintain good health, obviating the need for medicines. Thus, nutraceuticals that are indeed derived from food ingredients are believed to be potential alternative therapeutics.

Asymptomatic diseases/disorders necessitate proper diagnosis. Stressed circumstances have been reported to cause weight loss. Workplace stress is a key variable in the genesis and propagation of metabolic disorders. The nuances of the underlying mechanisms are still to be deciphered. Poor lifestyle trends have been attributed along with the consumption of junk foods in several such instances. Sugar-rich carbonated beverages, the use of contraband drugs, and the consumption of liquor in excess are assigned as risk factors. This book series covers advances and applications in addition to providing the basics of nutraceuticals.

The books in this series are valuable resources for industry professionals to design and develop quality products for end users. In addition, the book series is fortified by ideas of innovation, concept building, manufacturing aspects, quality control, and regulatory status of nutraceuticals.

Ostensibly, business has seen a rise in the nutraceutical consumption in recent years. Pure, safe, efficacious products are the need of the hour globally. There are a number of books on nutraceuticals in the market, yet these are only a few books presenting certain aspects of nutraceuticals therein. This book series offers a holistic view of this promising strategy, which is picking up pace with time. This book series is a unique endeavor to bring manufacturing, research and development, and marketing strategies under a single umbrella.

CURRENT BOOKS IN THE SERIES

- **Micronutrients and Macronutrients as Nutraceuticals**
  Editors: Prakash Chandra Gupta, PhD, Sayan Bhattacharyya, MBBS, MD, Nisha Sharma, PhD, MPharm, Rajesh K. Kesharwani, PhD, and Raj K. Keservani, PhD, MPharm
- **Formulations, Regulations, and Challenges of Nutraceuticals**
  Editors: Tingirikari Jagan Mohan Rao, PhD, Rajesh K. Kesharwani, PhD, Raj. K. Keservani, PhD, and Anil K. Sharma, PhD

- **Food Supplements and Dietary Fibers in Health and Disease**
  Editors: Bhushan R. Rane, PhD, MPharm, Raj K. Keservani, PhD, MPharm, Durgesh Singh, DPhil, Nayan A. Gujarathi, PhD, and Ashish S. Jain, PhD
- **Nutraceuticals in Cancer Prevention, Management, and Treatment**
  Editors: Raj K. Keservani, PhD, MPharm Bui Thanh Tung, PhD, Sippy Singh, DPhil, and Rajesh K. Kesharwani, PhD
- **Advances in Flavonoids for Human Health and Prevention of Diseases**
  Editors: Nisha Sharma, PhD, Deepika Saini, PhD, Rajesh K. Kesharwani, PhD, Prakash Chandra Gupta, and Raj. K. Keservani, PhD
- **The Flavonoids: Extraction and Applications**
  Editors: Deepika Saini, PhD, Rajesh K. Kesharwani, PhD, and Raj K. Keservani, PhD, MPharm
- **Immune-Boosting Nutraceuticals for Better Human Health: Novel Applications**
  Editors: Urmila Jarouliya, PhD, Raj K. Keservani, PhD, MPharm Rajesh K. Kesharwani, PhD, Virendra K. Patel, PhD, and Adi D. Bharti
- **Applications of Functional Foods in Disease Prevention**
  Editors: Raj K. Keservani, PhD, MPharm, and Eknath D. Ahire, MSPharm
- **Plant Metabolites and Vegetables as Nutraceuticals**
  Editors: Raj K. Keservani, PhD, MPharm, Bui Thanh Tung, PhD, Rajesh K. Kesharwani, PhD, MPharm, and Eknath D. Ahire
- **Preventive and Therapeutic Role of Vitamins as Nutraceuticals**
  Editors: Khemchand R. Surana, Eknath D. Ahire, Raj K. Keservani, PhD, MPharm, and Rajesh K. Kesharwani, PhD
- **Nutraceuticals and Bone Health**
  Editors: Deepak Sharma, PhD, Madan Mohan Gupta, PhD, Anil K. Sharma, PhD, MPharm, Raj K. Keservani, PhD, MPharm, and Rajesh K. Kesharwani, PhD
- **Flavonoids as Nutraceuticals**
  Editors: Rajesh K. Kesharwani, PhD, MTech, Deepika Saini, PhD, Raj K. Keservani, PhD, MPharm, and Anil Kumar Sharma, PhD
- **Herbals as Nutraceuticals: Their Role in Healthcare**
  Editors: Raj K. Keservani, PhD, MPharm, Rajeshwar Kamal Kant Arya, PhD, and Rajesh K. Kesharwani, PhD

- **Nutraceutical Fruits: Overview and Disease Prevention**
  Editors: Raj K. Keservani, PhD, MPharm
- **Nutrigenomics and Nutraceuticals**
  Editors: Raj K. Keservani, PhD, MPharm, Eknath D. Ahire, Shubham J. Khainar, PhD, Sanjay J. Kshirsagar, PhD, and Rajesh K. Kesharwani, PhD
- **Nutraceuticals in Cardiac Health Management**
  Editors: Raj K. Keservani, PhD, MPharm, Rajesh K. Kesharwani, PhD, Praveen Kumar Jain, PhD, Bhushan R. Rane, PhD, and Nayan A. Gujarathi, PhD
- **Nutraceuticals for the Treatment and Prevention of Sexual Disorders**
  Editors: Raj K. Keservani, PhD, MPharm, Sharangouda J. Patil, PhD, and Ivan Aranha, PhD
- **Nutraceuticals in Obesity Management and Control**
  Editors: Raj K. Keservani, PhD, MPharm, and Alka Lohani, PhD
- **The Nature of Nutraceuticals: History, Properties, Sources, and Nanotechnology**
  Editors: Rajesh K. Kesharwani, PhD, Prashant Kumar, PhD, and Raj K. Keservani, PhD, MPharm
- **Nutraceuticals in Insomnia and Sleep Problems**
  Editors: Raj K. Keservani, PhD, MPharm, Sayan Bhattacharyya, PhD, and Rajesh K. Kesharwani, PhD
- **Nutraceuticals in Respiratory and Pulmonary Diseases**
  Editors: Deepika Saini, PhD, Rajesh K. Kesharwani, PhD, and Raj K. Keservani, PhD, MPharm
- **Nutraceuticals in Arthritis and Psoriasis**
  Editors: Meenakshi Jaiswal, PhD, Raj K. Keservani, PhD, MPharm Rajesh K. Kesharwani, PhD, and Swati G. Talele, PhD
- **Nutraceuticals for the Treatment and Prevention of Sexual Disorders**
  Editors: Raj K. Keservani, PhD, Sharangouda J. Patil, PhD, and Ivan Aranha, PhD
- **Antioxidants as Nutraceuticals**
  Editors: Nayan A. Gujaratih, PhD, Raj K. Keservani, PhD, Rajesh K. Kesharwani, PhD, Bhushan R. Rane, PhD, and Yogeeta Sameer Goyal, PhD

- **Nutraceuticals in Management and Prevention of Diabetes**
  Editors: Raj K. Keservani, PhD, Prashant Kumar, PhD, and Dheeraj Chitara, PhD
- **Nutraceuticals in Mental Disorder and Brain Health**
  Editors: Raj K. Keservani, PhD, Eknath D. Ahire, PhD, and Shubham J. Khairnar, PhD

ABOUT THE EDITORS

Raj K. Keservani, PhD
Associate Professor, Faculty of BPharmacy, CSM Group of Institutions, Prayagraj, Uttar Pradesh, India

Raj K. Keservani, PhD, MPharm, is an Associate Professor in the Faculty of B. Pharmacy at CSM Group of Institutions, Prayagraj, India. He has more than 12 years of academic (teaching) experience from various institutes of India in pharmaceutical education. He has supervised more than 25 undergradate students for their research work and has published 31 peer-reviewed papers in the field of pharmaceutical sciences in national and international journals, one patent, 50 book chapters, three co-authored books, and 40 edited books. He is also active as a reviewer for several international scientific journals. Dr. Keservani is a life member of Society of Pharmaceutical Education and Research (SPER). His research interests include nutraceutical and functional foods, novel drug delivery systems (NDDS), transdermal drug delivery/drug delivery, health science, cancer biology, and neurobiology. Dr. Keservani graduated with a pharmacy degree from the Department of Pharmacy, Kumaun University, Nainital (Uttarakhand), India. He received his Master of Pharmacy (specialization in pharmaceutics) from the School of Pharmaceutical Sciences, Rajiv Gandhi Proudyogiki Vishwavidyalaya, Bhopal, India. He received his PhD degree from IKG Punjab Technical University, Jalandhar, Punjab, India.

Rajesh K. Kesharwani, PhD
Associate Professor, Department of Computer Application, Nehru Gram Bharati (Deemed to be University), Prayagraj, Uttar Pradesh, India

Rajesh K. Kesharwani, PhD, MTech, is working as an Associate Professor, Department of Computer Application, Nehru Gram Bharati (Deemed to be University), Prayagraj, India. He has more than 11 years of research and nine years of teaching experience at various institutes of India, imparting bioinformatics and biotechnology education. He has received several awards, including the NASI-Swarna Jayanti Puruskar by The National Academy of Sciences of India. He has supervised one PhD and more than 20 undergraduate and graduate students for their research work. Dr. Kesharwani has authored over 49 peer-reviewed articles, 20 book chapters, and 14 edited books with international publishers. He has been a member of many scientific communities as well as a reviewer for many international journals. He has presented many papers at various national and international conferences. He has been a recipient of a Ministry of Human Resource Development (India) Fellowship and a Senior Research Fellowship from the Indian Council of Medical Research, India. His research fields of interest are medical informatics, protein structure and function prediction, computer-aided drug designing, structural biology, drug delivery, cancer biology, nanobiotechnology, and biomedical sciences. Dr. Kesharwani received his PhD from the Indian Institute of Information Technology, Allahabad, and worked at NIT Warangal for two semesters.

Praveen Kumar Jain, PhD
Principal and Professor, Malhotra College of Pharmacy, Bhopal, Madhya Pradesh, India

Praveen Kumar Jain, PhD, MPharm, is working as a Principal and Professor at Malhotra College of Pharmacy, Airport Bypass Road, Bhopal, Madhya Pradesh, India. Dr. Jain has more than 15 years of teaching experience. He has published papers in national and international journals, presented papers at national and international seminars and conferences, and attended many workshops. Dr. Jain completed his graduation at the Institute of Pharmacy, Jiwaji University, M. P., India, in 2002 and earned a Master of Pharmacy from RGTU, Bhopal, India in 2007. His doctoral degree is from Suresh Gyan Vihar University, Jaipur, India, in 2019. His research interest includes nutraceuticals and novel drug delivery system.

Bhushan R. Rane, PhD
Professor and Head, Department of Pharmaceutics,
Shri D.D. Vispute College of Pharmacy & Research Centre,
New Panvel, Navi Mumbai, India, India

Bhushan R. Rane, PhD, MPharm, is presently working as a Professor and Head of the Department of Pharmaceutics, Shri D. D. Vispute College of

Pharmacy and Research Center, New Panvel, Navi Mumbai, India, which is affiliated with Mumbai University, Maharashtra, India. He has over 14 years of teaching experience at undergraduate and postgraduate levels, and, to date, he has guided more than 50 MPharm students. He has published more than 75 peer-reviewed research and review articles in national and international journals as well as co-authored eight books and more than 15 book chapters. He is a reviewer for several scientific and international journals. He has received grants from various APEX bodies for research, such as the All India Council for Technical Education, for his work. He is a lifetime member of several organizations. His research interests are focused on planning, improvement, and portrayal of vesicular, microparticulate, nanoparticulate systems, and advancement of different solid dosage forms for oral conveyance.

Nayan A. Gujarathi, PhD
Assistant Professor, Department of Pharmaceutics,
Shri Vile Parle Kelavani Mandal's Institute of Pharmacy, Dhule,
Maharashtra, India

Nayan A. Gujarathi, PhD, MPharm, is an Assistant Professor in the Department of Pharmaceutics at Shri Vile Parle Kelavani Mandal's Institute of Pharmacy, Dhule, India. He has 13 years of academic experience in pharmaceutical science. He has published over 30 peer-reviewed papers in the field of pharmaceutical sciences in national and international journals as well as several book chapters. He has presented his research work at an international conference organized by the Controlled Release Society and delivered several expert talks on outcome-based education for the accreditation process. His research interest encompasses novel drug delivery systems, polymer science, nanotechnology, and nutraceuticals.

CONTENTS

Contributors .... *xvii*
Preface .... *xxi*

PART I: Nutraceuticals and Functional Foods in Heart Disease........1

1. **Functional Foods in the Prevention of Cardiovascular Disease........3**
   Supriya Ray and Suresh B. Arakera

2. **Nutraceuticals for Cardiovascular Health and Diseases: Introduction and Overview........27**
   Bhushan R. Rane, Ashish S. Jain, Nidhi S. Kate, Samali S. Raut, Raj K. Keservani, Vinit S. Patil, Arvind Kumar Gupta, and Jaffar Shaik

PART II: Cardioprotective Activity of Different Nutrients........49

3. **Role of Probiotics and Dietary Fibers in Combating Heart Disease........51**
   Deepanshu Rana, Shrivardhan Dheeman, and Nidhi S. Belwal

4. **Benefits of Garlic in Cardiovascular Disease........69**
   Peeush Singhal, Ritu Vishnoi,Manisha,Vivek Srivastava, Somesh Thapliyal, and Vijay Jyoti Kumar

5. **Health Benefits of Green Tea: A Review........85**
   Niharika Dewangan

6. **Role of Vitamins in Heart Disease........103**
   Ababio Grace K.

7. **Nutraceutical Intervention of Tomato and Lycopene in Heart Disease........121**
   Tarkeshwar, Pradip Kumar Saini, Vikash Kumar Singh, Subash Chand Vimal, and Jitender Bhati

8. **Nutraceutical Potential of Lycopene and Tomatoes........139**
   Neha Saini, Ittishree Bhardwaj, and Ritu Kataria

9. **Role of Nutraceuticals in Dyslipidemia........151**
   Vipin Nautiyal and Deepanshu Rana

10. Role of Nutraceuticals in Hypertension 167
Ababio Grace K.

11. Dietary Supplementation and Cardiac Health 177
Bhushan R. Rane, Nidhi S. Kate, Akash J. Amkar, Jaffar Shaik, Amit Kumar Nayak, and Raj K. Keservani

12. Cardioprotective Effects of Bee Products: An Evidence-Based Review 201
Myrene Roselyn D'souza

PART III: Cardiotonic Activity of Polyphenols 219

13. Effects of Polyphenols on Hypertension 221
Ababio Grace K.

14. Cardioprotective Potential of Dietary Phytochemicals Present in the Medicinal Foods of Kerala, South India: A Review 233
S. R. Suja, Shobha Bhaskar, B. S. Bijukumar, and R. Prakashkumar

PART IV: Marine-Derived Nutrients in Cardiovascular 265

15. Role of Spirulina Supplementation and Other Nutraceuticals in Cardiovascular Disease 267
Charu Gupta

16. Endothelial Effects of Marine and Plant-Derived Omega-3 Fatty Acids 297
Deepanshu Rana and Vikash Singh Jadon

17. Marine-Derived Natural Flavonoids and Their Biological Activities 311
Aarti Tiwari, Vimal Kumar Yadav, Sandeep Kumar Singh, Ajay Kumar Shukla, and Manish Kumar

Index 327

CONTRIBUTORS

Akash J. Amkar
Shri D.D. Vispute College of Pharmacy and Research Center, Devad-Vichumbe, Panvel, Navi Mumbai, Maharashtra, India

Suresh B. Arakera
Department of Applied Genetics, Karnatak University Dharwad, Karnataka, India

Nidhi S. Belwal
Department of Microbiology, School of Life Sciences, Sardar Bhagwan Singh University, Balawala, Dehradun, Uttarakhand, India

Ittishree Bhardwaj
G.V.M. College of Pharmacy, Sonipat, Haryana, India

Shobha Bhaskar
Ethnomedicine and Ethnopharmacology Division, Jawaharlal Nehru Tropical Botanic Garden and Research Institute (JNTBGRI), Thiruvananthapuram, Kerala, India

Jitender Bhati
Assistant Professor, Department of Genetics and Plant Breeding, Chandra Shekhar Azad University of Agriculture and Technology, Kanpur, Uttar Pradesh, India

B. S. Bijukumar
Post-Graduate Department of Zoology and Research Center, Mahatma Gandhi College, Thiruvananthapuram, Kerala, India

Myrene Roselyn D'souza
Department of Biochemistry, Mount Carmel College Autonomous, Karnataka, India

Niharika Dewangan
Shri Shankaracharya Professional University, Bhilai, Chhattisgarh, India

Shrivardhan Dheeman
Department of Microbiology, School of Life Sciences, Sardar Bhagwan Singh University, Balawala, Dehradun, Uttarakhand, India

Arvind Kumar Gupta
Faculty of B. Pharmacy, CSM Group of Institutions, Prayagraj, Uttar Pradesh, India

Charu Gupta
Amity Institute of Herbal Research and Studies, Amity University, Noida, Uttar Pradesh, India

Vikash Singh Jadon
Department of Biochemistry and Biotechnology, School of Life Sciences, Sardar Bhagwan Singh University, Balawala, Dehradun, Uttarakhand, India

Ashish S. Jain
Shri D.D. Vispute College of Pharmacy and Research Center, Devad-Vichumbe, Panvel, Navi Mumbai, Maharashtra, India

Ababio Grace K.
University of Ghana Medical School, Medical Biochemistry, Ghana, Africa

Ritu Kataria
G.V.M. College of Pharmacy, Sonipat, Haryana, India

Nidhi S. Kate
Shri D.D. Vispute College of Pharmacy and Research Center, Devad-Vichumbe, Panvel, Navi Mumbai, Maharashtra, India

Raj K. Keservani
Faculty of B. Pharmacy, CSM Group of Institutions, Prayagraj, Uttar Pradesh, India

Manish Kumar
Department of Pharmacy, Madhav University, Pindwara, Rajasthan, India

Vijay Jyoti Kumar
Department of Pharmaceutical Sciences, H.N.B. Garhwal Central University, Srinagar, Uttarakhand, India

Manisha
Department of Botany, Chinmaya Degree College, Haridwar, Uttarakhand, India

Vipin Nautiyal
Assistant Professor, Department of Paramedical Sciences, Uttaranchal (P.G.) College of Biomedical Sciences and Hospital, Dehradun, Uttarakhand, India

Amit Kumar Nayak
Department of Pharmacy, School of Medical and Allied Sciences, GD Goenka University, Gurgaon, Haryana, India

Vinit S. Patil
Shri D.D. Vispute College of Pharmacy and Research Center, Devad-Vichumbe, Panvel, Navi Mumbai, Maharashtra, India

R. Prakashkumar
Ethnomedicine and Ethnopharmacology Division, Jawaharlal Nehru Tropical Botanic Garden and Research Institute (JNTBGRI), Thiruvananthapuram, Kerala, India

Deepanshu Rana
Assistant Professor, Department of Microbiology, School of Life Sciences, Sardar Bhagwan Singh University, Balawala, Dehradun, Uttarakhand, India

Bhushan R. Rane
Shri D.D. Vispute College of Pharmacy and Research Center, Devad-Vichumbe, Panvel, Navi Mumbai, Maharashtra, India

Samali S. Raut
Shri D.D. Vispute College of Pharmacy and Research Center, Devad-Vichumbe, Panvel, Navi Mumbai, Maharashtra, India

Supriya Ray
Department of Applied Genetics, Karnatak University Dharwad, Karnataka, India

Neha Saini
G.V.M. College of Pharmacy, Sonipat, Haryana, India

Pradip Kumar Saini
Research Scholar, Crop Physiology, Acharya Narendra Deva University of Agriculture and Technology, Ayodhya, Uttar Pradesh, India

Jaffar Shaik
Research Scholar, Department of Biochemistry, Acharya Nagarjuna University, Guntur, Andhra Pradesh, India

Ajay Kumar Shukla
Institute of Pharmacy, Dr. Ram Manohar Lohia Avadh University, Ayodhya, Uttar Pradesh, India

Sandeep Kumar Singh
Institute of Pharmacy, Dr. Ram Manohar Lohia Avadh University, Ayodhya, Uttar Pradesh, India

Vikash Kumar Singh
Research Scholar, Vegetable Science, Acharya Narendra Deva University of Agriculture and Technology, Ayodhya, Uttar Pradesh, India

Peeush Singhal
Department of Pharmaceutical Sciences, Gurukul Kangri Deemed University, Haridwar, Uttarakhand, India

Vivek Srivastava
Amity Institute of Pharmacy, Amity University Lucknow Campus, Malhaur, Gomti Nagar Extension, Lucknow, Uttar Pradesh, India

S. R. Suja
Ethnomedicine and Ethnopharmacology Division, Jawaharlal Nehru Tropical Botanic Garden and Research Institute (JNTBGRI), Thiruvananthapuram, Kerala, India

Tarkeshwar
Research Scholar, Department of Genetics and Plant Breeding, Acharya Narendra Deva University of Agriculture and Technology, Ayodhya, Uttar Pradesh, India

Somesh Thapliyal
Department of Pharmaceutical Sciences, H.N.B. Garhwal Central University, Srinagar, Uttarakhand, India

Aarti Tiwari
Institute of Pharmacy, Dr. Ram Manohar Lohia Avadh University, Ayodhya, Uttar Pradesh, India

Subash Chand Vimal
Professor and Head, Department of Genetics and Plant Breeding, Acharya Narendra Deva University of Agriculture and Technology, Ayodhya, Uttar Pradesh, India

Ritu Vishnoi
Department of Botany, Chinmaya Degree College, Haridwar, Uttarakhand, India

Vimal Kumar Yadav
Institute of Pharmacy, Dr. Ram Manohar Lohia Avadh University, Ayodhya, Uttar Pradesh, India

PREFACE

Nutraceuticals are natural nutritional substances that have been demonstrated to be effective in illness prevention or therapy. Multiple foods and nutraceuticals have been proven to reduce the risk of cardiovascular disease. This book presents an update on the most recent scientific evidence addressing the use of nutraceuticals in the prevention and management of heart disease.

Hypertension is the leading common cardiovascular disease risk factor, comprising coronary artery disease, cardiac arrest, infarction, strokes, final kidney problems, and sexual dysfunction. Worldwide, cardiovascular diseases (CVDs) constitute the major cause of death, and their etiology has multiple factors, including dietary patterns, that have been linked to their emergence. There has been increasing interest in research connecting the healthful benefits of food with the prevention and treatment of a diverse range of ailments.

This book, *Nutraceuticals in Cardiac Health Management,* comprises 17 chapters in four sections that demonstrates various nutraceutical components such as dietary fibers, garlic, green tea, vitamins, tomato, lycopene, bee products, and polyphenols used in the management and prevention of cardiovascular and hypertension of human being.

Chapter 1: Functional Foods in Prevention of Cardiovascular Disease, written by Supriya Ray and her colleagues, summarizes the various functional foods that are involved in preventing the risk of CVD (cardiovascular disease), the mechanism of the bioactive components that lower the risk of chronic illness as well as CVD and the dietary patterns that are involved in the prevention of CVD.

Chapter 2: Nutraceuticals for Cardiovascular Health and Diseases: Introduction and Overview, written by Bhushan R. Rane and his associates, provides an update on the most recent studies about the use of nutritional supplements in the prevention and treatment of cardiovascular disease.

Chapter 3: Role of Probiotics and Dietary Fibers in Heart Diseases, written by Deepanshu Rana and his associates, emphasizes the importance of both supplements as an alternative to maintaining a healthy lifestyle as prophylaxis to cardiovascular diseases.

Peeush Singhal et al. discusses that garlic is generally safe, but there have been a few reports of unusual adverse effects with little evidence of causality, in Chapter 4: Role of Garlic in Heart Diseases.

Increasing attention is being shown on the cardiovascular benefits of green tea due to the rising popularity of tea's health benefits and the huge increase in scientific research, as reported by Niharika Dewangan in Chapter 5: Health Benefits of Green Tea: A Review.

Grace K. Ababio wrote Chapter 6: Role of Vitamins in Heart Diseases and discusses antioxidant properties of vitamin C and presents a conceptual framework for vitamin E, which seems consistent with the literature.

Chapter 7: Nutraceutical Intervention of Tomato and Lycopene in Heart Disease, written by Tarkeshwar et al., summarizes what has been learned in recent years about lycopene's function in the prevention of cardiovascular diseases.

Chapter 8: Nutraceutical Potential of Lycopene and Tomatoes, written by Neha Saini and their coworkers, concludes that the use of lycopene decreases the incidence of heart disorders and also oxidative stress in an individual. Lycopene has acted to treat diseases in various mechanisms such as an antioxidant, photoprotection, anti-angiogenesis, immunomodulation, anti-inflammatory, induction, and apoptosis.

Vipin Nautiyal and Deepanshu Rana report on the lipid-lowering effects of nutraceutical bioactives in Chapter 9: Role of Nutraceuticals in Dyslipidemia.

As efforts are made to avoid toxicity, the ultimate choice includes the paradigm shift using nutraceuticals to promote long-term dietary compliance management of hypertension, which is discussed in Chapter 10: Role of Nutraceuticals in Hypertension, written by Grace K. Ababio.

Chapter 11: Dietary Supplementation and Cardiac Health, written by Bhushan R. Rane and their associates, discusses the significance of dietary supplements such as fish oil, ginseng, garlic, green tea, co-enzyme Q, omega-3 fatty acid, vitamin C, and vitamin E in heart health.

Chapter 12: Effects of Bee Products: An Evidence-Based Review,"written by Myrene Roselyn D'souza, discusses the composition of a variety of natural bee products, as well as the active biological effects in ameliorating symptoms of cardiovascular disease.

Chapter 13: Effects of Polyphenols in Hypertension, written by Grace K. Ababio, discusses the beneficial effects of polyphenols in hypertension.

Suja S. R. et al. highlights the dietary phytochemicals with cardioprotective potential present in the ingredients of some traditional foods of Kerala, their effects, and mechanisms of action, in Chapter 14: Cardioprotective Potential of Dietary Phytochemicals Present in the Medicinal Foods of Kerala, South India: A Review.

Charu Gupta and Dhan Prakash wrote Chapter 15: Role of Spirulina Supplementation and Other Nutraceuticals in Cardiovascular Disease, which provides an overview of the current knowledge of the health-promoting functions of spirulina and other nutraceuticals against cardiovascular disease, which are major health threats in the developed countries.

Deepanshu Rana and Vikash Singh Jadon discuss the potential effect of plant- and marine-derived omega-3 fatty acids as a source for ALA, which further elongates into EPA and DHA in Chapter 16: Endothelial Effects of Marine- and Plant-Derived Omega-3 Fatty Acids.

Ajay Kumar Shukla and his colleagues provide information about the biological activity of marine-derived natural flavonoids in Chapter 17: Marine-Derived Natural Flavonoids and Their Biological Activity.

PART I

NUTRACEUTICALS AND FUNCTIONAL FOODS IN HEART DISEASE

CHAPTER 1

FUNCTIONAL FOODS IN THE PREVENTION OF CARDIOVASCULAR DISEASE

SUPRIYA RAY and SURESH B. ARAKERA

Department of Applied Genetics, Karnatak University Dharwad, Karnataka, India

ABSTRACT

Cardiovascular diseases are the leading cause of high mortality rates globally and are a thriving health concern. Several lifestyle factors such as a healthy diet, proper nutrition, and regular exercise play a significant role in the pathogenesis, prevention, and treatment of cardiovascular diseases (CVD). Functional foods consist of active food components that impart health benefits beyond basic nutrition. Functional foods have been found to be beneficial in the prevention and treatment of CVD and other chronic diseases such as cancer, asthma, and many more. The protective mechanism of functional foods involves certain diets rich in fruits and vegetables, fish, whole grains, nuts, plant sterols and stanols, flaxseed, and diets low in saturated fat and sodium, which lower blood pressure, oxidation of low-density lipoprotein, inhibit platelet aggregation, and reduce blood lipid cholesterol, hence reducing the risk of CVD. This chapter summarizes the various functional foods that are involved in preventing the risk of CVD, the mechanism of the bioactive components that lower the risk of chronic illness as well as CVD, and the dietary patterns that are involved in the prevention of CVD.

Antioxidants as Nutraceuticals. Nayan A. Gujarathi, Raj K. Keservani, Rajesh K. Kesharwani, Bhushan R. Rane, Yogeeta Sameer Goyal (Eds.)

1.1 INTRODUCTION

Globally, cardiovascular diseases (CVD), diabetes, cancers, and respiratory illnesses, commonly non-communicable diseases, account for 60% of all deaths. Ischemic heart disease and stroke are the major causes of 17.7 million deaths. According to the World Health Organization (WHO), India accounts for one-fifth of the deaths in the younger population worldwide (WHO, 2016; Prabhakaran et al., 2016). In 2016, CVD alone led to 28.1% of deaths and 14.1% of disability-adjusted life years (DALYs) in India. The states with the highest rates of CVD, cholesterol levels, and blood pressure are Kerala, Tamil Nadu, and Punjab (Ruhil, 2018). The major risk factors for CVD include hypertension, diabetes, smoking, advancing age, obesity, hyperlipidemia, genetic risk factors, dietary habits, lack of exercise, and metabolic syndrome. Among all the risk factors investigated, dietary factors are playing a key role in leading to high CVD risk factors among people (Kumar & Sinha, 2020).

Poor dietary habits among people in urban areas of India have led to obesity, which is further associated with the development of hypertension, ischemic heart disease, diabetes, stroke, cancer, and arthritis. The prevalence of obesity, diabetes, and hypertension is increasing rapidly in urban areas. Studies have shown that Asians are less involved in regular physical activity and lead a sedentary lifestyle compared to Caucasian people (Kumar & Sinha, 2020). Several epidemiological studies have revealed that dietary habits and maintaining a healthy lifestyle can prevent the risk of cardiovascular diseases. In accordance with the report of WHO, people who consume more fruits and vegetables along with fish are less susceptible to the risk of having CVD rather than people who consume more junk foods containing saturated fats. These findings of WHO brought a revolution in people's dietary practices, choosing not only a healthy lifestyle by fulfilling the nutritional requirements but also reducing the level of cholesterol in their daily intake (Meier et al., 2019). The levels of sodium and saturated fats in people's diets led to an increase in the incidence of CVDs, which has been significantly explored in various studies (McGill, 1979).

Many studies have demonstrated that Nutraceuticals or Functional Foods (Keservani et al., 2010a, b) have a preventive effect on the incidence of CVD. The term "Functional Foods" still lacks a proper definition of its own and is still used in marketing (Bjelakovic & Gluud, 2007). The term functional food can be defined as foods that are not only important for the body but are also involved in solving the ailing state of the body through various action mechanisms that go beyond the supply of basic nutrition. The mechanisms involved in resolving the ill state of the body include lowering low-density lipoprotein cholesterol and total blood cholesterol (Boussageon et al., 2011). Therefore, this chapter highlights functional foods that are involved in the prevention of chronic illnesses such as CVD, the use and mechanism of different bioactive compounds that have a beneficial and protective role in CVD, and the dietary patterns that are involved in the prevention of CVD as well as other diseases (Keservani et al., 2016a).

1.2 FUNCTIONAL FOODS WITH PREVENTIVE EFFECTS

American Dietetic Association highlighted the beneficial effect of functional foods in 2014. It emphasized that functional foods must be included as fortified, enriched, enhanced, or in whole food forms. The major cause of CVD and other disorders like cancer is due to oxidative stress. The antioxidant property can be achieved endogenously or exogenously through food. Studies demonstrated that functional foods showed significant health benefits by releasing vitamins, minerals, and phytochemicals that will scavenge the free radicals produced in the body during oxidative stress. Thus, functional foods are known for reducing and preventing the risk of CVD (Keservani et al., 2017, 2020). The different functional foods involved in preventive effects are fruits and vegetables, fish, nuts and legumes, soy proteins, whole grains, coffee and tea, dark chocolates, flaxseed, mushrooms, ginger, and garlic (Lackland et al., 2014; Granato et al., 2020).

1.2.1 FRUITS AND VEGETABLES

A large number of studies have reported the beneficial effects of fruits and vegetables being included in the diet as a preventive measure for CVD. Simultaneously, studies have also reported a higher incidence of CVD cases as a result of lower consumption of fruits and vegetables. The protective effect of fruits and vegetables depends on their constituents. Fruits and vegetables contain certain bioactive components such as vitamin C, carotenoids, potassium, magnesium, and fiber which provide antioxidant properties and reduce the levels of Low-Density Lipoprotein (LDL) cholesterol. Plant foods contain phytochemicals as bioactive compounds such as phenolic compounds, carotenoids, tocotrienols, phytosterols, non-digestible carbohydrates like fiber, and organosulfur compounds which have shown significant health benefits in preventing CVD. The antioxidant properties of functional foods reduce reactive oxygen species, helping to prevent endothelial dysfunction in atherosclerotic conditions, reduce oxidized LDL cholesterol, and hinder the proliferation of vascular smooth muscle (Zhang et al., 2011; Song et al., 2010).

Vitamin E scavenges the free radicals by having an anti-inflammatory effect. Substantial evidence supports the inverse association of CVD and plasma vitamin E, which needs to be included in daily diet intake that can further lower the risk of CVD. Certain CVD risk factors including atherosclerosis, endothelial dysfunction, and platelet aggregation can be reduced by consuming berries which are rich in anthocyanin and procyanidin. Certain studies reported that consumption of citrus fruits, cherries, and berries can significantly reduce blood pressure and improve the lipid profile by reducing the cholesterol level. Apples contain phenolic compounds and fibers that have beneficial properties in reducing pulse rate, blood pressure level, total cholesterol level, and inflammation. Thus, a daily intake of 100 g to 150 g of apples can help in protection against CVD. Apples are also a rich source of vitamins B1, B2, A, C, and K, and minerals such as Iron, Phosphorus, Potassium, and Sugars (Boffetta et al., 2010; Basu et al., 2010; Wang et al., 2021; Sandoval-Ramírez et al., 2020).

1.2.2 FISH

Several studies have suggested that a high intake of fish and fish oil supplements has a significantly lower rate of CVD. Many oily fishes such as salmon, trout, tuna, and herring contain omega-3 fatty acids, which include plant-derived eicosapentaenoic acid (EPA), docosahexaenoic acid (DHA), and alpha-linolenic acid (ALA). Despite the beneficial effect of consuming fish on cardiovascular disease, the preparation, method of cooking, fish species, as well as the amount of fish consumption have an impact on CVD risk. Due to the lower intake of omega-3 fatty acids in our daily diet, certain formulations have been developed, such as incorporating fatty acids in cow's milk. This kind of incorporation meets the daily allowance of omega-3 fatty acids (He et al., 2004; Carrero et al., 2004; Bjerregaard et al., 2010).

Fish oil supplements provide a protective effect by lowering blood pressure, heart rate, and lipid profile levels through the mechanisms of anti-inflammatory, antiarrhythmic, and antithrombotic effects. Consumption of fish has also been related to reducing the risk of myocardial infarction. EPA and DHA lower LDL cholesterol and oxidative vulnerability in post-menopausal women, which can help reduce the risk of cardiovascular disease. A study of 65 meta-analyses showed that omega-3 fatty acids have lowered the level of triglycerides in a dose-dependent manner (Dyerberg et al., 2004; Lee & Wander, 2005).

1.2.3 NUTS AND LEGUMES

Almonds, walnuts, hazelnuts, olive oil, and pecans are the types of nuts that are studied as functional foods. Nuts are often considered to be a complex food comprising cholesterol-lowering mono- and polyunsaturated fatty acids, antioxidant polyphenols, arginine, and soluble fiber. Several studies have shown the cardioprotective effect of nuts. A study was conducted on 772 participants for 3 months while feeding them a diet enriched with almonds, olive oil, and walnuts. The results showed that an almond-enriched diet reduces LDL cholesterol levels more than the other two nuts. Walnuts have a high content of Polyunsaturated Fatty Acids (PUFAs) containing mainly omega-3 fatty acids, linoleic, and α-linolenic acid, whereas almonds have a high content of MUFAs (Monounsaturated Fatty Acids) (Sabaté & Ang, 2009; Choudhury et al., 2014).

The intake of a diet rich in nuts protects against CVD through certain mechanisms such as improving the lipid profile and apolipoprotein profile. Other mechanisms such as oxidative stress reduction, decreased inflammation, and improved endothelial cell function can also protect against CVD. In addition to nuts, other bioactive components such as phenolic compounds, phytosterols, L-arginine, and unsaturated fatty acids present in nuts also contribute to protection against CVD (Estruch et al., 2018).

Legumes are also complex foods that contain certain bioactive compounds such as polyphenols, folic acid, phytosterols, soluble and insoluble fibers, which have a combined effect in lowering cholesterol and reducing the risk of CVD (Martins et al., 2005).

1.2.4 SOY PROTEINS

Food and Drug Administration (FDA) approved soy protein as a functional food for lowering the risk of CVD a long time ago. An observation was conducted on the Chinese and Japanese populations who ingested soy protein in their diets, showing lower rates of ischemic and cerebrovascular events, low cholesterol levels, and lower LDL levels. A meta-analysis of 46 adult populations demonstrated that soy protein plays a protective role in decreasing total cholesterol and LDL levels in the blood. The chemicals found in soy proteins, such as saponins, isoflavones, globulins, trypsin inhibitors, soluble fibers, and phytic acids, are responsible for reducing cholesterol levels, making it a beneficial functional food that reduces LDL oxidation, lowers lipid metabolism, blood lipids, and improves arterial function (Blanco Mejia et al., 2019; Gil-Izquierdo et al., 2012).

A study reported a significant decrease in cholesterol levels due to isoflavones. Additionally, a high intake of isoflavones significantly lowered LDL cholesterol. The FDA has established the daily dose of soy protein as 25 mg/day. Enriching food with soy protein in soybeans can lower the lipid profile, thus reducing the risk of obesity and CVD. The bioactive components present in soybeans and soy-based products include phytosterols, antioxidant compounds, oligosaccharides, and globulins such as glycinin and beta-glycinin. These compounds have been reported to have a beneficial effect on human and animal health (Hodis et al., 2011; Basharat, 2020).

1.2.5 WHOLE GRAINS

Whole grains contain phytoprotective substances which work synergistically in reducing cardiovascular risk. A meta-analysis based on seven prospective cohort studies focused on the consumption of whole grains has shown that the association between dietary whole grains and the incidence of CVD is inverse, strong, and consistent across the trials. Effects on insulin sensitivity, lipids, blood pressure, and inflammation are the underlying mechanisms for the protective role of whole grains on CVD risk. After the consumption of whole grains, it has been shown to have a reduced glycemic response and reduced postprandial glucose surges when compared to refined grains. It has also been reported to have an association with reduced reactive oxygen, CVD risk, and reduced postprandial inflammation. The anti-inflammatory mechanism is unclear (Mellen et al., 2008; McKeown et al., 2002).

1.2.6 COFFEE AND TEA

The constituents in coffee responsible for the cardioprotective effect are kahweol and cafestol. Consumption of coffee may reduce the risk of myocardial infarction. A study reported that daily intake of caffeine in patients with type 2 diabetes has led to a decrease in heart disease and cardiovascular mortality (Bidel et al., 2006).

Tea is widely used as a beverage after water. The major bioactive components of green tea are catechins, which include Catechin (EC), Epigallocatechin (EGC), Epigallocatechin-3-Gallate (EGCG), Epicatechin-3-Gallate (ECG). A study of 340 cases reported that intake of 1 cup of tea per day may reduce the risk of myocardial infarction by 44% and may also reduce aortic atherosclerosis. Few epidemiological studies have shown the protective effect of tea in reducing CVD risk. A cohort study done on 700 Dutch men aged 65–84 years demonstrated that intake of epicatechin was associated with a reduced death rate due to heart diseases among CVD patients (Cao et al., 2019; Hartley et al., 2013; Dower et al., 2016).

Green tea, rich in glutamine, polyphenols, caffeine, and theanine, reduces oxidative stress and has been shown to reduce post-stroke depression in mice. The four major bioactive compounds, i.e., EC, ECG, EGC, and EGCG, have been found to reduce oxidative stress in myocardial muscles and blood, which further reduced the heart failure rate in mice. All different types of tea, such as black tea, white tea, and green tea, along with their bioactive compounds, possess excellent protective effects against CVD by mechanisms involving a decrease in lipid levels, lowering oxidative damage and associated inflammation, improvement in the functions of endothelial cells, and ischemia injury (Di Lorenzo et al., 2016; Oyama et al., 2017).

1.2.7 DARK CHOCOLATE

Cocoa is fortified with flavonoids (Keservani et al., 2016b) which are responsible for the prevention and treatment of cardiovascular disease. Flavonoids reduce the serum cholesterol level, LDL level, and blood pressure, and improve artery dilation and nitric oxide-dependent vasorelaxation. Flavonoids are responsible for raising the High-Density Lipoprotein (HDL) cholesterol by reducing LDL oxidation. Besides reducing the risk of CVD, a study showed that consuming dark chocolate made 81% of people look younger with fewer chronic illnesses and be more physically active. In contrast, white chocolate doesn't contain any flavonoids and thus shows no protective, preventive, or treatment effects in reducing the risk of CVD. A study reported that daily chocolate intake is inversely associated with insulin resistance and liver enzymes, which are risk factors for cardiometabolic disorders (Ried et al., 2017; Katz et al., 2011; Alkerwi et al., 2016).

Dark chocolate has been shown to have low bioavailability and a low degree of absorption into the intestine; hence, the lysosomal formulation in dark chocolate and Astaxanthin have shown signs of improvement in hypoxia and oxidative stress in the aging population. Raw cocoa powder and dark chocolate have proven to be most beneficial to health compared to milk chocolates, as milk chocolates reduce the bioavailability of flavanols. Various supporting pieces of evidence are emerging regarding the health benefits of dark chocolate. Besides protection against CVD, dark chocolate also regulates homeostasis and aids in cognitive and brain development. Most scientific research focuses on dark chocolate due to its presence of bioactive components such as alkaloids, flavanols, polyphenols, microelements, fatty acids, and amino acids (Katz et al., 2011; Petyaev et al., 2018).

1.2.8 FLAXSEED

Flaxseed is a distinctive plant with unique properties. It contains two components, namely α-linolenic acid and lignans. The α-linolenic acid content of flaxseed is 57% higher than any other seed oil, and the lignan content is 800 times higher than in 66 other plant foods, making flaxseed a functional food with unique properties. Flaxseed has antiestrogenic activity, which can be used by cancer patients as a therapeutic treatment and can also be used as hormone replacement therapy. Flaxseed provides protective health benefits for cardiovascular disease, cancer, hypertension, and hormone replacement therapy. Some studies have shown that flaxseed can be used as a treatment for cardiovascular disease as it reduces blood pressure, total cholesterol, and LDL cholesterol levels (Khalesi et al., 2015; Rodriguez-Leyva et al., 2013).

1.2.9 MUSHROOMS

Mushrooms are considered to be nutraceutical and functional food for medical health benefits. Mushrooms are a very good source of antioxidants that can promote health and prevent heart diseases. The antioxidant compounds of mushrooms responsible for the prevention of heart diseases are phenolic compounds, carotenoids, vitamin C, and vitamin E. Mushrooms also have proteins, unsaturated fatty acids, amino acids like valine, lectin, leucine, and carbohydrates mainly polysaccharides. Studies suggest the use of mushrooms and their extract as a natural source of antioxidants in human food and the use of mushrooms in formulations as a functional food (Reis et al., 2017; Giavasis, 2014; Kimatu et al., 2017).

Several studies of mushrooms as a potential for health benefit are based on *in-vitro* assays, although many *in vivo* studies showed the antioxidant potential of mushrooms in health benefits. Such a study is done on the ethanol extract of mushrooms, where bioactive components such as caffeic acid, catechin, gallic acid, ferulic acid, myricetin, and protocatechuic acid are present. The ethanol extract was used to feed the mice for 30 days regularly. The result showed an increase in antioxidant enzyme activity in the liver, serum, and heart of the mice and a decrease in malondialdehyde in the blood serum and vital organs of mice. Besides antioxidants, anti-tumor and immune-modulatory properties (Keservani et al., 2015), mushrooms can also provide anti-inflammatory, hypercholesterolemic, and anti-diabetic effects which will provide a cardio-protective role in human health. Therefore, based on these studies, mushrooms have great potential as functional foods in the food market (Liu et al., 2013; Valverde et al., 2015).

1.2.10 GINGER

Ginger is known to have many valuable compounds and is cultivated for cooking and medicinal purposes. Ginger inhibits the production of cyclooxygenases (COX), lipoxygenases (LOX), inflammatory cytokines, and nitric oxide and can potentially reduce the risk of CVD. Ginger possesses antioxidant properties that protect the lipids of the cell membrane from oxidation and scavenge free radicals. A study revealed that intake of ginger oil and garlic by post-menopausal women can lead to a reduction in cholesterol levels, triglycerides, LDL, body fat, and body mass index. Daily intake of 4 g of garlic can raise HDL and reduce phospholipids, serum total cholesterol levels, and atherosclerotic lesions. Thus, ginger shows a safer therapeutic effect than any other conventional drugs, since the side effects of ginger are negligible to date (Mojani et al., 2014; Basharat et al., 2019; Saptarini, 2013).

1.2.11 GARLIC

Garlic is used all over the world and is ranked top in herbal products (Sharma et al., 2020; Rane et al., 2020a, b, c). Garlic is beneficial for the treatment of heart disease and atherosclerosis. The garlic bulb contains the alliin amino acid which, when crushed, releases the alliinase enzyme which then converts alliin into allicin. The compound allicin gives the odor to garlic, which then decomposes into various sulfur-containing compounds. These compounds in garlic have the ability to lower blood pressure and serum cholesterol levels in CVD patients. Besides lowering blood pressure and cholesterol levels, it also has the ability to reduce LDL oxidation, decrease fibrinogen levels in the blood, maintain lipid profiles, and increase fibrinolysis (Beato et al., 2011; Omar & Al-Wabel, 2010; Sobenin et al., 2019).

Intake of 2 garlic capsules by 60 cardiac patients has shown a significant reduction in triglycerides and serum total cholesterol, an increase in HDL cholesterol levels, and an increase in fibrinolytic activity. The bioactive component of garlic oil, diallyl disulfide, has been demonstrated to inhibit the 3-Hydroxy-3-Methylglutaryl CoA (HMG CoA) reductase enzyme. In another study, the combination of garlic oil and onion oil on lipid profiles was studied in hyperlipidemic rats and showed a significant reduction in total fats, LDL cholesterol, body weight, and an improvement in HDL cholesterol levels in the blood. Besides garlic having hyperlipidemic effects, it also provides anti-hypertensive effects by reducing prostanoids that cause vasoconstriction and by inhibiting the enzyme that converts angiotensin. Therefore, all these studies suggest the therapeutic use of garlic in the prevention and treatment of heart disease and atherosclerosis (Ried et al., 2013; Badr et al., 2020; Yang et al., 2018).

1.3 BIOACTIVE COMPONENTS WITH PROTECTIVE EFFECTS IN CARDIOVASCULAR DISEASE

Epidemiological evidence suggests that early research was focused on plant-derived foods like carotenoids, vitamin C, and vitamin E for the prevention of many diseases such as cancers and cardiovascular disease. Current research focuses on finding the correlation between the individual components and their potential health benefits. Although there are certain studies that showed the combined effects of two bioactive compounds such as vitamin A and beta-carotene in the prevention and treatment of lung cancer and cardiovascular disease, there still lies uncertainty on whether the foods need to be consumed as a whole or need to be taken as supplements (Block et al., 1992; Prior & Cao, 2000; Omenn et al., 1996). There are certain members in the bioactive compounds which are as follows:

1.3.1 PHYTOCHEMICALS

Phytochemicals are the bioactive compounds that can be found in plant foods. Some of the compounds such as phytosterols, carotenoids, dietary fiber and prebiotics, organosulfur compounds, phenolic compounds including phenolic acids, phytoestrogens, and flavonoids exert potential health benefits in reducing blood pressure and LDL oxidation, which leads to reducing the risk of cardiovascular disease.

1.3.1.1 FLAVONOIDS

Flavonoids are derived from fruits and vegetables, cocoa, wine, and tea. Plant-derived flavonoids are mostly polyphenols that are commonly found in the human diet. Isoflavones like phytoestrogens and lignans often induce an estrogen-like response. Phytoestrogens have antioxidant activity and can increase vascular activity and influence the metabolism of lipoproteins. An association between decreased cardiovascular motility and general motility has been shown among elderly Dutch people after the consumption of flavonoids in their diet. The protective mechanism of flavonoids, as well as the mechanism of the anti-inflammatory properties of flavonoids, include their properties as metal chelators such as iron and copper that catalyze lipid oxidation, lowering the production of superoxide, platelet aggregation inhibitors, modulation of proinflammatory gene expression, and health beneficial effects on the lipid profile (Geleijnse et al., 2002; Mink et al., 2007; García-Lafuente et al., 2009).

Various flavonoid-rich foods such as chocolate, cocoa, wine, green, or black tea have demonstrated potential health benefits in reducing the risk of CVD by reducing blood pressure and the function of endothelial cells. Whether flavonoids are the only bioactive compound mediating the increase in vascular activity is still a mystery. No evidence has emerged so far about the therapeutic effect of isoflavones in reducing breast cancer, loss of bone mineral density in post-menopausal women, and in reducing CVD (Hooper et al., 2008).

1.3.1.2 CAROTENOIDS

Carotenoids have been known for their health-promoting effects such as reducing the risk of developing CVD, and cancer, and enhancing the immune system. Carotenoids such as beta-carotene and lycopene have antioxidant properties that function in reducing oxidative stress by extinguishing singlet oxygen and interacting with free radicals. Studies have established the association of lowering the risk of CVD by consuming fruits and vegetables.

Another study demonstrated the phytochemical properties of tomatoes, which have outstanding antioxidant activity in the cardiovascular system, showing that women are less prone to develop CVD when eating a large amount of lycopene from tomatoes regularly. Despite having astounding evidence in epidemiological studies about the role of carotenoids in reducing the risk of CVD, clinical trials are unsuccessful in demonstrating the beneficial effect (Krinsky & Johnson, 2005; Engelhard et al., 2006; Liu et al., 2001; Agarwal & Rao, 2000).

1.3.1.3 VITAMIN C

The antioxidant function of vitamin C is to reduce the concentrations of reactive oxygen species in atherosclerotic conditions, which helps in inhibiting the proliferation of vascular smooth muscles, reducing LDL cholesterol, and preventing endothelial dysfunction. Several studies have shown mixed results when assessing both the dietary and supplemental roles of vitamin C in CVD. Besides the role of vitamin C as an antioxidant, vitamin C has also been recognized as a pro-oxidant under high oxidative stress conditions. In most trials, vitamin C has been incorporated with beta-carotene and vitamin E and showed void results in relation to CVD. To deliver the health benefits of food, the bioactive compounds and nutrients act synergistically in the matrix of complex food (Aguirre & May, 2008; Ye & Song, 2008; Cook et al., 2007).

1.3.1.4 VITAMIN E

Besides having the free radicals scavenging property, Vitamin E exhibits anti-inflammatory activity at high doses. Studies have shown a strong inverse association between intake of vitamin E and coronary heart disease and between CVD and vitamin E. Other than failed clinical trials of vitamin C, in vitamin E supplementation, the clinical trials were also unsuccessful in preventing CVD. Meta-analysis of 90 trials showed void results (Singh et al., 2005; Gey et al., 1991; Bolton-Smith et al., 1992; Shekelle et al., 2004).

1.3.1.5 PLANT STEROLS AND STANOLS

Plant sterols are known for their cholesterol-lowering effect and were first identified in the 1950s. The efficacy of plant sterols such as campesterol, β-sitosterol, and stigmasterol has been found. Plant stanol, i.e., sitostanol, has the ability to reduce the intestinal absorption of cholesterol, leading to lower levels of cholesterol compared to plant sterols. Plant sterols and stanols structurally resemble cholesterol, allowing them to compete with cholesterol during absorption in the digestive tract. The mechanism of action of plant sterols has shown that their hydrophobicity differs from that of cholesterol, preventing cholesterol from entering micelles and causing it to precipitate in the lumen along with the cholesterol, thereby reducing cholesterol absorption into the bloodstream (Mensink et al., 2010; Bai, 2019).

A clinical trial in mildly hypercholesterolemic patients with plant sterol esters demonstrated a significant reduction in both LDL and total cholesterol by 14% and 10%, respectively. Consuming 0.65 g of plant sterols twice a day with meals as part of a diet low in cholesterol and saturated fat has been shown to reduce the risk of CVD. No side effects have been observed in studies following the intake of plant sterols or stanols in the daily diet, but a minor decrease in serum carotenoid concentration has been noted (Ras et al., 2014; Smet et al., 2012).

1.3.1.6 POLYPHENOL COMPOUNDS

Several *in vivo* studies have shown that polyphenols modulate lipid metabolism and inflammation, increase the release of nitric oxide and improve endothelial function, improve antioxidant properties, protect against episodes of atherothrombotic events which include platelet aggregation and myocardial ischemia, decrease LDL oxidation which reduces the potential risk of CVD (Perez-Jimenez & Saura-Calixto, 2008).

1.4 DIETARY PATTERNS IN PREVENTION OF CARDIOVASCULAR DISEASE

Eating habits have an impact on social, environmental, and health factors. In nutritional epidemiology, the traditional approach has mainly focused on the effects of individual foods or nutrients. However, an individual does not consume a single food in isolation; rather, they consume a whole meal consisting of a variety of foods. In fact, the dietary patterns of an individual have been less focused on due to their complex nature. The mechanism by which diets reduce inflammation is still unclear. The dietary patterns are as follows.

1.4.1 DASH DIET

A diet rich in whole grains, fruits, vegetables, nuts, fish, and low in dairy fat foods significantly lowers the systolic blood pressure in patients as reported by the Dietary Approaches to Stop Hypertension (DASH) trial. This dietary pattern consists of a very low-calorie diet that limits sweets, red meat, sugar-containing beverages, and saturated fat, which improves vasodilatation-mediated blood flow. Along with the DASH diet, decreasing salt intake in the diet, regular physical activity, and increasing potassium are the strategies that can reduce blood pressure (Moore et al., 2001; Blumenthal et al., 2010).

Associations between a DASH dietary pattern and the incidence of CVD events have been examined by several studies. The DASH diet possesses beneficial effects on various CVD risk factors, which include LDL cholesterol, total cholesterol, and inflammation. Therefore, the evidence is strong for the protective role of the DASH diet in the prevention of CVD (Parikh et al., 2009).

1.4.2 MEDITERRANEAN DIET

The Mediterranean diet consists of cereals, fruits, vegetables, oilseeds, nuts, beans, a small quantity of dairy products, and red meat. Intake of poultry and fish is in low to moderate amounts. Many studies have reported a lower rate of diseases among populations consuming this diet. Clinical trials have demonstrated the protective effect of the Mediterranean diet against CVD, which also reduces inflammatory markers and serum homocysteine concentrations in some high-risk populations. Besides the protective role against CVD, several Mediterranean diets consist of legumes, whole grains, low glycemic index starchy foods, fruits, vegetables, and polyunsaturated fatty acids, which provide protection against type 2 diabetes. A recent study reported that not all the components of this diet are equally protective. Olive oil and plant foods contain high antioxidants that benefit the health of the vascular system and offer protection against hypertension (Kushi et al., 1995; Esposito et al., 2006; Riccardi et al., 2005; Psaltopoulou et al., 2004).

1.4.3 PORTFOLIO DIET

The portfolio diet consists of two-step diets recommended for the management of high cholesterol levels in the blood. The Step I diet consists of saturated fats with less than 10% of total calories, less than 300 mg/day of cholesterol, and less than 30% of total calorie intake from fat. Step II diet consists of less than 200 mg of cholesterol and saturated fats with less than 7% of total calories. Current research suggests focusing on lowering low-density lipoprotein cholesterol, which can reduce the risk of CVD. Lowering low-density lipoprotein cholesterol can be achieved by adding dietary components such as soy protein, viscous fibers, almonds, and plant sterols. This combination of dietary compounds has been classified as the Portfolio Diet. This diet has also been shown to be effective in predicting cardiovascular risk and lowering C-reactive protein (DeWitt Goodman et al., 1988; Jenkins et al., 2002).

1.4.4 OKINAWAN DIET

The Okinawan Diet is a diet that is high in carbohydrates and low in fat, particularly saturated fat. A nutrient-dense and low-energy diet has been suggested to be beneficial in reducing the risk of CVD and many other chronic diseases. The mechanisms involved in the decreased risk of CVD and cancers include the intake of a high-antioxidant and low-calorie diet, which includes sweet potatoes and green leafy vegetables, high phytochemical content, low glycemic load, and reduced oxidative stress. Studies have also suggested that the Okinawan diet increases longevity by slowing the aging process in Okinawan populations (Willcox et al., 2006, 2007; Suzuki et al., 2001).

1.4.5 VEGETARIAN DIET

A vegetarian diet lacks meat and fish but is high in fruits, nuts, and vegetables, which are rich sources of polyphenols, antioxidants, and phytochemicals that have an anti-inflammatory effect. Vegetarian diets are lower in calcium, zinc, vitamin D, vitamin B-12, and omega-3 fatty acids but higher in vitamin C, folic acid, magnesium, vitamin E, and iron, which benefit in lowering cholesterol levels, blood pressure, and body weight due to lesser consumption of cholesterol, calories, and saturated fat in diets. Studies have reported a reduced mortality rate and ischemic heart disease in people consuming a vegetarian diet (Key et al., 1998; Genkinger et al., 2004).

1.5 CONCLUSION

Cardiovascular diseases are the leading cause of high mortality rates globally. Therefore, new alternative therapies and treatments are needed for the prevention of CVD. Several clinical and epidemiological studies have reported that consuming a diet rich in fish, fresh fruits and vegetables, whole grains, nuts, flaxseed, garlic, mushrooms, ginger, chocolate, coffee, and tea, and a diet low in saturated fat and low-fat dairy products can reduce the risk of CVD. Other prospective studies have also shown that bioactive compounds in foods alone or combination, such as flavonoids, carotenoids, vitamin C, vitamin E, plant sterols and stanols, and other antioxidant supplementation, can lower blood cholesterol levels as well as blood pressure, acting as a protective barrier against CVD.

Functional foods besides reducing the risk of CVD, also reduce certain diseases such as cancer, asthma, diabetes, obesity, hepatitis, and many other chronic diseases. Several studies have shown that functional foods have antioxidant and anti-inflammatory properties, which suggests incorporating those functional foods into a healthy diet to lower the risk of CVD. The detailed and extensive knowledge of various diseases as well as the dietary components has opened up new horizons in developing numerous dietary strategies for preventing and treating CVD. Future studies should focus on clinical trials using individual bioactive components or using these components in combination to assess the beneficial effect on health.

KEYWORDS

- **alpha-linolenic acid**
- **bioactive components**
- **cardiovascular disease**
- **docosahexaenoic acid**
- **eicosapentaenoic acid**
- **functional food**

REFERENCES

Agarwal, S., & Rao, A. V. (2000). Tomato lycopene and its role in human health and chronic diseases. *Canadian Medical Association Journal, 163*(6), 739–744.

Aguirre, R., & May, J. M. (2008). Inflammation in the vascular bed: importance of vitamin C. *Pharmacology and Therapeutics, 119*(1), 96–103.

Alkerwi, A. A., Sauvageot, N., Crichton, G. E., Elias, M. F., & Stranges, S. (2016). Daily chocolate consumption is inversely associated with insulin resistance and liver enzymes in the Observation of Cardiovascular Risk Factors in Luxembourg study. *British Journal of Nutrition, 115*(9), 1661–1668.

Badr, G. M., & Arafa, N. S. (2020). Synergetic effect of aged garlic extracts and methotrexate on rheumatoid arthritis induced by collagen in male albino rats. *Indian Journal of Experimental Biology, 58*(1), 33–38.

Bai, N. (2019). Advances in the prevention of cardiovascular diseases by phytosterol. In *Proceedings of the Third International Conference on Medical and Health Informatics* (pp. 110–114).

Basharat, A., Qamar, M. M., Basharat, N., Aslam, S., Rasul, A., & Naqvi, F. (2019). Effect of garlic, ginger and exercise on lipid profile in healthy postmenopausal women. *Annals of King Edward Medical University, 25*(4), 1.

Basharat, S. (2020). Therapeutic effect of Glycine max (soybean) bioactive components in CVD and obesity. *J. Food Nutr., 6*, 1–7.

Basu, A., Rhone, M., & Lyons, T. J. (2010). Berries: emerging impact on cardiovascular health. *Nutrition Reviews, 68*(3), 168–177.

Beato, V. M., Orgaz, F., Mansilla, F., & Montaño, A. (2011). Changes in phenolic compounds in garlic (*Allium sativum* L.) owing to the cultivar and location of growth. *Plant Foods for Human Nutrition, 66*(3), 218–223.

Bidel, S., Hu, G., Qiao, Q., Jousilahti, P., Antikainen, R., & Tuomilehto, J. (2006). Coffee consumption and risk of total and cardiovascular mortality among patients with type 2 diabetes. *Diabetologia, 49*(11), 2618–2626.

Bjelakovic, G., & Gluud, C. (2007). Surviving antioxidant supplements. *Journal of the National Cancer Institute, 99*(10), 742–743.

Bjerregaard, L. J., Joensen, A. M., Dethlefsen, C., Jensen, M. K., Johnsen, S. P., Tjønneland, A., Rasmussen, L. H., Overvad, K., & Schmidt, E. B. (2010). Fish intake and acute coronary syndrome. *European Heart Journal, 31*(1), 29–34.

Blanco Mejia, S., Messina, M., Li, S. S., Viguiliouk, E., Chiavaroli, L., Khan, T. A., Srichaikul, K., Mirrahimi, A., Sievenpiper, J. L., Kris-Etherton, P., & Jenkins, D. J. A. (2019). A meta-analysis of 46 studies identified by the FDA demonstrates that soy protein decreases circulating LDL and total cholesterol concentrations in adults. *The Journal of Nutrition, 149*(6), 968–981.

Block, G., Patterson, B., & Subar, A. (1992). Fruit, vegetables, and cancer prevention: a review of the epidemiological evidence. *Nutrition and Cancer, 18*(1), 1–29.

Blumenthal, J. A., Babyak, M. A., Sherwood, A., Craighead, L., Lin, P. H., Johnson, J., Watkins, L. L., Wang, J. T., Kuhn, C., Feinglos, M., & Hinderliter, A. (2010). Effects of the dietary approaches to stop hypertension diet alone and in combination with exercise and caloric restriction on insulin sensitivity and lipids. *Hypertension, 55*(5), 1199–1205.

Boffetta, P., Couto, E., Wichmann, J., Ferrari, P., Trichopoulos, D., Bueno-de-Mesquita, H. B., van Duijnhoven, F. J., Büchner, F. L., Key, T., Boeing, H., Nöthlings, U., Linseisen, J.,

Gonzalez, C. A., Overvad, K., Nielsen, M. R., Tjønneland, A., Olsen, A., Clavel-Chapelon, F., Boutron-Ruault, M. C., Morois, S., Lagiou, P., Naska, A., Benetou, V., Kaaks, R., Rohrmann, S., Panico, S., Sieri, S., Vineis, P., Palli, D., van Gils, C. H., Peeters, P. H., Lund, E., Brustad, M., Engeset, D., Huerta, J. M., Rodríguez, L., Sánchez, M. J., Dorronsoro, M., Barricarte, A., Hallmans, G., Johansson, I., Manjer, J., Sonestedt, E., Allen, N. E., Bingham, S., Khaw, K. T., Slimani, N., Jenab, M., Mouw, T., Norat, T., Riboli, E., & Trichopoulou, A. (2010). Fruit and vegetable intake and overall cancer risk in the European Prospective Investigation into Cancer and Nutrition (EPIC). *Journal of the National Cancer Institute, 102*(8), 529–537.

Bolton-Smith, C., Woodward, M., & Tunstall-Pedoe, H. (1992). The Scottish Heart Health Study. Dietary intake by food frequency questionnaire and odds ratios for coronary heart disease risk—II. The antioxidant vitamins and fibre. *European Journal of Clinical Nutrition, 46*(2), 85–93.

Boussageon, R., Bejan-Angoulvant, T., Saadatian-Elahi, M., Lafont, S., Bergeonneau, C., Kassaï, B., Erpeldinger, S., Wright, J. M., Gueyffier, F., & Cornu, C. (2011). Effect of intensive glucose lowering treatment on all-cause mortality, cardiovascular death and microvascular events in type 2 diabetes: meta-analysis of randomized controlled trials. *BMJ, 343*, d4169.

Cao, S. Y., Zhao, C. N., Gan, R. Y., Xu, X. Y., Wei, X. L., Corke, H., Atanasov, A. G., & Li, H. B. (2019). Effects and mechanisms of tea and its bioactive compounds for the prevention and treatment of cardiovascular diseases: An updated review. *Antioxidants, 8*(6), 166.

Carrero, J. J., Baró, L., Fonollá, J., González-Santiago, M., Martínez-Férez, A., Castillo, R., Jiménez, J., Boza, J. J., & López-Huertas, E. (2004). Cardiovascular effects of milk enriched with ω-3 polyunsaturated fatty acids, oleic acid, folic acid, and vitamins E and B6 in volunteers with mild hyperlipidemia. *Nutrition, 20*(6), 521–527.

Choudhury, K., Clark, J., & Griffiths, H. R. (2014). An almond-enriched diet increases plasma α-tocopherol and improves vascular function but does not affect oxidative stress markers or lipid levels. *Free Radical Research, 48*(5), 599–606.

Cook, N. R., Albert, C. M., Gaziano, J. M., Zaharris, E., MacFadyen, J., Danielson, E., Buring, J. E., & Manson, J. E. (2007). A randomized factorial trial of vitamins C and E and beta carotene in the secondary prevention of cardiovascular events in women: Results from the Women's Antioxidant Cardiovascular Study. *Archives of Internal Medicine, 167*(15), 1610–1618.

DeWitt Goodman, S., Hulley, S. B., & Clark, L. T. (1988). Report of the National Cholesterol Education Program Expert Panel on detection, evaluation, and treatment of high blood cholesterol in adults. *Archives of Internal Medicine, 148*(1), 36–69.

Di Lorenzo, A., Nabavi, S. F., Sureda, A., Moghaddam, A. H., Khanjani, S., Arcidiaco, P., Nabavi, S. M., & Daglia, M. (2016). Antidepressive-like effects and antioxidant activity of green tea and GABA green tea in a mouse model of post-stroke depression. *Molecular Nutrition & Food Research, 60*(3), 566–579.

Dower, J. I., Geleijnse, J. M., Hollman, P. C., Soedamah-Muthu, S. S., & Kromhout, D. (2016). Dietary epicatechin intake and 25-y risk of cardiovascular mortality: The Zutphen Elderly Study. *The American Journal of Clinical Nutrition, 104*(1), 58–64.

Dyerberg, J., Eskesen, D. C., Andersen, P. W., Astrup, A., Buemann, B., Christensen, J. H., Clausen, P., Rasmussen, B. F., Schmidt, E. B., Tholstrup, T., Toft, E., Toubro, S., & Stender, S. (2004). Effects of trans- and n-3 unsaturated fatty acids on cardiovascular risk markers in healthy males: An 8 weeks dietary intervention study. *European Journal of Clinical Nutrition, 58*(7), 1062–1070.

Engelhard, Y. N., Gazer, B., & Paran, E. (2006). Natural antioxidants from tomato extract reduce blood pressure in patients with grade-1 hypertension: A double-blind, placebo-controlled pilot study. *American Heart Journal, 151*(1), 100.e1–100.e6.

Esposito, K., Ciotola, M., & Giugliano, D. (2006). Mediterranean diet, endothelial function and vascular inflammatory markers. *Public Health Nutrition, 9*(8), 1073–1076.

Estruch, R., Ros, E., Salas-Salvadó, J., Covas, M. I., Corella, D., Arós, F., Gómez-Gracia, E., Ruiz-Gutiérrez, V., Fiol, M., Lapetra, J., Lamuela-Raventos, R. M., Serra-Majem, L., Pintó, X., Basora, J., Muñoz, M. A., Sorlí, J. V., Martínez, J. A., Fitó, M., Gea, A., Hernán, M. A., & Martínez-González, M. A. (2018). Primary prevention of cardiovascular disease with a Mediterranean diet supplemented with extra-virgin olive oil or nuts. *New England Journal of Medicine, 378*(25), e34.

García-Lafuente, A., Guillamón, E., Villares, A., Rostagno, M. A., & Martínez, J. A. (2009). Flavonoids as anti-inflammatory agents: Implications in cancer and cardiovascular disease. *Inflammation Research, 58*(9), 537–552.

Geleijnse, J. M., Launer, L. J., Van der Kuip, D. A., Hofman, A., & Witteman, J. C. (2002). Inverse association of tea and flavonoid intakes with incident myocardial infarction: The Rotterdam study. *American Journal of Clinical Nutrition, 75*(5), 880–886.

Genkinger, J. M., Platz, E. A., Hoffman, S. C., Comstock, G. W., & Helzlsouer, K. J. (2004). Fruit, vegetable, and antioxidant intake and all-cause, cancer, and cardiovascular disease mortality in a community-dwelling population in Washington County, Maryland. *American Journal of Epidemiology, 160*(12), 1223–1233.

Gey, K. F., Puska, P., Jordan, P., & Moser, U. K. (1991). Inverse correlation between plasma vitamin E and mortality from ischemic heart disease in cross-cultural epidemiology. *American Journal of Clinical Nutrition, 53*(1), 326S–334S.

Giavasis, I. (2014). Bioactive fungal polysaccharides as potential functional ingredients in food and nutraceuticals. *Current Opinion in Biotechnology, 26*, 162–173.

Gil-Izquierdo, A., Penalvo, J. L., Gil, J. I., Medina, S., Horcajada, M. N., Lafay, S., Silberberg, M., Llorach, R., Zafrilla, P., Garcia-Mora, P., & Ferreres, F. (2012). Soy isoflavones and cardiovascular disease: Epidemiological, clinical and – omics perspectives. *Current Pharmaceutical Biotechnology, 13*(5), 624–631.

Granato, D., Barba, F. J., Bursać Kovačević, D., Lorenzo, J. M., Cruz, A. G., & Putnik, P. (2020). Functional foods: Product development, technological trends, efficacy testing and safety. *Annual Review of Food Science and Technology, 11*, 93–118.

Hartley, L., Flowers, N., Holmes, J., Clarke, A., Stranges, S., Hooper, L., & Rees, K. (2013). Green and black tea for the primary prevention of cardiovascular disease. *Cochrane Database of Systematic Reviews, 6*, 1–48.

He, K., Song, Y., Daviglus, M. L., Liu, K., Van Horn, L., Dyer, A. R., & Greenland, P. (2004). Accumulated evidence on fish consumption and coronary heart disease mortality: A meta-analysis of cohort studies. *Circulation, 109*(22), 2705–2711.

Hodis, H. N., Mack, W. J., Kono, N., Azen, S. P., Shoupe, D., Hwang-Levine, J., Petitti, D., Whitfield-Maxwell, L., Yan, M., Franke, A. A., & Selzer, R. H. (2011). Isoflavone soy protein supplementation and atherosclerosis progression in healthy postmenopausal women: A randomized controlled trial. *Stroke, 42*(11), 3168–3175.

Hooper, L., Kroon, P. A., Rimm, E. B., Cohn, J. S., Harvey, I., Le Cornu, K. A., Ryder, J. J., Hall, W. L., & Cassidy, A. (2008). Flavonoids, flavonoid-rich foods, and cardiovascular risk: A meta-analysis of randomized controlled trials. *American Journal of Clinical Nutrition, 88*(1), 38–50.

Jenkins, D. J., Kendall, C. W., Faulkner, D., Vidgen, E., Trautwein, E. A., Parker, T. L., Marchie, A., Koumbridis, G., Lapsley, K. G., Josse, R. G., Leiter, L. A., & Connelly, P. W. (2002). A dietary portfolio approach to cholesterol reduction: Combined effects of plant sterols, vegetable proteins, and viscous fibers in hypercholesterolemia. *Metabolism, 51*(12), 1596–1604.

Katz, D. L., Doughty, K., & Ali, A. (2011). Cocoa and chocolate in human health and disease. *Antioxidants & Redox Signaling, 15*(10), 2779–2811.

Keservani, R. K., Kesharwani, R. K., Sharma, A. K., Vyas, N., & Chadoker, A. (2010b). Nutritional Supplements: An Overview. *International Journal of Current Pharmaceutical Review and Research, 1*(1), 59–75.

Keservani, R. K., Kesharwani, R. K., Vyas, N., Jain, S., Raghuvanshi, R., & Sharma, A. K. (2010a). Nutraceutical and functional food as future food: A review. *Der. Pharmacia. Lettre, 2*(1), 106–116.

Keservani, R. K., Sharma, A. K., & Kesharwani, R. K. (2016a). Nutraceutical and Functional Foods for Cardiovascular Health. In *Food Process Engineering* (pp. 291–312). Apple Academic Press, CRC Press. ISBN: 9781771884020.

Keservani, R. K., Sharma, A. K., & Kesharwani, R. K. (2016b). Medicinal effect of nutraceutical fruits for the cognition and brain health. *Scientifica, 2016,* Article ID 3109254, 10 pages. https://doi.org/10.1155/2016/3109254.

Keservani, R. K., Sharma, A. K., & Kesharwani, R. K. (2017). An overview and therapeutic applications of nutraceutical and functional foods. *Recent Advances in Drug Delivery Technology*, 160–201. ISBN: 9781522507543.

Keservani, R. K., Sharma, A. K., & Kesharwani, R. K. (Eds.). (2020). Nutraceuticals and Dietary Supplements: Applications in Health Improvement and Disease Management, Apple Academic Press, CRC Press. Pp. 1–344. ISBN: 9781771888738.

Key, T. J., Fraser, G. E., Thorogood, M., Appleby, P. N., Beral, V., Reeves, G., Burr, M. L., Chang-Claude, J., Frentzel-Beyme, R., Kuzma, J. W., Mann, J., & McPherson, K. (1998). Mortality in vegetarians and non-vegetarians: A collaborative analysis of 8300 deaths among 76,000 men and women in five prospective studies. *Public Health Nutrition, 1*(1), 33–41.

Khalesi, S., Irwin, C., & Schubert, M. (2015). Flaxseed consumption may reduce blood pressure: A systematic review and meta-analysis of controlled trials. *The Journal of Nutrition, 145*(4), 758–765.

Kimatu, B. M., Zhao, L., Biao, Y., Ma, G., Yang, W., Pei, F., & Hu, Q. (2017). Antioxidant potential of edible mushroom (*Agaricus bisporus*) protein hydrolysates and their ultrafiltration fractions. *Food Chemistry, 230*, 58–67.

Krinsky, N. I., & Johnson, E. J. (2005). Carotenoid actions and their relation to health and disease. *Molecular Aspects of Medicine, 26*(6), 459–516.

Kumar, A. S., & Sinha, N. (2020). Cardiovascular disease in India: A 360-degree overview. *Medical Journal Armed Forces India, 76*(1), 1–3. https://doi.org/10.1016/j.mjafi.2019.12.005.

Kushi, L. H., Lenart, E. B., & Willett, W. C. (1995). Health implications of Mediterranean diets in light of contemporary knowledge—1. Plant foods and dairy products. *American Journal of Clinical Nutrition, 61*(6), 1407S–1415S.

Lackland, D. T., Roccella, E. J., Deutsch, A. F., Fornage, M., George, M. G., Howard, G., Kissela, B. M., Kittner, S. J., Lichtman, J. H., Lisabeth, L. D., Schwamm, L. H., & Smith, E. E. (2014). Factors influencing the decline in stroke mortality: A statement from the American Heart Association/American Stroke Association. *Stroke, 45*(1), 315–353.

Lee, Y. S., & Wander, R. C. (2005). Reduced effect on apoptosis of 4-hydroxyhexenal and oxidized LDL enriched with n-3 fatty acids from postmenopausal women. *Journal of Nutritional Biochemistry, 16*(4), 213–221.

Liu, J., Jia, L., Kan, J., & Jin, C. H. (2013). In vitro and in vivo antioxidant activity of ethanolic extract of white button mushroom (*Agaricus bisporus*). *Food and Chemical Toxicology, 51*, 310–316.

Liu, S., Lee, I. M., Ajani, U., Cole, S. R., Buring, J. E., & Manson, J. E. (2001). Intake of vegetables rich in carotenoids and risk of coronary heart disease in men: The Physicians' Health Study. *International Journal of Epidemiology, 30*(1), 130–135.

Martins, J. M., Riottot, M., de Abreu, M. C., Viegas-Crespo, A. M., Lança, M. J., Almeida, J. A., Freire, J. B., & Bento, O. P. (2005). Cholesterol-lowering effects of dietary blue lupin (*Lupinus angustifolius* L.) in intact and ileorectal anastomosed pigs. *Journal of Lipid Research, 46*(7), 1539–1547.

McGill, H. C. (1979). The relationship of dietary cholesterol to serum cholesterol concentration and to atherosclerosis in man. *American Journal of Clinical Nutrition, 32*(12), 2664–2702.

McKeown, N. M., Meigs, J. B., Liu, S., Wilson, P. W. F., & Jacques, P. F. (2002). Whole-grain intake is favorably associated with metabolic risk factors for type 2 diabetes and cardiovascular disease in the Framingham Offspring Study. *American Journal of Clinical Nutrition, 76*(2), 390–398.

Meier, T., Gräfe, K., Senn, F., Sur, P., Stangl, G. I., Dawczynski, C., März, W., Kleber, M. E., & Lorkowski, S. (2019). Cardiovascular mortality attributable to dietary risk factors in 51 countries in the WHO European Region from 1990 to 2016: A systematic analysis of the Global Burden of Disease Study. *European Journal of Epidemiology, 34*(1), 37–55.

Mellen, P. B., Walsh, T. F., & Herrington, D. M. (2008). Whole grain intake and cardiovascular disease: A meta-analysis. *Nutrition, Metabolism and Cardiovascular Diseases, 18*(4), 283–290.

Mensink, R. P., de Jong, A., Lütjohann, D., Haenen, G. R., & Plat, J. (2010). Plant stanols dose-dependently decrease LDL-cholesterol concentrations, but not cholesterol-standardized fat-soluble antioxidant concentrations, at intakes up to 9 g/d. *The American Journal of Clinical Nutrition, 92*(1), 24–33.

Mink, P. J., Scrafford, C. G., Barraj, L. M., Harnack, L., Hong, C. P., Nettleton, J. A., & Jacobs, D. R. Jr. (2007). Flavonoid intake and cardiovascular disease mortality: A prospective study in postmenopausal women. *American Journal of Clinical Nutrition, 85*(3), 895–909.

Mojani, M. S., Ghasemzadeh, A., Rahmat, A., Loh, S. P., & Ramasamy, R. (2014). Assessment of bioactive compounds, nutritional composition and antioxidant activity of Malaysian young ginger (*Zingiber officinale* Roscoe). *International Food Research Journal, 21*(5), 1931.

Moore, T. J., Conlin, P. R., Ard, J., & Svetkey, L. P. (2001). DASH (Dietary Approaches to Stop Hypertension) diet is effective treatment for stage 1 isolated systolic hypertension. *Hypertension, 38*(2), 155–158.

Omar, S. H., & Al-Wabel, N. A. (2010). Organosulfur compounds and possible mechanism of garlic in cancer. *Saudi Pharmaceutical Journal, 18*(1), 51–58.

Omenn, G. S., Goodman, G. E., Thornquist, M. D., Balmes, J., Cullen, M. R., Glass, A., Keogh, J. P., Meyskens, F. L., Valanis, B., Williams, J. H., Barnhart, S., & Hammar, S. (1996). Effects of a combination of beta carotene and vitamin A on lung cancer and cardiovascular disease. *New England Journal of Medicine, 334*(18), 1150–1155.

Oyama, J. I., Shiraki, A., Nishikido, T., Maeda, T., Komoda, H., Shimizu, T., Makino, N., & Node, K. (2017). EGCG, a green tea catechin, attenuates the progression of heart failure induced by the heart/muscle-specific deletion of MnSOD in mice. *Journal of Cardiology, 69*(2), 417–427.

Parikh, A., Lipsitz, S. R., & Natarajan, S. (2009). Association between a DASH-like diet and mortality in adults with hypertension: Findings from a population-based follow-up study. *American Journal of Hypertension, 22*(4), 409–416.

Perez-Jimenez, J., & Saura-Calixto, F. (2008). Grape products and cardiovascular disease risk factors. *Nutrition Research Reviews, 21*(2), 158–173.

Petyaev, I. M., Klochkov, V. A., Chalyk, N. E., Pristensky, D. V., Chernyshova, M. P., Kyle, N. H., & Bashmakov, Y. K. (2018). Markers of hypoxia and oxidative stress in aging volunteers ingesting lycosomal formulation of dark chocolate containing astaxanthin. *The Journal of Nutrition, Health & Aging, 22*(9), 1092–1098.

Prabhakaran, D., Jeemon, P., & Roy, A. (2016). Cardiovascular diseases in India. *Circulation, 133*, 1605–1620.

Prior, R. L., & Cao, G. (2000). Antioxidant phytochemicals in fruits and vegetables: Diet and health implications. *HortScience, 35*(4), 588–592.

Psaltopoulou, T., Naska, A., Orfanos, P., Trichopoulos, D., Mountokalakis, T., & Trichopoulou, A. (2004). Olive oil, the Mediterranean diet, and arterial blood pressure: The Greek European Prospective Investigation into Cancer and Nutrition (EPIC) study. *The American Journal of Clinical Nutrition, 80*(4), 1012–1018.

Raj, K., Kesharwani, R. K., Sharma, A. K., & Jarouliya, U. (2015). Dietary Supplements, Nutraceutical and Functional Foods in Immune Response (Immunomodulators). In D. Bagchi, H. G. Preuss, & A. Swaroop (Eds.), *Nutraceutical and Functional Foods in Human Life and Disease Prevention* (pp. 343–358). CRC Press, Taylor and Francis. ISBN: 9781482237214.

Rane, B. R., Bharath, M. S., Patil, R. R., Keservani, R. K., & Jain, A. S. (2020b). Novel Approaches in Nutraceuticals. In R. K. Kesharwani, R. K. Keservani, & A. K. Sharma (Eds.), *Enhancing the Therapeutic Efficacy of Herbal Formulations through Novel Drug Delivery Systems* (pp. 241–266). IGI Global International Publisher. ISBN: 9781799844532.

Rane, B. R., Patil, A. S., Keservani, R. K., & Jain, A. S. (2020a). Novel Approaches in Herbal Formulation. In R. K. Kesharwani, R. K. Keservani, & A. K. Sharma (Eds.), *Enhancing the Therapeutic Efficacy of Herbal Formulations through Novel Drug Delivery Systems* (pp. 43–68). IGI Global International Publisher. ISBN: 9781799844532.

Rane, B. R., Tadavi, S. A., & Keservani, R. K. (2020c). Naturopathy. In A. K. Sharma, R. K. Keservani, & S. P. Gautam (Eds.), *Herbal Product Development* (pp. 321–347). Apple Academic Press, CRC Press, Taylor & Francis Group. ISBN: 9781771888776.

Ras, R. T., Geleijnse, J. M., & Trautwein, E. A. (2014). LDL-cholesterol-lowering effect of plant sterols and stanols across different dose ranges: A meta-analysis of randomized controlled studies. *British Journal of Nutrition, 112*(2), 214–219.

Reis, F. S., Martins, A., Vasconcelos, M. H., Morales, P., & Ferreira, I. C. (2017). Functional foods based on extracts or compounds derived from mushrooms. *Trends in Food Science & Technology, 66*, 48–62.

Riccardi, G., Capaldo, B., & Vaccaro, O. (2005). Functional foods in the management of obesity and type 2 diabetes. *Current Opinion in Clinical Nutrition and Metabolic Care, 8*(6), 630–635.
Ried, K., Fakler, P., & Stocks, N. P. (2017). Effect of cocoa on blood pressure. *The Cochrane Database of Systematic Reviews, 8*, 1465–1858.
Ried, K., Frank, O. R., & Stocks, N. P. (2013). Aged garlic extract reduces blood pressure in hypertensives: A dose–response trial. *European Journal of Clinical Nutrition, 67*(1), 64–70.
Rodriguez-Leyva, D., Weighell, W., Edel, A. L., LaVallee, R., Dibrov, E., Pinneker, R., Maddaford, T. G., Ramjiawan, B., Aliani, M., Guzman, R., & Pierce, G. N. (2013). Potent antihypertensive action of dietary flaxseed in hypertensive patients. *Hypertension, 62*(6), 1081–1089.
Ruhil, R. (2018). India has reached on the descending limb of tobacco epidemic. *Indian Journal of Community Medicine, 43*, 153–156.
Sabaté, J., & Ang, Y. (2009). Nuts and health outcomes: New epidemiologic evidence. *American Journal of Clinical Nutrition, 89*(5), 1643S–1648S.
Sandoval-Ramírez, B. A., Catalán, Ú., Calderón-Pérez, L., Companys, J., Pla-Pagà, L., Ludwig, I. A., Romero, M. P., & Solà, R. (2020). The effects and associations of whole-apple intake on diverse cardiovascular risk factors: A narrative review. *Critical Reviews in Food Science and Nutrition, 60*(22), 3862–3875.
Saptarini, N. M. (2013). Structure-based in silico study of 6-gingerol, 6-ghogaol and 6-paradol, active compounds of ginger (Zingiber officinale) as COX_2 inhibitors. *International Journal of Chemistry, 5*(3), 12–18.
Sharma, A. K., Keservani, R. K., & Gautam, S. P. (2020). Herbal Product Development: Formulation and Applications, Apple Academic Press, CRC Press, Taylor & Francis Group. Pp. 1–376. ISBN: 9781771888776.
Shekelle, P. G., Morton, S. C., Jungvig, L. K., Udani, J., Spar, M., Tu, W., Suttorp, M. J., Coulter, I., Newberry, S. J., & Hardy, M. (2004). Effect of supplemental vitamin E for the prevention and treatment of cardiovascular disease. *Journal of General Internal Medicine, 19*(4), 380–389.
Singh, U., Devaraj, S., & Jialal, I. (2005). Vitamin E, oxidative stress, and inflammation. *Annual Review of Nutrition, 25*, 151–174.
Smet, E. D., Mensink, R. P., & Plat, J. (2012). Effects of plant sterols and stanols on intestinal cholesterol metabolism: Suggested mechanisms from past to present. *Molecular Nutrition & Food Research, 56*(7), 1058–1072.
Sobenin, I. A., Myasoedova, V. A., Iltchuk, M. I., Zhang, D. W., & Orekhov, A. N. (2019). Therapeutic effects of garlic in cardiovascular atherosclerotic disease. *Chinese Journal of Natural Medicines, 17*(10), 721–728.
Song, W., Derito, C. M., Liu, M. K., He, X., Dong, M., & Liu, R. H. (2010). Cellular antioxidant activity of common vegetables. *Journal of Agricultural and Food Chemistry, 58*(11), 6621–6629.
Suzuki, M., Wilcox, B. J., & Wilcox, C. D. (2001). Implications from and for food cultures for cardiovascular disease: Longevity. *Asia Pacific Journal of Clinical Nutrition, 10*(2), 165–171.
Valverde, M. E., Hernández-Pérez, T., & Paredes-López, O. (2015). Edible mushrooms: Improving human health and promoting quality life. *International Journal of Microbiology, 2015*, 1–14.

Wang, Y., Gallegos, J. L., Haskell-Ramsay, C., & Lodge, J. K. (2021). Effects of chronic consumption of specific fruit (berries, citrus and cherries) on CVD risk factors: A systematic review and meta-analysis of randomized controlled trials. *European Journal of Nutrition, 60*(2), 615–639.

WHO. (2016). World Health Organization; Geneva: Global Health Estimates 2015: Deaths by Cause, Age, Sex, by Country and by region (2000–2015). https://www.who.int/data/global-health-estimates.

Willcox, B. J., Willcox, D. C., Todoriki, H., Fujiyoshi, A., Yano, K., He, Q., Curb, J. D., & Suzuki, M. (2007). Caloric restriction, the traditional Okinawan diet, and healthy aging: The diet of the world's longest-lived people and its potential impact on morbidity and lifespan. *Annals of the New York Academy of Sciences, 1114*, 434–455.

Willcox, D. C., Willcox, B. J., Todoriki, H., Curb, J. D., & Suzuki, M. (2006). Caloric restriction and human longevity: What can we learn from the Okinawans? *Biogerontology, 7*(3), 173–177.

Yang, C., Li, L., Yang, L., Lǚ, H., Wang, S., & Sun, G. (2018). Anti-obesity and hypolipidemic effects of garlic oil and onion oil in rats fed a high-fat diet. *Nutrition & Metabolism, 15*(1), 43.

Ye, Z., & Song, H. (2008). Antioxidant vitamins intake and the risk of coronary heart disease: Meta-analysis of cohort studies. *European Journal of Cardiovascular Prevention and Rehabilitation, 15*(1), 26–34.

Zhang, X., Shu, X. O., Xiang, Y. B., Yang, G., Li, H., Gao, J., & Zheng, W. (2011). Cruciferous vegetable consumption is associated with a reduced risk of total and cardiovascular disease mortality. *The American Journal of Clinical Nutrition, 94*(1), 240–246.

CHAPTER 2

NUTRACEUTICALS FOR CARDIOVASCULAR HEALTH AND DISEASES: INTRODUCTION AND OVERVIEW

BHUSHAN R. RANE,[1] ASHISH S. JAIN,[1] NIDHI S. KATE,[1] SAMALI S. RAUT,[1] RAJ K. KESERVANI,[2] VINIT S. PATIL,[1] ARVIND KUMAR GUPTA,[2] and JAFFAR SHAIK[3]

[1]*Shri D.D. Vispute College of Pharmacy and Research Center, Devad-Vichumbe, Panvel, Navi Mumbai, Maharashtra, India*

[2]*Faculty of B. Pharmacy, CSM Group of Institutions, Prayagraj, Uttar Pradesh, India*

[3]*Research Scholar, Department of Biochemistry, Acharya Nagarjuna University, Guntur, Andhra Pradesh, India*

ABSTRACT

Cardiovascular disease (CVD) is among the most prevalent health and global economic issues. Dietary factors influence cardiovascular risk either directly or indirectly through their effects on other risk factors such as hypertension and dyslipidemia. There has been a lot of research interest that links the beneficial effects of food to disease prevention and treatment. Nutraceuticals are natural nutritional compounds that are beneficial in illness therapy and disease prevention. Several foods and dietary supplements have been demonstrated to help prevent cardiovascular disease. Dietary treatments offer new, potentially simple, and economical options for population-based CVD risk reduction initiatives, and the opportunity to use nutraceuticals to positively

Antioxidants as Nutraceuticals. Nayan A. Gujarathi, Raj K. Keservani, Rajesh K. Kesharwani, Bhushan R. Rane, Yogeeta Sameer Goyal (Eds.)

influence CV risk variables should be acknowledged as a huge opportunity. The goal of this article is to provide an overview of the most recent evidence regarding the use of nutraceuticals in the diagnosis, mitigation, and therapy of cardiovascular disease.

2.1 INTRODUCTION

In recent years, a new diet-health model has emerged, emphasizing the positive aspects of eating. People's basic eating habits have changed due to their new lifestyles. Junk food consumption has increased significantly, leading to various disorders caused by poor nutrition. Obesity is now widely recognized as a global issue. In many developing countries, heart disease remains the leading cause of death, followed by osteoporosis, cancer, arthritis, and other conditions (Raut et al., 2021; Padmavathi et al., 2018). Nutraceuticals are utilized for the treatment and prevention of conditions such as cardiovascular disease (Keservani et al., 2016a), cancer, obesity, and diabetes mellitus. Specific nutraceuticals play a crucial role in various physical activities and help reduce the risk of numerous illnesses in individuals. These dietary supplements are used to boost immunity, treat and prevent a wide range of illnesses (Keservani et al., 2015b), and maintain health. According to recent studies, these nutraceuticals are particularly effective in preventing and healing a variety of diseases (Ghani et al., 2019). The most common reason for death worldwide is cardiovascular disease (CVD). According to the WHO, 17.9 million people died from CVDs globally in 2019, which accounted for 32% of all deaths. Stroke and heart attacks were responsible for 85% of these fatalities. Around 75% of CVD mortality occurs in low- and middle-income countries. CVDs were responsible for 38% of the 17 million deaths (under the age of 70) caused by noncommunicable diseases in 2019. The majority of cardiovascular disorders can be avoided by managing behavioral risk factors such as tobacco use, smoking, obesity and poor diet, physical inactivity, and alcohol abuse. It's crucial to diagnose cardiovascular disease as early as possible so that counseling and medication can begin. WHO Member States agreed on global methods to minimize the avoidable non-communicable disease (NCD) burden in 2013, including a plan for the control and prevention of NCDs from the year 2013–2020, globally. This mission aims to reduce the number of premature deaths related to NCDs by 25% by 2025 through nine voluntary targets. Two of the goals are directly related to CVD prevention and control. Target 6 states that between 2010 and 2025, it aims to reduce the global prevalence of high blood pressure by 25%.

By 2025, at least half of those eligible for medication therapy and counseling (including glycemic regulation) should receive it to prevent heart attacks and strokes. Additionally, target 9 specifies that in both public and private facilities, 80% of the affordable basic technologies and essential medicines, including generics, needed to treat major NCDs should be accessible. Health systems will need significant improvements to achieve these goals. Various nutraceuticals have been suggested to provide potential benefits in treating CVD, and some of them are outlined in this study.

2.2 DEFINITION

The words "nutraceutical" and "pharmaceutical" were combined in 1989 by Stephen DeFelice, MD, chairman and founder in New Jersey. Nutraceuticals, according to DeFelice, are "foods or components of foods that give medicinal or health advantages, such as the prevention of a disease." But the phrase "nutraceutical," as it is frequently used in marketing, lacks a legal definition. He suggests that functional foods and nutraceuticals should be redefined. Food is referred to as "functional food" when it is cooked or prepared to utilize "scientific intelligence," with or without an understanding of how it will be employed. Functional food provides the vitamins, lipids, proteins, carbs, and other nutrients it requires for optimal existence. A nutraceutical is a functional food that aids in the prevention and/or treatment of disease and/or disorder (Keservani et al., 2010; Ekta et al., 2003). Since the initial definition of nutraceuticals was given, a variety of other definitions have been presented; by either limiting the dose types covered by the phrase (e.g., pills, capsules), enforcing some sort of processing constraints limiting the health benefits criteria, or establishing their relationship to other product categories (Palthur et al., 2010). Several definitions concur or cross-reference the original DeFelice definition. Some of them are as follows: Any food or fruit component that has health advantages, including the ability to prevent and treat disease, is referred to as a nutraceutical. These goods might include everything from isolated nutrients, nutritional supplements, and particular diets to foods that have been genetically modified, and refined foods including cereals, soups, and drinks. Any nontoxic food ingredient with medically validated health advantages, such as the treatment and prevention of disease, is referred to as a nutraceutical. Products known as nutraceuticals are made from food sources and claim to have additional health advantages over and beyond the fundamental nutritional value of the food they are produced from. Products may make claims to slow the aging process, extend life expectancy, prevent chronic diseases, promote health, or enhance the function of the body, depending on the applicable laws (Keservani et al., 2017, 2020).

2.3 IMPORTANCE OF NUTRACEUTICALS

Nutraceuticals have an essential role in a variety of bodily activities, as well as lowering the risk of numerous diseases in humans. The use of certain dietary supplements to alleviate a variety of ailments, as well as to build immunity and control health. Based on recent studies, these nutraceuticals have been shown to be quite effective in preventing and treating various diseases (Ghani et al., 2019). Nutraceuticals are currently gaining popularity due to their beneficial nutritional and safety profiles, in addition to their therapeutic power. Pharmaceutical and nutritional firms are aware of the shifting patterns brought on by the benefits of these chemicals. The majority of nutraceuticals have several therapeutic advantages (Kalra et al., 2003). Modern work patterns have resulted in the emergence of a new class of ailments known colloquially as lifestyle disorders. Improper diet and reliance on fast foods are common causative agents of many problems, as are a lack of physical activity, wrong body posture, and excessive stress. Nutraceuticals are a unique combination of current technology and natural agents, and they may be the greatest potential answer for the management of lifestyle disorders. These lifestyle issues are also thought to be responsible for the predisposition to several complex clinical illnesses (Sharma et al., 2009). For more than two decades, scientists have attempted to link phytochemicals to their contribution to health benefits. According to statistics, the intake of vegetables and fruits reduces the likelihood of diseases in the esophagus, stomach, lungs, endometrium, oral cavity, pancreas, throat, and colon (Bradbury et al., 2014). Nutraceuticals are used as immunity boosters, cure Parkinson's and Alzheimer's disease (Keservani et al., 2015a), ability to cure metabolic disorders, i.e., obesity (Jarouliya & Keservani, 2019a), cardiovascular disease, etc., ability to prevent cancer and diabetes, manage chronic inflammatory disorders, ability to cure bone disorders such as osteoporosis, arthritis, etc. (Sachdeva et al., 2020).

2.4 VARIOUS CARDIOVASCULAR DISEASES

CVDs are heart and blood vessel disorders. Among them are:

2.4.1 STROKE

Stroke is the world's 2nd largest cause of mortality and a major cause of disability. A stroke is a neurological condition in which blood vessels get blocked. It can be classified as Ischemic and hemorrhagic strokes. Most deaths were caused due to Ischemic stroke. According to WHO, in India in the year 2019, stroke was the 3rd most common cause of death with 50.88 deaths per 1,00,000 population, and was the 4th top cause of death in the USA. Because of the effect of decreased blood flow to certain parts of the brain, ischemic strokes might appear in pre-determined syndromes. This enables clinicians to forecast which parts of the brain vasculature will be damaged. Ischemic cerebrovascular illness is caused primarily by thrombosis, embolism, and focal hypoperfusion, all of which can result in a decrease or disruption in cerebral blood flow (CBF), affecting neurological function owing to glucose and oxygen deprivation (Kuriakose et al., 2020; Hui et al., 2021; Kanyal et al., 2015). Hemorrhagic stroke occurs in 10–15% of all strokes and is associated with a high fatality rate. Blood vessels break due to stress and internal injury in the brain tissues. It produces vascular system toxicity, which contributes to infarction. Intracerebral and subarachnoid hemorrhage are the two types of hemorrhagic stroke. The main factors contributing to stroke are modifiable factors like smoking, hypertension, alcohol and drug abuse, and non-modifiable factors like Sex, Gender, and Genetics (Kuriakose et al., 2020).

2.4.2 RHEUMATIC HEART DISEASE

Acute rheumatic fever (ARF) is an autoimmune reaction in pharyngitis induced by group A Streptococcus infection. Rheumatic heart disease (RHD) is the long-term damage to cardiac valves caused by ARF, which can be caused by a single severe episode or numerous recurrent occurrences of ARF. The circulating autoantibodies bind to the endothelial surface of the mitral valves, causing an increase in the production of vascular cell adhesion protein 1 (VCAM-1). The infiltration of T lymphocytes into the valvular sub-endothelium is facilitated by the active endothelium, resulting in edema and elongation of the chordae tendineae. Anti-collagen antibodies are created in response to valvular tissue stretching that exposes extracellular matrix components. Antibodies can accumulate in the valve, adding to an inflammatory environment. The heart valves become a sensitive immune-privileged target for degeneration as a result of these modifications (Leal et al., 2019; Carapetis et al., 2016). According to WHO, in those under the age of 25, rheumatic heart disease is the most common type of heart disease. Rheumatic heart disease takes the lives of about 2,88,348 people each year, the majority of whom reside in low- and middle-income countries.

2.4.3 VALVULAR HEART DISEASE

Damage or defects in one of the four heart valves, the aortic, mitral, tricuspid, or pulmonary, cause valvular heart disease (VHD). These valve defects can be congenital or acquired. The risk of disease is influenced by age, gender, tobacco use, hypercholesterolemia, hypertension, and type II diabetes. VHD is a rapidly growing health problem in the United States, with an incidence of 2.5%. The incidence of acquired VHD is projected to rise due to the world's aging population (Zeng et al., 2016). The two most frequent kinds of valvular disease in Europe are aortic stenosis and mitral regurgitation. Because degenerative etiologies predominate, the frequency of valve disease rises dramatically with age. There is no universally accepted definition of valvular disease because the clinical significance of these disorders is determined by the severity of valve failure rather than structural impairment (Iung et al., 2011).

2.4.4 CONGESTIVE HEART FAILURE

Heart failure is a persistent and advancing clinical illness induced by anatomical or functional cardiac defects that result in either reduced (in Heart Failure with reduced ejection fraction) or preserved (in Heart Failure with preserved ejection fraction) ejection fraction (HFpEF) (Arrigo et al., 2020). Left ventricular ejection fraction (LVEF) is affected. Any disease that hinders the filling of the ventricles or the ejection of blood into the systemic circulation causes it. The most common symptoms of patients are fluid retention, dyspnea, and weariness (peripheral and pulmonary edema). Heart structural and functional problems, as well as additional triggering events, all contribute to congestive heart failure. This causes a decrease in cardiac output, which is consequently insufficient to supply the body's peripheral demands. The following are the four key factors that affect left ventricular (LV) functions: (i) muscle contractility is intrinsically reduced; (ii) an increase in pulmonary congestion and dyspnea is caused by preload or left atrial filling pressure; (iii) despite the fact that systemic blood pressure is frequently lowered, systemic vascular resistance (afterload) increases, which can lower cardiac output even further; and (iv) in general, heart rate increases as a defense response related to an increase in sympathetic stimulation and catecholamine levels. There is frequently a disparity in the quantity and demand of myocardial oxygen in patients with coronary disease. An increase in heart size could be harmful. An increase in catecholamines, which raises heart rate and contractility in an effort to maintain cardiac output, is one of the intrinsic compensating mechanisms. Another is cardiac muscle hyperplasia, which aids in cardiac function. An increase in left ventricle filling pressure can improve performance by increasing the extraction of peripheral arterial-venous oxygen. The Frank-Starling mechanism maximizes the amount of oxygen supplied for a specific cardiac output. Despite the fact that these compensating mechanisms are originally beneficial, many of them, such as an increase in catecholamines and vascular resistance throughout the body, may become excessive (Parmley et al., 1985).

2.4.5 DEEP VENOUS THROMBOSIS (DVT)

It is caused by blood clotting in a deep vein of an extremity (usually the calves or thighs) or the pelvis. It is the most common cause of pulmonary embolism. DVT is caused by conditions that limit venous return, cause endothelial damage or malfunction, or create hypercoagulability. DVT can be asymptomatic or produce discomfort and edema in an extremity; pulmonary embolism is an acute complication. The diagnosis is made based on the patient's history and physical examination, and it is confirmed by objective testing, most commonly duplex ultrasonography. When DVT is suspected, D-Dimer testing is utilized; a negative result helps to rule out deep venous thrombosis. A favorable result, on the other hand, is unspecific and necessitates further testing to confirm DVT. Anticoagulants are used in treatment. With quick and adequate treatment, the prognosis is generally favorable. Long-term problems that are common are venous incompetence accompanied or unaccompanied by post-phlebitic syndrome (Douketis et al., 2021). Thrombosis is a defense mechanism that closes off injured blood arteries and stops the loss of blood. The thrombosis is neutralized or stabilized by fibrinolysis. Vein thrombosis causes are typically complex, with each member of the Virchow triad playing a different role in each patient. However, all of these factors lead to early thrombus contact with the endothelium. Leukocyte adherence to the endothelium and local cytokine production are thus stimulated, both of which aid in venous thrombosis. Thrombus propagation depends on the relative equilibrium between both the clotting and thrombolytic pathways. The soleal sinuses and other low-flow locations, which are located behind venous valve pockets, are where deep venous thrombosis typically begins in the lower limb underneath the knee (Waheed et al., 2021; Kudaravalli et al., 2021; Hotwagner et al., 2021).

2.4.6 CORONARY ARTERY DISEASE (CAD)

The most severe form of cardiac disease that can cause sudden death is coronary artery disease (Mastoi et al., 2018; Gopal et al., 2018; Iqbal et al., 2018). However, CAD diagnoses are costly and time-consuming procedures that a patient must go through. Coronary artery diseases (CAD) are heart and blood vessel ailments that claim 17.1 million lives worldwide each year (World Health Organization, 2010). At the age of 40, men have a 50% lifetime risk of getting CAD while women have a 33% lifetime risk (Pheng et al., 2017). The European Heart Network and the European Society of Cardiology, on the other hand, estimate that over 4 million individuals died from CVDs in Europe, with 1.9 million dying in the European Union (EU), or 47% and 40% of all deaths, respectively. Older age, male gender, overweight, hypertension, current smoking, diabetes mellitus, hypertriglyceridemia, and hypercholesterolemia are all traditional risk factors for CAD. Coronary artery disease is usually the result of atheromatous constriction and subsequent vascular blockage. Early atheroma [from the Greek athera (porridge) and Oma (lump)] appears in young adulthood. A mature plaque is made up of two components, each of which is connected with a different cell population. The lipid core is primarily released by necrotic "foam cells"—monocyte-derived macrophages that move into the intima and consume lipids. Smooth muscle cells migrate from the media into the intima, where they proliferate and change phenotypically to create a fibrous capsule surrounding the lipid core. When a plaque causes a >50% diameter stenosis (or a >75% reduction in cross-sectional area), diminished blood flow through the coronary artery during exertion may result in angina. Acute coronary events typically occur as a result of thrombus development following plaque disruption. Intimal damage produces denudation of the thrombogenic matrix or lipid pool, which leads to thrombus development. Occlusion is more complete in acute myocardial infarction than in unstable angina, where arterial occlusion is typically partial. Microinfarcts may be caused by downstream embolism of thrombus (Grech et al., 2003).

2.4.7 CONGENITAL HEART DISEASE

Congenital abnormalities emerge in the growing fetus. Congenital heart disease is a prominent congenital anomaly characterized by cardiac abnormalities apparent at birth. Among all birth abnormalities, congenital heart disease is the leading cause of infant mortality. It is a structural anomaly of the heart or major vessels that can be discovered in infancy or subsequently in life (Dolk et al., 2011; Gilboa et al., 2010). Congenital cardiac disease is the greatest reason for death in children worldwide, particularly in underdeveloped nations (Chelo et al., 2016; Kouame et al., 2015). It also contributes to more than 20% of prenatal infant deaths (Sadowski et al., 2009; Hoffman et al., 2002). Congenital heart disease is expected to affect 8 out of every 1,000 live births. Congenital heart disease is divided into three categories: mild, severe, and uncomplicated. In each group, the predicted occurrence of moderate and severe congenital heart disease is reviewed at 1.5/1000 live births (van der Bom et al., 2011; Warnes et al., 2001; Bernier et al., 2010). Physical exams and clinical manifestations such as abnormal heart rhythms, cyanosis, chest discomfort, and palpitations can be used to diagnose congenital heart disease in patients (Sayasathid et al., 2012). Congenital cardiac abnormalities are caused by changes in the developing processes of embryonic structure or the inability of structure to form during an initial embryonic stage. It's an anatomical flaw that affects the organ system's structure and function. The cause of aberrant cardiac development in newborns is still unknown. Despite substantial advancements in recognizing the causes of congenital heart disease in the recent decade. Congenital malformations can be linked to genetic problems, while other deformities are caused by environmental teratogens or diet. A disruption in cell migration can disrupt heart development. These findings highlight the dynamic and complex pathophysiology of congenital heart disease. Additional research is required to discover the etiology of congenital heart disease, which will pave the way for healthcare professionals and health officers to understand prevention measures and treatment (Upadhyay et al., 2019).

2.4.7.1 TYPES OF CONGENITAL HEART DISEASE

- **Ventricular Septal Defect:** The breach in the wall that separates the heart's right and left ventricles is known as a ventricular septal defect.

- **Atrial Septal Defect:** An atrial septal defect is a cardiac birth abnormality defined by a hole in the wall that separates the heart's upper chambers.
- **Pulmonary Stenosis:** It occurs when the valve between the lower right heart chamber and the lung arteries narrows.
- **Patent Ductus Arteriosus:** The patent ductus arteriosus (PDA) is a gap between two blood arteries that lead from the heart.
- **Tetralogy of Fallot:** Tetralogy of Fallot abnormalities cause oxygen-depleted blood to flow from the heart and throughout the body.
- **Coarctation of Aorta:** It's a constriction of the aorta, a large blood vessel that extends from the heart to the rest of the body.
- **Transposition of Great Arteries:** It is a heart defect in which the two main arteries bringing blood from the heart, the pulmonary arteries and the aorta, are "transposed" in their positions.
- **Aortic Stenosis:** A significant blood vessel that leaves the heart has a narrowed valve. This constriction prevents the valve from fully opening, decreasing blood circulation in the system and putting more strain on the heart.

2.4.8 ARRHYTHMIA

Cardiac arrhythmias are characterized by a slow or rapid heartbeat with an erratic rhythm. Necrosis of heart cells can result from a long-term ischemic effect caused by a complete lack of oxygen. This results in an aberrant re-entry of electrical impulses, resulting in arrhythmia. In the case of fibrosis, aging, and cardiac channel mutation, an abnormal cardiac action potential develops, making the patient vulnerable to cardiac arrhythmias. An electrical device that generates, conducts, and distributes electrical signals toward the contractile myocardium in the presence of certain cardiac structures (Bhardwaj et al., 2012; Padeletti et al., 2017). Electric impulses are generated in the heart from the sinus node and directed to particular ionic channels that are explicitly located in cells and other parts of the heart. In a crisis, the secondary pacemaker shows activity. The ability to induce numerous depolarizations decreases the SA node and is minimal in the ventricle. The major pacemaker receives critical neurovegetative signals, where depolarization is frequently modulated to meet the metabolic needs of the organism (Rodrigo et al., 2015; Dhinakaran et al., 2019).

2.4.8.1 TYPES OF ARRHYTHMIAS

- **Atrial Flutter:** Rapid contractions of the heart's upper chambers spread to the lower chambers, resulting in a rapid heartbeat.
- **Atrial Fibrillation:** Atrial fibrillation is a cardiac rhythm that is abnormal and often very fast, which can cause blood clots in the heart. It raises the risk of stroke, heart failure, and other cardiovascular problems.
- **Supraventricular Tachycardia:** Supraventricular tachycardia is a fast heartbeat caused by a disruption in the heart's regular electrical impulses.
- **Ventricular Tachycardia (VT):** Unusual electrical impulses in the lower chambers of the heart lead to VT, a condition that affects the heart's rhythm.
- **Ventricular Fibrillation (VF):** VF is a life-threatening cardiac rhythm that begins in the heart's bottom chambers. A heart attack can cause it to happen. Sustained ventricular fibrillation can result in low blood pressure, unconsciousness, or death when the heart does not pump adequately.

2.4.9 MARFAN SYNDROME

This syndrome is a connective tissue disorder that is primarily caused by genetic mutations in the fibrillin-1 gene. Antoine Bernard-Jean Marfan, a French doctor, originally identified the illness in 1896. Different ophthalmic, skeletal, cardiovascular, respiratory, cutaneous, and neurological problems have been added to the diagnosis of this condition since then, resulting in what we now call Marfan syndrome (MFS). It can be difficult to diagnose since many of its symptoms are age-related, while others are widespread in the general population. There is a lot of phenotypic heterogeneity, and there is a significant overlap with other connective tissue disorders. Because untreated Marfan syndrome is linked to early death, it's critical to get a proper diagnosis as soon as possible (Cañadas et al., 2010). Those suffering from the illness are typically tall and skinny, with long limbs, legs, fingers, and toes. They are also prone to scoliosis and have extremely flexible joints. The heart and aorta are the most vulnerable, with a higher risk of the mitral valve and aortic aneurysm. The lungs, eyes, bones, and spinal cord covering are all typically impacted. The severity of MFS symptoms varies. MFS is caused by mutations in FBN1, one of the genes responsible for the production of fibrillin, which leads to aberrant connective tissue. It is an inherited dominant condition. Approximately 75% of the time, the ailment is genetically inherited, whereas 25% of the time it's a new mutation (Wikipedia).

2.5 NUTRACEUTICALS FOR CARDIOVASCULAR DISEASES

2.5.1 ALLICIN

Garlic contains the active component allicin. Garlic appears to work through a variety of pathways to accomplish a significant effect by lowering serum lipids and blood pressure, inhibiting platelet aggregation, and enhancing fibrinolytic antioxidant activity, according to evidence from several research studies (Qidwai et al., 2013). Garlic can treat moderate hypertension, lower cholesterol levels, and prevent atherosclerosis. More clinical trials are needed to fully comprehend the mechanisms underlying the therapy or prevention of certain cardiovascular diseases (Alali et al., 2017; Sobenin et al., 2019).

2.5.2 COCOA

Cocoa, which is high in oligomeric procyanidins, is one of the most researched nutraceuticals: chocolate flavonoids (Keservani & Sharma, 2014; Keservani et al., 2016b), in particular, appear to boost nitric oxide (NO) bioavailability, protect the vascular endothelium, and lower levels of various CVD risk factors (Carrizzo et al., 2020). Because of its antioxidant and anti-inflammatory properties, as well as the activation of nitric oxide, cocoa flavonol appears to offer potential benefits against hypertension, blood lipids, stroke, and CVD (Singh et al., 2022).

2.5.3 CURCUMIN

Turmeric's roots and rhizomes contain curcumin, which has been used as a traditional medicine to improve blood circulation and stasis. Curcumin possesses anti-inflammatory, antioxidant, and anti-infective properties

(Singh et al., 2021). Curcumin, in addition to calcium homeostatic capabilities, contains antioxidative, anti-inflammatory, and anti-proliferative activities. These functions are linked to lower blood pressure and the prevention of vascular smooth cell growth (Carrizzo et al., 2020).

2.5.4 VITAMINS

Vitamin C's significant antioxidant properties aid in lowering tissue reactive oxygen species levels, which helps to avoid endothelial dysfunction, decrease vascular smooth muscle proliferation, and lower oxidized LDL cholesterol in atherosclerosis. Vitamin E is a potent anti-inflammatory agent, especially at high dosages, in addition to its action as a free radical scavenger. A review of the literature points to a strong inverse relationship between plasma vitamin E and cardiovascular disease (Alissa et al., 2012). Vitamin D is best known for its involvement in calcium absorption and bone mineralization in the intestine. The discovery of the vitamin D receptor (VDR) and 1-hydroxylase in cardiomyocytes, endothelial cells, and vascular smooth muscle cells, as well as the observation of seasonal fluctuations in blood pressure, link vitamin D to the cardiovascular system and hence can help enhance the health of a patient suffering from CVD. Furthermore, observational studies have linked vitamin D insufficiency to an increased risk of hypertension, heart failure, and atherosclerosis (Latic et al., 2020).

2.5.5 STANOLS/STEROLS

Plant sterols/stanols consumption has been linked to reduced circulating total cholesterol levels in people. Their effect is mostly on LDL-C lowering, with little or no effect on HDL-C or triglycerides. It also was connected to lowering blood pressure but some studies have failed to prove so. Although the evidence is limited, these substances appear to have no antihypertensive effects in humans and no evidence of adverse blood pressure consequences (Sosnowska et al., 2017). Phytosterols and phytostanols stop cholesterol from being absorbed in the intestine (Alissa et al., 2012).

2.5.6 OMEGA-3 FATTY ACIDS

Omega-3 fatty acids (Ω3FAs) are among the most often prescribed supplements in the global market. They appear to reduce TG, inflammation, and platelet aggregation, induce vasodilation, and improve blood rheology, endothelial function, and myocardial function. Animal studies have indicated that adding Ω3FAs to the cell membrane increases cellular function through interacting with and modulating membrane channels, as well as changing the physicochemical properties of the cell membrane. The membrane-incorporated Ω3FAs may be able to influence membrane protein signaling positively (Jarouliya & Keservani, 2019b). Furthermore, in animal investigations, Ω3FA integration has been linked to alterations in the H-Ras signaling molecule and inhibited protein kinase C-theta signaling.

2.5.7 COENZYME Q10

Myocardial CoQ10 content tends to drop with age and myocardial dysfunction. To move electrons from complexes I and II to complex III, CoQ10 functions in the mitochondrial inner membrane. It also functions as a membrane antioxidant due to its redox activity. Several studies have shown that supplementary CoQ10 improves functional metrics like ejection fraction, stroke volume, and cardiac output and that long-term CoQ10 therapy lowers major adverse cardiovascular events, improves HF symptoms, and is safe and well tolerated.

2.5.8 SPIRULINA

Spirulina (*Cyanobacterium*) is high in protein, vitamins, minerals, carotenoids, and phycocyanins. Spirulina supplementation has been linked to improved blood lipid profiles. Spirulina maxima administered orally is related to considerable alterations in TC and LDL-C values. Preclinical studies discovered a considerable increase in lipase activity after spirulina consumption, which is thought to aid with hyperlipidemia. The precise mechanism of action for this effect, however, is still being researched. One interesting theory is that spirulina binds to cholesterol metabolites and bile acids, increasing their fecal excretion. In principle, this would lower serum cholesterol levels. According to some accounts, the cholesterol effects may have been caused by C-phycocyanin activities. Resveratrol's suggested mechanistic pathway has been demonstrated in Table 2.1.

TABLE 2.1 Nutraceutics and Their Effects on Cardiovascular Conditions

Sr. No.	Active Ingredients	Effects
1.	Resveratrol	Anti-inflammatory, decrease interstitial fibrosis, decrease cardiac hypertrophy, and reduce oxidative stress markers
2.	Stanols/Sterols	Decrease LDL Cholesterol, inhibits intestinal cholesterol absorption
3.	Vitamin C	Anti-oxidant inhibits vascular smooth muscle proliferation and reduces oxidized LDL cholesterol
4.	Vitamin E	Free-radical scavenger, anti-inflammatory
5.	Vitamin D	Increase HDL Cholesterol levels, anti-oxidant
6.	Lycopene	Anti-oxidants reduce oxidative stress *in vivo*
7.	Allicin	Antioxidant, antiapoptotic, and anti-inflammatory actions
8.	Cocoa	Decrease blood pressure and decrease LDL cholesterol levels
9.	Quercetin	Anti-inflammatory, antihypertensive
10.	Curcumin	Anti-inflammatory, antihypertensive, and decreases hypertrophy
11.	Calcium	Anti-hypertensive
12.	Sour tea	Anti-hypertensive
13.	Saffron	Anti-hypertensive
14.	Turmeric Curcumin	Anti-hypertensive
15.	Spirulina	Decreasing the risk of atherosclerosis
16.	Coenzyme Q10	Decreases atherosclerosis, anti-hypertensive Cardiovascular aging, in angina pectoris
17.	Omega 3 fatty acids	Decrease triglycerides, improve blood rheology and myocardial function

2.6 CONCLUSION

Following the recession, the worldwide market is currently entering a period of expansion. Even when the effects of the crisis fade, the nutraceutical business is expected to stay in a growth phase, led by growing markets such as India, China, and Brazil. Various Indian enterprises have established themselves as suppliers of phytoconstituents and phytochemicals both domestically and globally, which will aid the growing nutraceuticals sector in the near future (Shinde et al., 2014). Diabetic nephropathy, hypertension, and dyslipidemia are cardiovascular disease risk factors. Present healthcare therapies for diabetes management and dyslipidemia in certain patients, especially those at high risk, are insufficient, and recent research suggests that the use of nutraceuticals has the potential to improve therapy effectiveness. Many nutraceuticals being investigated for cardiovascular disease prevention and treatment are well tolerated by patients. However, there is frequently insufficient data on long-term safety and efficacy against clinical studies including cardiac disease and death rates. More clinical research is needed to identify nutraceuticals with the highest clinical expense in the treatment and prevention of cardiovascular disease (Sahebkar et al., 2016; Serban et al., 2015; Banach et al., 2014; Ursoniu et al., 2015).

2.7 FUTURE PERSPECTIVE

In clinical practice and research, novel dietary approaches to cardiovascular protection are extremely important. However, nutrition is a complicated research topic, and it's unclear if a single dietary component or a mix of nutrients and dietary behaviors is to blame for any cardioprotective effects. Advances in our understanding of disease processes and healthy dietary components have opened up new possibilities for developing dietary strategies to prevent and/or treat CVD. Nutraceuticals appear to be an essential resource for the prevention and maintenance of vascular health before or in conjunction with therapeutic therapy, based on their effects. Furthermore, a patient's best inclination to therapy with a natural substance may be the most effective way to improve the preventive strategy and lower the incidence of CVDs. Thus, to improve the patient's results, it is fair to consider the use of nutraceuticals as a supplement to "conventional" lifestyle adjustments and "common" pharmacological therapies.

KEYWORDS

- **cardiovascular**
- **functional foods**
- **Nutraceuticals**
- **prevention**
- **treatment**

REFERENCES

Abubakar, S. M., Ukeyima, M. T., Spencer, J. P. E., & Lovegrove, J. A. (2019). Acute effects of Hibiscus sabdariffa calyces on postprandial blood pressure, vascular function, blood lipids, biomarkers of insulin resistance and inflammation in humans. *Nutrients, 11*(2), 341. https://doi.org/10.3390/nu11020341.

Alali, F. Q., El-Elimat, T., Khalid, L., Hudaib, R., Al-Shehabi, T. S., & Eid, A. H. (2017). Garlic for cardiovascular disease: Prevention or treatment? *Current Pharmaceutical Design, 23*(7), 1028–1041. https://doi.org/10.2174/1381612822666161010124530.

Alissa, E. M., & Ferns, G. A. (2012). Functional foods and nutraceuticals in the primary prevention of cardiovascular diseases. *Journal of Nutrition and Metabolism, 2012*, 569486. https://doi.org/10.1155/2012/569486.

Arrigo, M., Jessup, M., Mullens, W., Reza, N., Shah, A. M., Sliwa, K., & Mebazaa, A. (2020). Acute heart failure. *Nature Reviews Disease Primers, 6*(1), 1–15. https://doi.org/10.1038/s41572-020-0151-7.

Aziz, Z., Wong, S. Y., & Chong, N. J. (2013). Effects of Hibiscus sabdariffa L. on serum lipids: A systematic review and meta-analysis. *Journal of Ethnopharmacology, 150*(2), 442–450. https://doi.org/10.1016/j.jep.2013.09.042.

Banach, M., Aronow, W. S., Serban, C., Sahabkar, A., Rysz, J., Voroneanu, L., & Covic, A. (2015). Lipids, blood pressure and kidney update 2014. *Pharmacological Research, 95–96*, 111–125. https://doi.org/10.1016/j.phrs.2015.03.009.

Bernier, P.-L., Stefanescu, A., Samoukovic, G., & Tchervenkov, C. I. (2010). The challenge of congenital heart disease worldwide: Epidemiologic and demographic facts. *Seminars in Thoracic and Cardiovascular Surgery: Pediatric Cardiac Surgery Annual, 13*(1), 26–34. https://doi.org/10.1053/j.pcsu.2010.02.005.

Bradbury, K. E., Appleby, P. N., & Key, T. J. (2014). Fruit, vegetable, and fiber intake in relation to cancer risk: Findings from the European Perspective Investigation into Cancer and Nutrition (EPIC). *The American Journal of Clinical Nutrition, 100*(suppl_1), 394S–398S. https://doi.org/10.3945/ajcn.113.071357.

Cañadas, V., Vilacosta, I., Bruna, I., & Fuster, V. (2010). Marfan syndrome. Part 1: Pathophysiology and diagnosis. *Nature Reviews Cardiology, 7*(5), 256–265. https://doi.org/10.1038/nrcardio.2010.30.

Carapetis, J. R., Beaton, A., Cunningham, M. W., Guilherme, L., Karthikeyan, G., Mayosi, B. M., Sable, C., Steer, A., Wilson, N., Wyber, R., & Zühlke, L. (2016). Acute rheumatic fever and rheumatic heart disease. *Nature Reviews Disease Primers, 2*, 15084. https://doi.org/10.1038/nrdp.2015.84.

Cardiovascular diseases (CVDs). (n.d.). Retrieved from: https://www.who.int/news-room/fact-sheets/detail/cardiovascular-diseases-(cvds) (accessed on 12 June 2024).

Chaudhari, S. P. (2017). Nutraceuticals: A review. *World Journal of Pharmacy and Pharmaceutical Sciences, 6,* Issue 8, 681–739. DOI : 10.20959/wjpps20178–9825.

Chelo, D., Nguefack, F., Menanga, A. P., Ngo Um, S., Gody, J. C., Tatah, S. A., & Koki Ndombo, P. O. (2016). Spectrum of heart diseases in children: An echocardiographic study of 1,666 subjects in a pediatric hospital, Yaounde, Cameroon. *Cardiovascular Diagnosis and Therapy, 6*(1), 10–19. https://doi.org/10.3978/j.issn.2223-3652.2015.11.04.

Cheng, H. M., Koutsidis, G., Lodge, J. K., Ashor, A., Siervo, M., & Lara, J. (2017). Tomato and lycopene supplementation and cardiovascular risk factors: A systematic review and meta-analysis. *Atherosclerosis, 257*, 100–108. https://doi.org/10.1016/j.atherosclerosis.2017.01.009.

Chung, M., Tang, A. M., Fu, Z., Wang, D. D., & Newberry, S. J. (2016). Calcium intake and cardiovascular disease risk. *Annals of Internal Medicine, 165*(12), 856. https://doi.org/10.7326/m16-1165.

Coffey, S., Roberts-Thomson, R., Brown, A., Carapetis, J., Chen, M., Enriquez-Sarano, M., Zühlke, L., & Prendergast, B. D. (2021). Global epidemiology of valvular heart disease. *Nature Reviews Cardiology, 18*(12), 853–864. https://doi.org/10.1038/s41569-021-00570-z.

da Costa, J. P. (2017). A current look at nutraceuticals – Key concepts and future prospects. *Trends in Food Science & Technology, 62*, 68–78. https://doi.org/10.1016/j.tifs.2017.02.010.

Deep venous thrombosis (DVT). (2015). In Encyclopedia of Trauma Care, (eds) Papadakos, P. J., Gestring, M. L., (p. 431). Springer Berlin Heidelberg. https://doi.org/10.1007/978–3-642–36226–4_421.

Dolk, H., Loane, M., & Garne, E. (2011). Congenital heart defects in Europe. *Circulation, 123*(8), 841–849. https://doi.org/10.1161/circulationaha.110.958405.

Ebrahimi, F., Aryaeian, N., Pahlavani, N., Abbasi, D., Hosseini, A. F., & Fallah, S. (2019). The effect of saffron (*Crocus sativus* L.) supplementation on blood pressure, and renal and liver function in patients with type 2 diabetes mellitus: A double-blinded, randomized clinical trial. *Avicenna Journal of Phytomedicine, 9*(4), 322–333.

Ferguson, J. J. A., Stojanovski, E., MacDonald-Wicks, L., & Garg, M. L. (2016). Fat type in phytosterol products influence their cholesterol-lowering potential: A systematic review and meta-analysis of RCTs. *Progress in Lipid Research, 64*, 16–29. https://doi.org/10.1016/j.plipres.2016.08.002.

Ghaffari, S., & Roshanravan, N. (2019). Saffron; an updated review on biological properties with special focus on cardiovascular effects. *Biomedicine & Pharmacotherapy, 109*, 21–27. https://doi.org/10.1016/j.biopha.2018.10.031.

Ghani, U. (2019). A review on nutraceuticals as therapeutic agents. *International Journal of Biosciences, 15*(5), 326–340.

Ghani, U., Naeem, M., Rafeeq, H., Imtiaz, U., Amjad, A., Ullah, S., Rehman, A., & Qasim, F. A. (2019). A novel approach towards nutraceuticals and biomedical applications. *Scholars International Journal of Biochemistry, 2*(10), 245–252. https://doi.org/10.36348/sijb.2019.v02i10.001.

Gilboa, S. M., Salemi, J. L., Nembhard, W. N., Fixler, D. E., & Correa, A. (2010). Mortality resulting from congenital heart disease among children and adults in the United States, 1999 to 2006. *Circulation, 122*(22), 2254–2263. https://doi.org/10.1161/circulationaha.110.947002.

Global health estimates: Leading causes of death. (n.d.). Retrieved from: https://www.who.int/data/gho/data/themes/mortality-and-global-health-estimates/ghe-leading-causes-of-death (accessed on 12 June 2024).

Grech, E. D. (2003). ABC of interventional cardiology: Pathophysiology and investigation of coronary artery disease. *BMJ, 326*(7397), 1027–1030. https://doi.org/10.1136/bmj.326.7397.1027.

Hoffman, J. I. E., & Kaplan, S. (2002). The incidence of congenital heart disease. *Journal of the American College of Cardiology, 39*(12), 1890–1900. https://doi.org/10.1016/s0735-1097(02)01886-7.

Hopkins, A. L., Lamm, M. G., Funk, J. L., & Ritenbaugh, C. (2013). Hibiscus sabdariffa L. in the treatment of hypertension and hyperlipidemia: A comprehensive review of animal and human studies. *Fitoterapia, 85*, 84–94. https://doi.org/10.1016/j.fitote.2013.01.003.

Hui, C., Tadi, P., Khan Suheb, M. Z., & Patti, L. (2024). Ischemic Stroke. In *StatPearls*. StatPearls Publishing. pp. 1–2.

Iung, B., & Vahanian, A. (2011). Epidemiology of valvular heart disease in the adult. *Nature Reviews Cardiology, 8*(3), 162–172. https://doi.org/10.1038/nrcardio.2010.202.

Jarouliya, U., & Keservani, R. K. (2019a). Pathways leading to child obesity. In D. Bagchi (Ed.), *Global Perspectives on Childhood Obesity: Current Status, Consequences and Prevention* (2nd ed., pp. 137–146). Academic Press. ISBN: 9780128128404.

Jarouliya, U., & Keservani, R. K. (2019b). Protein function as cell surface and nuclear receptor in human diseases. In S. Bharti & D. K. Mahapatra (Eds.), *Medicinal Chemistry with Pharmaceutical Product Development* (pp. 1–32). Apple Academic Press, CRC Press, Taylor & Francis Group. ISBN: 9781771887106.

Kalra, E. K. (2003). Nutraceutical-definition and introduction. *AAPS PharmSci, 5*(3), 27–28. https://doi.org/10.1208/ps050325.

Kanyal, N. (2015). The science of ischemic stroke: Pathophysiology & pharmacological treatment. *International Journal of Pharma Research & Review, 4*(10), 65–84.

Keservani, R. K., & Sharma, A. K. (2014). Flavonoids: Emerging trends and potential health benefits. *Journal of Chinese Pharmaceutical Sciences, 23*(12), 815.

Keservani, R. K., Kesharwani, R. K., Sharma, A. K., & Ahmad, M. F. (2015). Stress, Parkinson's, Alzheimer's disease: Role of dietary supplements. In D. Bagchi, H. G. Preuss, & A. Swaroop (Eds.), *Nutraceutical and Functional Foods in Human Life and Disease Prevention* (pp. 241–253). CRC Press, Taylor & Francis. ISBN: 9781482237214.

Keservani, R. K., Kesharwani, R. K., Sharma, A. K., & Jarouliya, U. (2015). Dietary supplements, nutraceutical and functional foods in immune response (Immunomodulators). In D. Bagchi, H. G. Preuss, & A. Swaroop (Eds.), *Nutraceutical and Functional Foods in Human Life and Disease Prevention* (pp. 343–358). CRC Press, Taylor & Francis. ISBN: 9781482237214.

Keservani, R. K., Kesharwani, R. K., Sharma, A. K., Vyas, N., & Chadoker, A. (2010). Nutritional supplements: An overview. *International Journal of Current Pharmaceutical Review and Research, 1*(1), 59–75.

Keservani, R. K., Kesharwani, R. K., Vyas, N., Jain, S., Raghuvanshi, R., & Sharma, A. K. (2010). Nutraceutical and functional food as future food: A review. *Der Pharmacia Lettre, 2*(1), 106–116.

Keservani, R. K., Sharma, A. K., & Kesharwani, R. K. (2016a). Nutraceutical and functional foods for cardiovascular health. In *Food Process Engineering* (pp. 291–312). Apple Academic Press, CRC Press. ISBN: 9781771884020.

Keservani, R. K., Sharma, A. K., & Kesharwani, R. K. (2016b). Medicinal effect of nutraceutical fruits for the cognition and brain health. *Scientifica, 1,* Article ID 3109254, 10 pp. https://doi.org/10.1155/2016/3109254.

Keservani, R. K., Sharma, A. K., & Kesharwani, R. K. (2017). An overview and therapeutic applications of nutraceutical and functional foods. In *Recent Advances in Drug Delivery Technology* (pp. 160–201). ISBN: 9781522507543.

Keservani, R. K., Sharma, A. K., & Kesharwani, R. K. (Eds.). (2020). Nutraceuticals and Dietary Supplements: Applications in Health Improvement and Disease Management, Apple Academic Press, CRC Press. Pp. 1–344. ISBN: 9781771888738.

Kouame, B., N'guetta-Brou, I., Kouame, G. Y., Koffi, M., Odehouri-Koudou, T., Dieth, G., Dick, R., Sounkere, M., Yaokreh, J., Tembely, S., & Ouattara, O. (2015). Epidemiology of congenital abnormalities in West Africa: Results of a descriptive study in teaching hospitals in Abidjan: Cote D'Ivoire. *African Journal of Paediatric Surgery, 12*(1), 51. https://doi.org/10.4103/0189-6725.150983.

Kuriakose, D., & Xiao, Z. (2020). Pathophysiology and treatment of stroke: Present status and future perspectives. *International Journal of Molecular Sciences, 21*(20). https://doi.org/10.3390/ijms21207609.

Latic, N., & Erben, R. G. (2020). Vitamin D and cardiovascular disease, with emphasis on hypertension, atherosclerosis, and heart failure. *International Journal of Molecular Sciences, 21*(18), 6483. https://doi.org/10.3390/ijms21186483.

Leal, M. T. B. C., Passos, L. S. A., Guarçoni, F. V., Aguiar, J. M. de S., Silva, R. B. R. da, Paula, T. M. N. de, Santos, R. F. D., Nassif, M. C. L., Gomes, N. F. A., Tan, T. C., & Nunes, M. C. P. (2019). Rheumatic heart disease in the modern era: Recent developments and current challenges. *Revista da Sociedade Brasileira de Medicina Tropical, 52*, e20180041. https://doi.org/10.1590/0037-8682-0041-2019.

Lennon, S. L., DellaValle, D. M., Rodder, S. G., Prest, M., Sinley, R. C., Hoy, M. K., & Papoutsakis, C. (2017). 2015 evidence analysis library evidence-based nutrition practice guideline for the management of hypertension in adults. *Journal of the Academy of Nutrition and Dietetics, 117*(9), 1445–1458.e1417. https://doi.org/10.1016/j.jand.2017.04.008.

Marijon, E., Mirabel, M., Celermajer, D. S., & Jouven, X. (2012). Rheumatic heart disease. *Lancet, 379*(9819), 953–964. https://doi.org/10.1016/s0140-6736(11)61171-9.

Mehta, D. (2017). Integrative medicine and cardiovascular disorders. *Primary Care, 44*(2), 351–367. https://doi.org/10.1016/j.pop.2017.02.005.

Noale, M., Limongi, F., & Maggi, S. (2020). Epidemiology of cardiovascular diseases in the elderly. *Advances in Experimental Medicine and Biology, 1216*, 29–38. https://doi.org/10.1007/978-3-030-33330-0_4.

Padmavathi, D. (2018). A general review on "nutraceuticals": Its golden health impact over human community. *International Journal of Food Science and Nutrition, 3*(2), 214–217.

Kuriakose, D., & Xiao, Z. (2020). Pathophysiology and treatment of stroke: Present status and future perspectives. *International Journal of Molecular Sciences, 21*(20), 7609. https://doi.org/10.3390/ijms21207609.

Parmley, W. W. (1985). Pathophysiology of congestive heart failure. *The American Journal of Cardiology, 56*(2), A7–A11. https://doi.org/10.1016/0002-9149(85)91199-3.

Pourmasoumi, M., Hadi, A., Najafgholizadeh, A., Kafeshani, M., & Sahebkar, A. (2019). Clinical evidence on the effects of saffron (*Crocus sativus* L.) on cardiovascular risk factors: A systematic review and meta-analysis. *Pharmacological Research, 139*, 348–359. https://doi.org/10.1016/j.phrs.2018.11.038.

Qidwai, W., & Ashfaq, T. (2013). Role of garlic usage in cardiovascular disease prevention: An evidence-based approach. *Evidence-Based Complementary and Alternative Medicine, 2013*, 125649. https://doi.org/10.1155/2013/125649.

Quiara Lovatti, A., Samuel Barbosa, C., & Darízy Flávia, S. (2019). Role of nutraceuticals in the prevention and treatment of hypertension and cardiovascular diseases. *Journal of Hypertension Management, 2*(3), 19–27. https://doi.org/10.23937/2474-3690/1510037.

Raut, I. H., Lodhi, N. G., & Kalode, P. D. (2021). A general review on nutraceuticals: Its golden health impact over human community. *International Journal of Advanced Research, 9*(01), 1121–1125. https://doi.org/10.21474/IJAR01/12399.

Ried, K., Fakler, P., & Stocks, N. P. (2017). Effect of cocoa on blood pressure. *The Cochrane Database of Systematic Reviews, 2017*(4), 1–10. https://doi.org/10.1002/14651858.CD008893.pub3.

Ried, K., Sullivan, T. R., Fakler, P., Frank, O. R., & Stocks, N. P. (2012). Effect of cocoa on blood pressure. *Cochrane Database of Systematic Reviews, 4,* 1–8. https://doi.org/10.1002/14651858.cd008893.pub2.

Rivellese, A. A., Ciciola, P., Costabile, G., Vetrani, C., & Vitale, M. (2019). The possible role of nutraceuticals in the prevention of cardiovascular disease. *High Blood Pressure & Cardiovascular Prevention, 26*(2), 101–111. https://doi.org/10.1007/s40292-019-00309-5.

Rusconi, M., & Conti, A. (2010). *Theobroma cacao* L., the food of the gods: A scientific approach beyond myths and claims. *Pharmacological Research, 61*(1), 5–13. https://doi.org/10.1016/j.phrs.2009.08.008.

Sachdeva, V., Roy, A., & Bharadvaja, N. (2020). Current prospects of nutraceuticals: A review. *Current Pharmaceutical Biotechnology, 21*(10), 884–896. https://doi.org/10.2174/1389201021666200130113441.

Sadowski, S. L. (2009). Congenital cardiac disease in the newborn infant: Past, present, and future. *Critical Care Nursing Clinics of North America, 21*(1), 37–48. https://doi.org/10.1016/j.ccell.2008.10.001.

Sahebkar, A., Serban, C., Ursoniu, S., & Banach, M. (2016). Effect of garlic on plasma lipoprotein(A) concentrations: A systematic review and meta-analysis of randomized controlled clinical trials. *Nutrition, 32*(1), 33–40. https://doi.org/10.1016/j.nut.2015.06.009.

Sayasathid, J., Sukonpan, K., & Somboo, N. (2012). Epidemiology and Etiology of Congenital Heart Diseases. InTech. Vol. 1, pp. 47–84.

Serban, C., Sahebkar, A., Antal, D., Ursoniu, S., & Banach, M. (2015). Effects of supplementation with green tea catechins on plasma C-reactive protein concentrations: A systematic review and meta-analysis of randomized controlled trials. *Nutrition, 31*(9), 1061–1071. https://doi.org/10.1016/j.nut.2015.02.004.

Sharma, M., & Majumdar, P. (2009). Occupational lifestyle diseases: An emerging issue. *Indian Journal of Occupational and Environmental Medicine, 13*(3), 109. https://doi.org/10.4103/0019-5278.58912.

Shinde, N., Bangar, B., Deshmukh, S., & Kumbhar, P. (2014). Nutraceuticals: A review on current status. *Research Journal of Pharmacy and Technology, 7*(1), 110–111.

Singh, L., Sharma, S., Xu, S., Tewari, D., & Fang, J. (2021). Curcumin as a natural remedy for atherosclerosis: A pharmacological review. *Molecules, 26*(13), 4036. https://doi.org/10.3390/molecules26134036.

Singh, R., Singh, R. B., Mojto, V., Pella, D., Fedacko, J., Vargova, V., Hristova, K., Wilczynska, A., Mojtova, M., & Gvozdjáková, A. (2022). Cocoa and chocolate consumption and prevention of cardiovascular diseases and other chronic diseases. In *Functional Foods and Nutraceuticals in Metabolic and Non-Communicable Diseases* (pp. 279–299). Elsevier.

Sobenin, I. A., Myasoedova, V. A., Iltchuk, M. I., Zhang, D.-W., & Orekhov, A. N. (2019). Therapeutic effects of garlic in cardiovascular atherosclerotic disease. *Chinese Journal of Natural Medicines, 17*(10), 721–728. https://doi.org/10.1016/S1875-5364(19)30088-3.

Sosnowska, B., Penson, P., & Banach, M. (2017). The role of nutraceuticals in the prevention of cardiovascular disease. *Cardiovascular Diagnosis and Therapy, 67*(1), S21–S31. https://doi.org/10.21037/cdt.2017.03.20.

Thies, F., Mills, L. M., Moir, S., & Masson, L. F. (2016). Cardiovascular benefits of lycopene: Fantasy or reality? *Proceedings of the Nutrition Society, 76*(2), 122–129. https://doi.org/10.1017/s0029665116000744.

Upadhyay, J., Tiwari, N., Rana, M., Rana, A., Durgapal, S., & Bisht, S. (2019). Pathophysiology, etiology, and recent advancement in the treatment of congenital heart disease. *Journal of Indian College of Cardiology, 9*(2), 67. https://doi.org/10.4103/jicc.jicc_11_19.

Ursoniu, S., Sahebkar, A., Serban, M.-C., & Banach, M. (2015). Lipid profile and glucose changes after supplementation with astaxanthin: A systematic review and meta-analysis of randomized controlled trials. *Archives of Medical Science, 2*, 253–266. https://doi.org/10.5114/aoms.2015.50960.

van der Bom, T., Zomer, A. C., Zwinderman, A. H., Meijboom, F. J., Bouma, B. J., & Mulder, B. J. M. (2011). The changing epidemiology of congenital heart disease. *Nature Reviews Cardiology, 8*(1), 50–60. https://doi.org/10.1038/nrcardio.2010.166.

Vlachopoulos, C., Alexopoulos, N., & Stefanadis, C. (2006). Effect of dark chocolate on arterial function in healthy individuals: Cocoa instead of ambrosia? *Current Hypertension Reports, 8*(3), 205–211.

Waheed, S. M., Kudaravalli, P., & Hotwagner, D. T. (2021). Deep vein thrombosis. In *StatPearls* [Internet], 1–2. StatPearls Publishing.

Warnes, C. A., Liberthson, R., Danielson, G. K., Dore, A., Harris, L., Hoffman, J. I. E., Somerville, J., Williams, R. G., & Webb, G. D. (2001). Task force 1: The changing profile of congenital heart disease in adult life. *Journal of the American College of Cardiology, 37*(5), 1170–1175. https://doi.org/10.1016/s0735-1097(01)01272-4.

Yifan, W., Maria Fides, O., Bianca, R., & Jiwang, C. (2020). Resveratrol and spirulina: Nutraceuticals that potentially improve cardiovascular disease. *Journal of Cardiovascular Medicine and Cardiology, 7*(2), 138–145. https://doi.org/10.17352/2455-2976.000129.

Zeng, Y. I., Sun, R., Li, X., Liu, M., Chen, S., & Zhang, P. (2016). Pathophysiology of valvular heart disease. *Experimental and Therapeutic Medicine, 11*(4), 1184–1188. https://doi.org/10.3892/etm.2016.3048.

PART II

CARDIOPROTECTIVE ACTIVITY OF DIFFERENT NUTRIENTS

CHAPTER 3

ROLE OF PROBIOTICS AND DIETARY FIBERS IN COMBATING HEART DISEASE

DEEPANSHU RANA, SHRIVARDHAN DHEEMAN, and NIDHI S. BELWAL

Department of Microbiology, School of Life Sciences, Sardar Bhagwan Singh University, Balawala, Dehradun, Uttarakhand, India

ABSTRACT

Cardiovascular diseases may arise due to various factors and have emerged as a major challenge to be controlled by medications and a healthy lifestyle. Specifically, probiotics and dietary fibers have become alternative management options for coronary heart disease (CHDs), thus reducing the death toll, which has been on the rise worldwide. Various factors and pathways in which the products of probiotics may intertwine and contribute to managing cholesterol have been extensively reviewed in this article. This review is not limited to but extends its focus to discussing the benefits of dietary fibers in controlling cholesterol levels and the severity of CHD among patients. This further emphasizes the importance of both supplements as alternatives to maintaining a healthy lifestyle and as prophylaxis for cardiovascular diseases. Although various aspects are explored, this article calls for more studies to be conducted on this alternative management of CHDs.

3.1 INTRODUCTION

Cholesterol, as one of the several important basic building blocks, is also known as a risk factor for heart disease when its concentration rises in the bloodstream.

Antioxidants as Nutraceuticals. Nayan A. Gujarathi, Raj K. Keservani, Rajesh K. Kesharwani, Bhushan R. Rane, Yogeeta Sameer Goyal (Eds.)

Thus, cholesterol is observed as a cause and sin (Yubero-Serrano et al., 2021; Kumar et al., 2012; Aloglu & Oner, 2006). At present, world populations face acute to chronic risks of cardiovascular diseases, which are the primary causes of mortality and morbidity worldwide (Sadeghzadeh et al., 2017; Nichols et al., 2014). A number of risk factors are known which may endorse heart diseases such as hyperlipidemia (high levels of lipids in the blood), hypertension (high blood pressure), obesity, cigarette smoking, and lack of exercise (Akbarzadeh & Homayouni, 2012; Ghaffari et al., 2010; Akbarzadeh et al., 2003, 2010; Ranjbar et al., 2007). The situation of an obstacle in coronary arteries, which reduces oxygenated blood supply to the myocardium, is referred to as heart disease. Precisely, atherosclerosis is a condition of similar dysfunction of arteries due to intima, accumulation of plaques, and thereby reduction in blood flow (Akbarzadeh & Homayouni, 2012; Akbarzadeh & Toufan, 2008). According to a report, coronary and cardiovascular heart diseases are rapidly increasing and becoming one of the major causes of the high death toll in adults, not only in low- and middle-income countries but also in developed countries (De Hert et al., 2022; Akbarzadeh & Homayouni, 2012; Mendis et al., 2011). For example, in the United States, 10 in 30 deaths occur due to cardiovascular heart diseases, and five are due to coronary heart disease (Peters et al., 2021; DiRienzo, 2014) (Figure 3.1). Hyperlipidemia may arise due to an imbalanced intake of food enriched and fortified with fats, oils, etc. Among high-density lipids (HDL) and low-density lipids (LDL), cholesterol of the LDL class, LDL-C concentration increase in the bloodstream causes the progression of heart diseases via the formation, growth, destabilization, and rupture of atherosclerotic plaques. Additional risk factors include elevated levels of serum triacylglycerol (TAG) and triglyceride-rich lipoproteins, low levels of high-density lipoprotein cholesterol (HDL-C), and non-lipid-related risk factors, such as markers for inflammation (DiRienzo, 2014). On the other hand, congenital heart disease represents the most common group of congenital anomalies with an incidence of 4 to 10 per 1,000 live births (Tsintoni et al., 2019; Hoffman et al., 2004; Hoffman & Kaplan, 2002). In concern to cardio-vascular disease, WHO has estimated 17.9 million deaths representing 32% of all deaths worldwide (WHO, 2021) Figure 3.2.

Pharmacological agents that effectively scale back cholesterol levels are available for the treatment of high cholesterol; however, they are expensive and are known to have other side effects (Kumar et al., 2012; Bliznakov, 2002). Probiotics and fermented foods have played important roles in human diets for thousands of years and are safely consumed on a large scale (DiRienzo, 2014; Hotel & Cordoba, 2001; Parvez et al., 2006). Probiotics are known to have advantageous functions not only in the restoration of natural

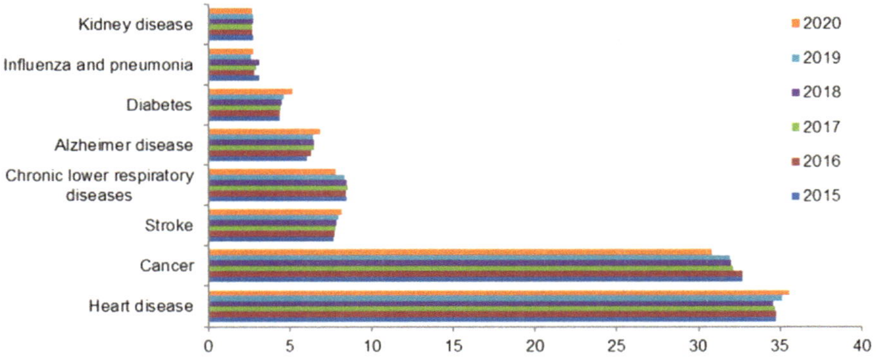

FIGURE 3.1 Estimated total deaths in the United States from leading diseases. The data shown is coverage of the year from 2015 to 2020. Data does not include the death toll caused by COVID-19.

Source: Adapted from Ahmad & Anderson (2021).

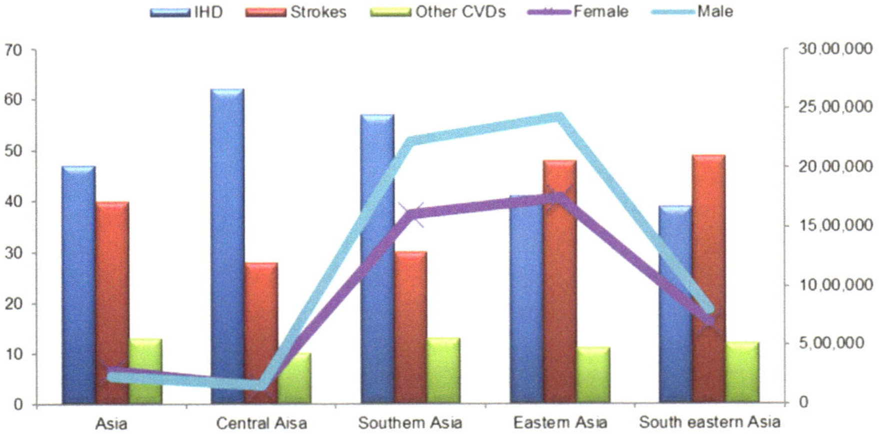

FIGURE 3.2 All-age deaths are related to different heart diseases.

Source: Adapted from Roth et al. (2017); Zhao (2021).

microflora but also play a major role in cholesterol reduction (Akbarzadeh & Homayouni, 2012). Probiotics were first used by Lilly & Stillwell in 1965, where the two authors described probiotics as a "growth-promoting factor produced by microorganisms" (Lilly & Stillwell, 1965). Fuller (1989) defined probiotics as "live microorganisms which when administered in adequate amounts confer a health benefit on the host" (Fuller, 1989) but Ilya Ilyich Mechnikov (Élie Metchnikoff) was the Nobel prize winner who first stated the relationship between probiotics and their direct health benefits (Metchnikoff,

1910). The Nobel, however, was not a token of honor for his contribution to probiotics, but rather for work in immunity, which was also shared with Paul Ehrlich. Probiotics are very common nutraceutical products (Keservani et al., 2010a, b), often administered to critically ill (Barraud et al., 2010), surgically operated cancer patients (Ohigashi et al., 2011) and in the downregulation of pro-inflammatory cytokines (Tarhani & Nezami, 2019; Asahara et al., 2001). In recent years, probiotics have emerged in dairy foods, and their consumption via dairy products has been observed as an ideal way to re-establish microflora balance in the gastrointestinal tract (GIT) (Patil et al., 2021; Homayouni, 2008). Effective applications of probiotics as immunomodulatory, anticarcinogenic, antidiabetic, hypocholesterolemia, and hypotensive have been widely discussed (Patil et al., 2021; Akbarzadeh & Homayouni, 2012; Lye et al., 2009; Mai & Draganov, 2009; Shah, 2007). As understood by definition, probiotics are live microorganisms, which include lactic acid bacteria (LAB), especially lactobacilli, due to their beneficial impacts on human health and culminating disorders caused by the pathogenic attack of microbes, cholesterol imbalance, diabetes, cancer, and immunity dysfunction (Kumar et al., 2010, 2011, 2012; Manoj et al., 2009; Nagpal et al., 2007; Yadav et al., 2007a, b; Mack et al., 1999; Bengmark et al., 1998). Lactic acid bacteria (LAB) with active bile salt hydrolase (BSH) or products containing them have been suggested to lower cholesterol levels by producing deconjugated bile salts which are less absorbed in comparison with conjugated counterparts and finally excreted through fecal matter, controlling the serum cholesterol level (Kumar et al., 2012; De Smet et al., 1998) (Figure 3.3).

Healthy metabolism is the key to a healthy gut, which depends on the nutrient-rich dish 'Thali.' Dietary fiber is another component of a good diet and a good life. Dietary fibers (Keservani et al., 2017, 2020) possess several protective benefits, including protection against cardiovascular disease (Keservani et al., 2016a) because insoluble fibers bind to toxins, prevent their absorption, and target them for elimination (Adams et al., 2018; Kumar et al., 2012; Kritchevsky, 2001). The term "dietary fiber" was first used in 1953 by Eben Hipsley in his research while observing populations provided with high-fiber diets tended to have lower rates of pregnancy toxemia (Hipsley, 1953). Previously, the term "crude fiber" was used to identify a fractional component of plant-based foods that escaped solvent, acid, and alkali extractions (Trowell, 1976). The pioneers observed "dietary fiber" as "unavailable" plant material, i.e., that which escaped digestion and absorption in the human upper GIT (Brownlee, 2011; Asp, 1987). Chemically, dietary fibers are a complex cluster of carbohydrates and polymers that are not hydrolyzed by human enzymes and, therefore, are not digestible or absorbed in

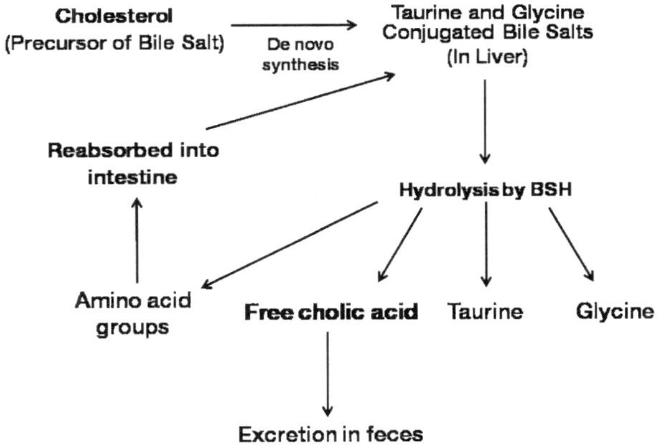

FIGURE 3.3 Cholesterol as the precursor for the synthesis of new bile acids and the hypercholesterolemia role of bile salt hydrolase (BSH)s.

the body (Soliman, 2019; Eastwood & Kay, 1979). These are endogenous components of plant materials, predominantly non-starch polysaccharides, and lignin, which show resistance to human enzymatic digestion (Pilch, 1987). Though these are distinguished by their physiological properties and systemic effects, chemically they are grouped into two categories, water-soluble and water-insoluble (Anderson, 1985). Water-soluble fiber dissolves in hot water but remains insoluble in cold water. Examples of soluble fibers include pectin, gums, certain hemicelluloses, and storage polysaccharides. Fruits (Keservani et al., 2016b), oats, barley, and legumes contain more soluble fibers than other foods. Insoluble fiber includes cellulose, lignin, and many hemicelluloses. Vegetables, wheat, and most grain products contain primarily insoluble fibers (American Diabetes Association, 2000; Butrum et al., 1988; Anderson & Bridges, 1988; Anderson, 1985, 1986, 1987; James, 1981) (Table 3.1). Dietary fiber functions as a matrix in food which may stimulate some specific kinds of gastrointestinal conditions (Dikeman & Fahey, 2006; Englyst & Englyst, 2005; Jenkins et al., 2000; McDougall et al., 1996). Some studies on rats have elucidated that administration of iso-maltodextrin decreases fat absorption for up to 6 hours. The mechanism was postulated as increased micelle stabilization (Takagaki et al., 2018). In different studies on guinea pigs, pectin, guar gum, and Plantago psyllium exhibited redoubled LDL-ApoB a 100 turnover, and upregulation of internal organ low-density lipoprotein receptors, resulting in quicker destructive metabolism and clearance (Wood et al., 2007; Fernandez et al., 1997; Fernandez et al., 1992, 1994; Fernandez et al., 1990). Studies conducted in many animal models showed the useful effects of dietary fibers within the reduction of cardiopathy risk or reduction in disorder mortality. For instance, Lo et al. (1987) showed that dietary fiber isolated from soybean was effective in preventing induration of the arteries in rabbits. The systemic emergence of dietary fibers is important for human health as illustrated in Figure 3.4.

In this review, we summarized the potential role of probiotics and dietary fibers in the management of heart diseases as their administration not only alters the intestinal microflora but also reduces the absorption of lipid molecules which by a large reduces the accumulation of fat molecules in the human body.

TABLE 3.1 Different Food Groups as Sources of Fibers in the Asian Region

Food Items	Fiber Content (g/100 g of Serve)
Grain	
Wheat bran	24
Rice bran	24.8
Oats	16
Pulses	
Beans	45.8
Peas	43
Lentils	20
Chickpeas	10.6
Fruits	
Peaches	13
Plums	12.4
Guava	8.9
Oranges	7.7
Vegetables	
Potato	14.2
Tomato	6.6
Corn	5.8
Carrot	4.8

Source: Adapted from Soliman, 2019.

3.2 RISK FACTORS ASSOCIATED WITH CORONARY HEART DISEASE

Coronary heart diseases in wealthy societies emerged in a large proportion whereas; rheumatic heart disease is common in developing countries (Akbar-Zadeh et al., 2003; Akbarzadeh & Toufan, 2008). The known risk factors of CHD can be classified into four categories. The first include being male, increasing age, genetic traits, lipid metabolism abnormalities, body build,

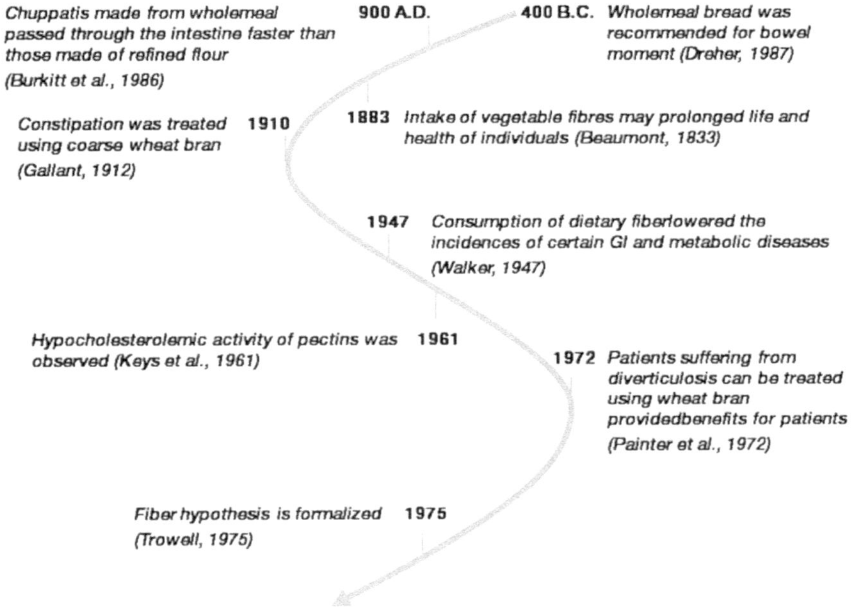

FIGURE 3.4 Historical development in the discovery of dietary fiber.

Source: Adapted from Anderson et al. (1990).

and ethnic origin, which can't be modified. The second category includes cigarette smoking, hyperlipidemia, low levels of high-density lipoprotein (Singh et al., 2017b), obesity (Jarouliya & Keservani, 2019), hypertension, low physical activity, increased thrombosis, stress, and alcohol consumption, which can't be changed. The third is associated with disease states, which include diabetes and glucose intolerance. The last and fourth are related to geographic distribution like climate and season, cold weather, soft drinking water, etc. (Akbarzadeh et al., 2009a; Lovegrove & Jackson, 2003). It has been incontestable that there's a robust and consistent relationship between total plasma sterol (Poli et al., 2021; Martin et al., 1986). Accumulation of LDL in the plasma leads to cholesterol deposition in the arterial wall via LDL oxidation. Followed by change lipoprotein is haunted by macrophages, that finally become foam cells and kind the premise of the first hardening of the arteries plaque. It's been calculated that every 1% increase in cholesterol level results in a 2–3% increase in CHD risk (Akbarzadeh et al., 2009b; Gensini et al., 1998). A higher level of HDL is often reported in women than in men due to low physical activity, not smoking, and diabetes (Akbarzadeh et al., 2009c; Assmann et al., 1998).

3.3 MECHANISMS OF PROBIOTIC ACTION

Diet is taken into account to manage the chance of CHD through its effects on certain risk factors including blood lipids, blood pressure, and possibly also through thrombogenic mechanisms. New evidence suggests a protective role for dietary antioxidants (Singh et al., 2017a) such as vitamins E and C and carotenes, possibly through a mechanism that prevents the oxidation of LDL cholesterol particles (Lovegrove & Jackson, 2003). Due to low consumer compliance with low-fat diets, attempts are made to identify other dietary components that can reduce blood cholesterol levels (Mann & Spoerry, 1974).

The mechanisms of action of probiotics on cholesterol reduction are physiological actions of the end products of fermentation of short-chain fatty acids (SCFAs), cholesterol assimilation, deconjugation of bile acids, and cholesterol binding to bacterial cell walls. The SCFAs that are produced by bacteria using anaerobic breakdown of carbohydrates are acetic acid, propionic, and butyric acids. The deconjugation reaction is catalyzed by the conjugated bile hydrolase enzyme, which is produced exclusively by bacteria. Deconjugation ability is widely found in many intestinal bacteria including the genera *Enterococcus, Peptostreptococcus, Bifidobacterium, Fusobacterium, Clostridium, Bacteroides,* and *Lactobacillus* (Hylemond, 1985). This reaction releases the amino acid moiety and the deconjugated bile, thereby reducing cholesterol absorption, by increasing fecal excretion of the deconjugated bile acids.

Grill et al. (1995) reported *Bifidobacterium longum* as the most efficient bacterium when tested against 6 different bile salts. Another study reports that *Lactobacillus* sp. had varying abilities to deconjugate glycocholate and taurocholate and generate cholic acid which is excreted through fecal matter (Habib et al., 2022; Gilliland et al., 1985). Intervention studies on animals and ostomy patients have shown that oral administration of bound microorganism species junction rectifier augmented the excretion of free and secondary digestive juice salts (De Smet et al., 1998; Marteau et al., 1995). A few pieces of evidence are from the *in-vitro* studies that support the hypothesis that certain bacteria can assimilate (take up) cholesterol. It was reported earlier that *L. acidophilus* and *B. bifidum* had the ability to assimilate cholesterol, but only in the presence of bile and under anaerobic conditions (Rasic et al., 1992; Gilliland et al., 1985). Also, Klaver, & Meer (1993) have concluded that *L. acidophilus* and a *Bifidobacterium* sp. alleviate cholesterol from their growth media *via* assimilation and enzyme, bile salt deconjugase activity. The same mechanism was identified by Tahri and co-workers (1995) with some conflicting results and concluded removal of cholesterol, assimilation in the cell, and bile acid deconjugase activity occur simultaneously. Followed by the mechanism of cholesterol binding to bacterial cell walls, a possible explanation for the hypocholesterolemic effects of probiotics was suggested. Hosono (1995) reported that *Lactococcus lactis* subsp. biovar shows the highest binding capacity for cholesterol. It was further speculated that the binding differences were due to the chemical and structural properties of the cell walls. It was also interesting in the study that even killed cells may have the ability to bind cholesterol in the intestine.

3.4 MECHANISMS OF DIETARY FIBERS' ACTION

One well-established way to reduce the risk of developing cardiovascular disease (CVD) is to lower serum LDL cholesterol levels by reducing saturated fat intake. However, the importance of different dietary approaches, such as increasing the intake of soluble dietary fibers, is increasingly recognized. Well-controlled intervention studies have now shown that four major soluble fiber types – β-glucan, psyllium, pectin, and Cyamopsis tetragonolobus gum – effectively lower serum LDL cholesterol concentrations without affecting HDL cholesterol or triacylglycerol concentrations. The exact mechanism by which soluble fibers lower serum LDL cholesterol levels is not known. Evidence suggests that soluble fibers may interfere with protein and/or steroid metabolism. Other suggested mechanisms include the inhibition of hepatic cholesterol synthesis by fermentation products and delayed absorption of macronutrients leading to increased insulin sensitivity (Theuwissen & Mensink, 2008).

Evidence suggests that some water-soluble fibers bind bile acids during the formation of micelles in the intestinal lumen (Kritchevsky & Story, 1974; Eastwood & Hamilton, 1968). These observations led to the hypothesis that soluble fibers could increase the excretion of digestive juice acids. Instead, it's been proposed that soluble fibers could form a thick unagitated water layer within the intestinal lumen. This layer could act as a physical barrier, thereby decreasing the (re)absorption of fats, including cholesterol and digestive juice acids. This may cause an increased fecal output of these two components. As a result, intestinal conversion of cholesterol into digestive juice acids increases, intestinal pools of free cholesterol decrease, and—to reach a new steady-state—endogenous cholesterol synthesis can increase. This results in increased activities of 7-α-hydroxylase and reductase to compensate for the losses of digestive juice acids and cholesterol from the liver stores. Furthermore, intestinal LDL cholesterol receptors become upregulated to restore intestinal cholesterol stores, which can lead to lower blood cholesterol concentrations. Several human studies have explored the effects of soluble fibers on steroid excretion. In hypercholesterolemic men, who got 100 g of oat bran for 10 days, a reduction in blood cholesterol levels and an increase in fecal sterol excretion were observed (Kirby et al., 1981). In another study, ileostomy subjects were given 4 different pieces of bread on 2 consecutive days in random order. The bread was mainly made from oat bran, oat bran treated with β-glucanase, barley, or wheat flour. The 24-hour excretion of bile acids was significantly higher during the oat bran period than in the other 3 periods (Lia et al., 1995).

Water-soluble fibers escape absorption in the small intestine and are fermented in the large intestine by colonic bacteria. This fermentation results in the production of short-chain fatty acids (SCFA), such as acetate, propionate, and butyrate. Butyrate is primarily metabolized by colonic epithelial cells, while acetate and propionate are rapidly absorbed. It has been hypothesized that the production of SCFA and changes in the propionate and acetate ratio may impact lipid metabolism. However, this hypothesis mainly comes from animal studies, while well-controlled intervention studies in humans are limited (Theuwissen & Mensink, 2008).

3.5 FUTURE ASPECTS

Coronary Heart Diseases are known to affect an individual through different clinical conditions like hyperlipidemia, hypertension, and obesity which result in great mortality and morbidity. In recent years, several probiotic foods have been produced industrially. These foods have received attention for their beneficial effects on the gut microflora and their links to systemic effects on the lowering of lipids known to be risk factors for heart diseases. On the other hand, dietary fibers impacting all aspects of gut physiology are vital to a healthy diet. Initial observations linking dietary fiber to health extolled the benefits of consumption of fiber-rich foods rather than dietary supplementation with fibers. Probiotics may prevent coronary heart disease by reducing cholesterol and impacting microbial bile acid metabolism, having systemic effects on notably lowering cholesterol and TAG. Although the exact mechanism of water-soluble fiber action is still unknown, water-soluble fibers lower the (re)absorption of bile acids and have been considered the most likely mechanisms. In order to completely confirm probiotic bacteria and dietary fibers as safe and potent treatments for heart diseases, further multi-centered, large-scale, randomized controlled clinical studies need to be conducted. Additionally, more specific data should be gathered to properly understand their effects in high-risk populations of patients.

Risk factors known to affect an individual's risk of CHD have been categorized as hyperlipidemia, hypertension, obesity, cigarette smoking, and lack of exercise. Probiotics may prevent coronary heart disease through cholesterol reduction and microbial bile acid metabolism. Probiotics have beneficial effects on the gut microbiome and are linked to their systemic effects on the lowering of lipids known to be risk factors for CHD, notably cholesterol and TAG.

3.6 CONCLUSION

Although the exact mechanism of water-soluble fiber's action is still unknown, water-soluble fibers lower the (re)absorption of bile acids have been considered as the most likely mechanisms. As a result, hepatic conversion of cholesterol into bile acids increases, and hepatic pools of free cholesterol decrease—to reach a new steady state—endogenous cholesterol synthesis will increase. This leads to increased activities of 7-α-hydroxylase and HMG-CoA reductase to compensate for the losses of bile acids and cholesterol from the liver stores. Furthermore, hepatic LDL cholesterol receptors become upregulated to re-establish hepatic cholesterol stores, which will lead to decreased serum LDL cholesterol concentrations. Furthermore, epidemiological studies suggest that a diet high in probiotics and water-soluble fiber protects against CVD, and underlies current dietary recommendations to further increase their intake.

ACKNOWLEDGMENT

The author (s) are thankful to the Administration of Sardar Bhagwan Singh University, Dehradun (UK), India.

CONFLICT OF INTEREST

The author(s) declares no conflict of interest.

KEYWORDS

- **CHDs**
- **Cholesterol**
- **Dietary fibers**
- **Healthy lifestyle**
- **Probiotics**

REFERENCES

Adams, S., Che, D., Qin, G., Rui, H., Sello, C. T., & Hailong, J. (2018). Interactions of dietary fibre with nutritional components on gut microbial composition, function and health in monogastrics. *Current Protein & Peptide Science, 19*, 1011–1023.

Ahmad, F. B., & Anderson, R. N. (2021). The leading causes of death in the US for 2020. *JAMA, 325*(18), 1829–1830.

Akbarzadeh, F., & Homayouni, A. (2012). Dairy probiotic foods and coronary heart disease: A review on mechanism of action. In *Probiotics* (pp. 121–128). InTech.

Akbarzadeh, F., & Toufan, M. (2008). Atrioventricular delays, cardiac output and diastolic function in patients with implanted dual chamber pacing and sensing pacemakers. *Pakistan Journal of Biological Sciences, 11*(20), 2407–2412.

Akbar-Zadeh, F., Hejazi, E., Kooshavar, H., & Pezeshkian, M. (2003). Prevalence of cardiovascular diseases and cardiac risk factors in northwestern Tabriz. *Medical Journal of Tabriz University of Medical Sciences and Health Services, 59*(11), 1–4.

Akbarzadeh, F., Kazemi, B., & Pourafkari, L. (2009a). Supraventricular arrhythmia induction by an implantable cardioverter defibrillator in a patient with hypertrophic cardiomyopathy. *Pacing and Clinical Electrophysiology, 33*(3), 372–376.

Akbarzadeh, F., Kazemi-Arbat, B., Golmohammadi, A., & Pourafkari, L. (2009b). Biatrial pacing vs. intravenous amiodarone in prevention of atrial fibrillation after coronary artery bypass surgery. *Pakistan Journal of Biological Sciences, 12*(19), 1325.

Akbarzadeh, F., Pourafkari, L., Mohammad Hashemi Jazi, S., Hesami, L., & Habibi, H. (2010). Prevalence and severity of CAD among hypertensive and normotensive patients undergoing elective coronary angiography in Tabriz Madani Heart Center. *ARYA Atherosclerosis Journal, 5*, 1–5.

Akbarzadeh, F., Ranjbar Kouchaksaraei, F., Bagheri, Z., & Ghezel, M. (2009c). Effect of preoperative information and reassurance in decreasing anxiety of patients who are candidates for coronary artery bypass graft surgery. *Journal of Cardiovascular and Thoracic Research, 1, 25–28.*

Aloğlu, H., & Öner, Z. (2006). Assimilation of cholesterol in broth, cream, and butter by probiotic bacteria. *European Journal of Lipid Science and Technology, 108*(9), 709–713.

American Diabetes Association. (2000). Nutrition recommendations and principles for people with diabetes mellitus. *Diabetes Care, 23*, S43.

Anderson, J. W. (1985, November). Physiological and metabolic effects of dietary fiber. In *Federation Proceedings* (Vol. 44, No. 14, pp. 2902–2906).

Anderson, J. W. (1986). Plant fiber in foods. *HCF Diabetes Research Foundation*, 1–3, Lexington, KY.

Anderson, J. W. (1987). About fiber. In *The HCF Nutrition Program: The HCF Guidebook* (pp. 11). HCF Diabetes Foundation, Lexington, KY.

Anderson, J. W., & Bridges, S. R. (1988). Dietary fiber content of selected foods. *American Journal of Clinical Nutrition, 47*(3), 440–447.

Anderson, J. W., Deakins, D. A., Floore, T. L., Smith, B. M., & Whitis, S. E. (1990). Dietary fiber and coronary heart disease. *Critical Reviews in Food Science and Nutrition, 29*(2), 95–147.

Asahara, T., Nomoto, K., Shimizu, K., Watanuki, M., & Tanaka, R. (2001). Increased resistance of mice to Salmonella enterica serovar Typhimurium infection by synbiotic administration of Bifidobacteria and transgalactosylated oligosaccharides. *Journal of Applied Microbiology, 91*(6), 985–996.

Asp, N. G. (1987). Definition and analysis of dietary fibre. *Scandinavian Journal of Gastroenterology, 22*(sup129), 16–20.

Assmann, G., Cullen, P., & Schulte, H. (1998). The Münster Heart Study (PROCAM). Results of follow-up at 8 years. *European Heart Journal, 19*, A2–11.

Barraud, D., Blard, C., Hein, F., Marçon, O., Cravoisy, A., Nace, L., Alla, F., Bollaert, P. E., & Gibot, S. (2010). Probiotics in the critically ill patient: A double-blind, randomized, placebo-controlled trial. *Intensive Care Medicine, 36*(9), 1540–1547.

Bengmark, S., Ahrne, S., Molin, G., & Jeppsson, B. (1998). Intestinal colonizing lactobacilli. *Journal of Nutrition, 14*(8), 585–594.

Bliznakov, E. G. (2002). Lipid-lowering drugs (statins), cholesterol, and coenzyme Q10. The Baycol case-a modern Pandora's box. *Biomedicine & Pharmacotherapy, 56*(1), 56–59.

Brownlee, I. A. (2011). The physiological roles of dietary fibre. *Food Hydrocolloids, 25*(2), 238–250.

Butrum, R. R., Clifford, C. K., & Lanza, E. (1988). NCI dietary guidelines: Rationale. *American Journal of Clinical Nutrition, 48*(3), 888–895.

Corzo, G., & Gilliland, S. E. (1999a). Measurement of bile salt hydrolase activity from Lactobacillus acidophilus based on disappearance of conjugated bile salts. *Journal of Dairy Science, 82*(3), 466–471.

Corzo, G., & Gilliland, S. E. (1999b). Bile salt hydrolase activity of three strains of Lactobacillus acidophilus. *Journal of Dairy Science, 82*(3), 472–480.

De Hert, M., Detraux, J., & Vancampfort, D. (2022). The intriguing relationship between coronary heart disease and mental disorders. *Dialogues in Clinical Neuroscience*. *20*(1), 31–40.

De Smet, I., De Boever, P., & Verstraete, W. (1998). Cholesterol lowering in pigs through enhanced bacterial bile salt hydrolase activity. *British Journal of Nutrition, 79*(2), 185–194.

Dikeman, C. L., & Fahey Jr, G. C. (2006). Viscosity as related to dietary fiber: A review. *Critical Reviews in Food Science and Nutrition, 46*(8), 649–663.

DiRienzo, D. B. (2014). Effect of probiotics on biomarkers of cardiovascular disease: Implications for heart-healthy diets. *Nutrition Reviews, 72*(1), 18–29.

Eastwood, M. A., & Hamilton, D. (1968). Studies on the adsorption of bile salts to nonabsorbed components of diet. *Biochimica et Biophysica Acta, 152*, 165–173.

Eastwood, M. A., & Kay, R. M. (1979). A hypothesis for the action of dietary fiber along the gastrointestinal tract. *American Journal of Clinical Nutrition, 32*(2), 364–367.

Englyst, K. N., & Englyst, H. N. (2005). Carbohydrate bioavailability. *British Journal of Nutrition, 94*(1), 1–11.

Fernandez, M. L., Lin, E. C., Trejo, A., & McNamara, D. J. (1992). Prickly pear (Opuntia sp.) pectin reverses low density lipoprotein receptor suppression induced by a hypercholesterolemic diet in guinea pigs. *Journal of Nutrition, 122*, 2330–2340.

Fernandez, M. L., Trejo, A., & McNamara, D. J. (1990). Pectin isolated from prickly pear (Opuntia sp.) modifies low density lipoprotein metabolism in cholesterol-fed guinea pigs. *Journal of Nutrition, 120*, 1283–1290.

Fernandez, M. L., Vergara-Jimenez, M., Conde, K., Behr, T., & Abdel-Fattah, G. (1997). Regulation of apolipoprotein B-containing lipoproteins by dietary soluble fiber in guinea pigs. *American Journal of Clinical Nutrition, 65*, 814–822.

Fuller, R. (1989). Probiotics in man and animals. *Journal of Applied Bacteriology, 66*(5), 365–378.

Gensini, G. F., Comeglio, M., & Colella, A. (1998). Classical risk factors and emerging elements in the risk profile for coronary artery disease. *European Heart Journal, 19*, A53–A61.

Ghaffari, S., Akbarzadeh, F., & Pourafkari, L. (2011). Aneurysmal coronary arteriovenous fistula closing with covered stent deployment: A case report and review of literature. *Cardiology Journal, 18*(5), 556–559.

Gilliland, S. E., Nelson, C. R., & Maxwell, C. (1985). Assimilation of cholesterol by Lactobacillus acidophilus. *Applied and Environmental Microbiology, 49*(2), 377–381.

Grill, J. P., Cayuela, C., Antoine, J. M., & Schneider, F. (2000). Isolation and characterization of a Lactobacillus amylovorus mutant depleted in conjugated bile salt hydrolase activity: Relation between activity and bile salt resistance. *Journal of Applied Microbiology, 89*(4), 553–563.

Habib, B., Vaid, S., Bangotra, R., Sharma, S., & Bajaj, B. K. (2022). Bioprospecting of probiotic lactic acid bacteria for cholesterol lowering and exopolysaccharide producing potential. *Biologia, 77*(7), 1931–1951.

Hipsley, E. H. (1953). Dietary "fibre" and pregnancy toxaemia. *British Medical Journal, 2*(4833), 420.

Hoffman, J. I., & Kaplan, S. (2002). The incidence of congenital heart disease. *Journal of the American College of Cardiology, 39*(12), 1890–1900.

Hoffman, J. I., Kaplan, S., & Liberthson, R. R. (2004). Prevalence of congenital heart disease. *American Heart Journal, 147*(3), 425–439.

Homayouni, A. (2008). Therapeutical effects of functional probiotic, prebiotic and symbiotic foods (1st ed.). *Tabriz University of Medical Sciences*, pp. 33–37. Tabriz, Iran.

Hosono, A. (1995). Binding of cholesterol with lactic acid bacteria cells. *Milchwissenschaft, 50*, 556–560.

Hotel, A. C. P., & Cordoba, A. (2001). Health and nutritional properties of probiotics in food including powder milk with live lactic acid bacteria. *Preventive, 5*(1), 1–10.

Hylemon, P. B. (1985). Metabolism of bile acids in intestinal microflora. In *New Comprehensive Biochemistry* (Vol. 12, pp. 331–343). Elsevier.

James, W. P. T. (1981). Nutritional guidelines for health education in Britain. *Nutrition Today, 21*, 21–22.

Jarouliya, U., & Keservani, R. K. (2019). Pathways leading to child obesity. In D. Bagchi (Ed.), *Global Perspectives on Childhood Obesity: Current Status, Consequences and Prevention* (2nd ed., pp. 137–146). Academic Press, Elsevier.

Jenkins, D. J., Kendall, C. W., Axelsen, M., Augustin, L. S., & Vuksan, V. (2000). Viscous and nonviscous fibres, nonabsorbable and low glycaemic index carbohydrates, blood lipids and coronary heart disease. *Current Opinion in Lipidology, 11*(1), 49–56.

Keservani, R. K., Kesharwani, R. K., Sharma, A. K., Vyas, N., & Chadoker, A. (2010b). Nutritional supplements: An overview. *International Journal of Current Pharmaceutical Review and Research, 1*(1), 59–75.

Keservani, R. K., Kesharwani, R. K., Vyas, N., Jain, S., Raghuvanshi, R., & Sharma, A. K. (2010a). Nutraceutical and functional food as future food: A review. *Der Pharmacia Lettre, 2*(1), 106–116.

Keservani, R. K., Sharma, A. K., & Kesharwani, R. K. (2016a). Nutraceutical and functional foods for cardiovascular health. In *Food Process Engineering* (pp. 291–312). Apple Academic Press, CRC Press.

Keservani, R. K., Sharma, A. K., & Kesharwani, R. K. (2016b). Medicinal effect of nutraceutical fruits for the cognition and brain health. *Scientifica*, Article ID 3109254. https://doi.org/10.1155/2016/3109254.

Keservani, R. K., Sharma, A. K., & Kesharwani, R. K. (2017). An overview and therapeutic applications of nutraceutical and functional foods. In *Recent Advances in Drug Delivery Technology* (pp. 160–201). IGI Global.

Keservani, R. K., Sharma, A. K., & Kesharwani, R. K. (Eds.). (2020). *Nutraceuticals and Dietary Supplements: Applications in Health Improvement and Disease Management*. pp. 1–344. CRC Press.

Kirby, R. W., Anderson, J. W., Sieling, B., Rees, E. D., Chen, W. J., Miller, R. E., & Kay, R. M. (1981). Oat-bran intake selectively lowers serum low-density lipoprotein cholesterol concentrations of hypercholesterolemic men. *American Journal of Clinical Nutrition, 34*(5), 824–829.

Klaver, F. A., & Van der Meer, R. (1993). The assumed assimilation of cholesterol by lactobacilli and Bifidobacterium bifidum is due to their bile salt-deconjugating activity. *Applied and Environmental Microbiology, 59*(4), 1120–1124.

Kritchevsky, D. (2001). Diet and atherosclerosis. *Journal of Nutrition, Health & Aging, 5*(3), 155–159.

Kritchevsky, D., & Story, J. A. (1974). Binding of bile salts in vitro by non-nutritive fiber. *Journal of Nutrition, 104*(4), 458–462.

Kumar, M., Kumar, A., Nagpal, R., Mohania, D., Behare, P., Verma, V., Kumar, P., Poddar, D., Aggarwal, P. K., Henry, C. J. K., & Jain, S. (2010). Cancer-preventing attributes of probiotics: An update. *International Journal of Food Sciences and Nutrition, 61*(5), 473–496.

Kumar, M., Nagpal, R., Kumar, R., Hemalatha, R., Verma, V., Kumar, A., Chakraborty, C., Singh, B., Marotta, F., Jain, S., & Yadav, H. (2012). Cholesterol-lowering probiotics as potential biotherapeutics for metabolic diseases. *Experimental Diabetes Research, 2012*, Article ID 902154. https://doi.org/10.1155/2012/902154.

Kumar, M., Verma, V., Nagpal, R., Kumar, A., Behare, P. V., Singh, B., & Aggarwal, P. K. (2010). Anticarcinogenic effect of probiotic fermented milk and chlorophyllin on aflatoxin-B1-induced liver carcinogenesis in rats. *British Journal of Nutrition, 107*(7), 1006–1016.

Kumar, M., Verma, V., Nagpal, R., Kumar, A., Gautam, S. K., Behare, P. V., Grover, C. R., & Aggarwal, P. K. (2011). Effect of probiotic fermented milk and chlorophyllin on gene expressions and genotoxicity during AFB1-induced hepatocellular carcinoma. *Gene, 490*(1–2), 54–59.

Kumar, V., Sinha, A. K., Makkar, H. P., de Boeck, G., & Becker, K. (2012). Dietary roles of non-starch polysaccharides in human nutrition: A review. *Critical Reviews in Food Science and Nutrition, 52*(10), 899–935.

Lia, A., Hallmans, G., Sandberg, A. S., Sundberg, B., Aman, P., & Andersson, H. (1995). Oat beta-glucan increases bile acid excretion and a fiber-rich barley fraction increases cholesterol excretion in ileostomy subjects. *American Journal of Clinical Nutrition, 62*(6), 1245–1251.

Lilly, D. M., & Stillwell, R. H. (1965). Probiotics: Growth-promoting factors produced by microorganisms. *Science, 147*(3659), 747–748.

Lo, G. S., Evans, R. H., Phillips, K. S., Dahlgren, R. R., & Steinke, F. H. (1987). Effect of soy fiber and soy protein on cholesterol metabolism and atherosclerosis in rabbits. *Atherosclerosis, 64*(1–2), 47–54.

Lovegrove, J., & Jackson, K. (2003). Coronary heart disease. In T. Mattila-Sandholm & M. Saarela (Eds.), *Functional Dairy Products* (pp. 54–93). Woodhead Publishing and CRC Press.

Lye, H. S., Kuan, C. Y., Ewe, J. A., Fung, W. Y., & Liong, M. T. (2009). The improvement of hypertension by probiotics: Effects on cholesterol, diabetes, renin and phytoestrogens. *International Journal of Dairy Science, 10*, 3755–3775.

Mack, D. R., Michail, S., Wei, S., McDougall, L., & Hollingsworth, M. A. (1999). Probiotics inhibit enteropathogenic E. coli adherence in vitro by inducing intestinal mucin gene expression. *American Journal of Physiology – Gastrointestinal and Liver Physiology, 276*(4), G941–G950.

Mai, V., & Draganov, P. V. (2009). Recent advances and remaining gaps in our knowledge of associations between gut microbiota and human health. *World Journal of Gastroenterology, 15*(1), 81–85.

Mann, G. V., & Spoerry, A. (1974). Studies of a surfactant and cholesteremia in the Maasai. *American Journal of Clinical Nutrition, 27*(5), 464–469.

Manoj, K., Dheeraj, M., Devastotra, P., Behare, P. V., Ravinder, N., Ashok, K., & Aggarwal, P. K. (2009). A probiotic fermented milk prepared by mixed culture reduces pathogen shedding and alleviates disease signs in rats challenged with pathogens. *International Journal of Probiotics and Prebiotics, 4*(3), 211–218.

Marteau, T. M. (1995). Towards informed decisions about prenatal testing: A review. *Prenatal Diagnosis, 15*(13), 1215–1226.

Martin, M., Browner, W., Hulley, S., Kuller, L., & Wentworth, D. (1986). Serum cholesterol, blood pressure, and mortality: Implications from a cohort of 361 662 men. *The Lancet, 328*(8513), 933–936.

McDougall, G. J., Morrison, I. M., Stewart, D., & Hillman, J. R. (1996). Plant cell walls as dietary fibre: Range, structure, processing and function. *Journal of the Science of Food and Agriculture, 70*(2), 133–150.

Mendis, S., Puska, P., & Norrving, B. E. (2011). Global Atlas on Cardiovascular Disease Prevention and Control. World Health Organization. pp.155. ISBN: 978–92–4-156437–3.

Metchnikoff, E. (1910). Etudes sur la flore intestinale-Deuxieme memoire. *Annales de l'Institut Pasteur (Paris), 24*, 755–770.

Moser, S. A., & Savage, D. C. (2001). Bile salt hydrolase activity and resistance to toxicity of conjugated bile salts are unrelated properties in lactobacilli. *Applied and Environmental Microbiology, 67*(8), 3476–3480.

Nagpal, R., Yadav, H., Puniya, A. K., Singh, K., Jain, S., & Marotta, F. (2007). Potential of probiotics and prebiotics for synbiotic functional dairy foods: An overview. *International Journal of Probiotics and Prebiotics, 2*(2/3), 75.

Nichols, M., Townsend, N., Scarborough, P., & Rayner, M. (2014). Cardiovascular disease in Europe 2014: Epidemiological update. *European Heart Journal, 35*(42), 2950–2959.

Ohigashi, S., Hoshino, Y., Ohde, S., Onodera, H. (2011). Functional outcome, quality of life, and efficacy of probiotics in postoperative patients with colorectal cancer. *Surgery Today, 41*(9), 1200–1206.

Parvez, S., Malik, K. A., Ah Kang, S., & Kim, H. Y. (2006). Probiotics and their fermented food products are beneficial for health. *Journal of Applied Microbiology, 100*(6), 1171–1185.

Patil, Y. M., Patwardhan, R. B., & Abhyankar, P. S. (2021). Improving the gut microbiota with probiotics and faecal microbiota transplantation. *Journal of Pure and Applied Microbiology, 15*(3), 1111–1125.

Peters, S. A., Colantonio, L. D., Dai, Y., Zhao, H., Bittner, V., Farkouh, M. E., Dluzniewski, P., Poudel, B., Muntner, P., & Woodward, M. (2021). Trends in recurrent coronary heart disease after myocardial infarction among US women and men between 2008 and 2017. *Circulation, 143*(7), 650–660.

Pilch, S. M. (1987). Physiologic effects and health consequences of dietary fiber. *Federation of American Societies for Experimental Biology, Life Sciences Research Office, Bethesda, MD, 36*, 1–251.

Poli, A., Marangoni, F., Corsini, A., Manzato, E., Marrocco, W., Martini, D., Medea, G., & Visioli, F. (2021). Phytosterols, cholesterol control, and cardiovascular disease. *Nutrients, 13*(8), 2810.

Ranjbar, F., Akbarzadeh, F., Kazemi, B., & Safaeiya, A. (2007). Relaxation therapy in the background of standard antihypertensive drug treatment is effective in management of moderate to severe essential hypertension. *Saudi Medical Journal, 28*(9), 1353–1356.

Rašić, J. L., Vujičić, I. F., Škrinjar, M., & Vulić, M. (1992). Assimilation of cholesterol by some cultures of lactic acid bacteria and bifidobacteria. *Biotechnology Letters, 14*(1), 39–44.

Roth, G. A., Johnson, C., Abajobir, A., Abd-Allah, F., Abera, S. F., Abyu, G., Ahmed, M., Aksut, B., Alam, T., Alam, K., & Alla, F. (2017). Global, regional, and national burden of cardiovascular diseases for 10 causes, 1990 to 2015. *Journal of the American College of Cardiology, 70*(1), 1–25.

Sadeghzadeh, J., Vakili, A., Sameni, H. R., Shadnoush, M., Bandegi, A. R., & Khorasani, M. Z. (2017). The effect of oral consumption of probiotics in prevention of heart injury in a rat myocardial infarction model: A histopathological, hemodynamic and biochemical evaluation. *Iranian Biomedical Journal, 21*(3), 174.

Shah, N. P. (2007). Functional cultures and health benefits. *International Dairy Journal, 17*(11), 1262–1277.

Singh, P., Kesharwani, R. K., & Keservani, R. K. (2017a). Antioxidants and vitamins: Roles in cellular function and metabolism. In *Sustained Energy for Enhanced Human Functions and Activity* (pp. 385–407). Academic Press.

Singh, P., Kesharwani, R. K., & Keservani, R. K. (2017b). Protein, carbohydrates, and fats: Energy metabolism. In *Sustained Energy for Enhanced Human Functions and Activity* (pp. 103–115). Academic Press.

Soliman, G. A. (2019). Dietary fiber, atherosclerosis, and cardiovascular disease. *Nutrients, 11*(5), 1155.

Tahri, K., Crociani, J., Ballongue, J., & Schneider, F. (1995). Effects of three strains of bifidobacteria on cholesterol. *Letters in Applied Microbiology, 21*(3), 149–151.

Takagaki, R., Ishida, Y., Sadakiyo, T., Taniguchi, Y., Sakurai, T., Mitsuzumi, H., Watanabe, H., Fukuda, S., & Ushio, S. (2018). Effects of isomaltodextrin in postprandial lipid kinetics: Rat study and human randomized crossover study. *PLoS ONE, 13*, e0196802.

Tanaka, H., Doesburg, K., Iwasaki, T., & Mierau, I. (1999). Screening of lactic acid bacteria for bile salt hydrolase activity. *Journal of Dairy Science, 82*(12), 2530–2535.

Tanaka, H., Hashiba, H., Kok, J., & Mierau, I. (2000). Bile salt hydrolase of Bifidobacterium longum—biochemical and genetic characterization. *Applied and Environmental Microbiology, 66*(6), 2502–2512.

Tarhani, F., & Nezami, A. (2019). Role of probiotics in treatment of congenital heart disease and necrotizing enterocolitis. *PharmaNutrition, 8*, 100144.

Theuwissen, E., & Mensink, R. P. (2008). Water-soluble dietary fibers and cardiovascular disease. *Physiology & Behavior, 94*(2), 285–292.

Trowell, H. (1976). Definition of dietary fiber and hypotheses that it is a protective factor in certain diseases. *American Journal of Clinical Nutrition, 29*(4), 417–427.

Trowell, H. C. (1975). Dietary-fiber hypothesis of the etiology of diabetes mellitus. *Diabetes, 24*(8), 762–765.

Tsintoni, A., Dimitriou, G., & Karatza, A. A. (2020). Nutrition of neonates with congenital heart disease: existing evidence, conflicts and concerns. *Journal of Maternal-Fetal & Neonatal Medicine, 33*(14), 2487–2492.

Wood, B. J., & Holzapfel, W. H. N. (Eds.). (1992). *The Genera of Lactic Acid Bacteria* (Vol. 2). Springer Science & Business Media.

Wood, R. J., Fernandez, M. L., Sharman, M. J., Silvestre, R., Greene, C. M., Zern, T. L., Shrestha, S., Judelson, D. A., Gomez, A. L., Kraemer, W. J., & Volek, J. S. (2007). Effects of a carbohydrate-restricted diet with and without supplemental soluble fiber on plasma low-density lipoprotein cholesterol and other clinical markers of cardiovascular risk. *Metabolism, 56*(1), 58–67.

World Health Organization. (2009). Cardiovascular Disease. Fact sheet no. 317. Retrieved from: https://www.who.int/europe/news-room/fact-sheets/item/cardiovascular-diseases.

World Health Organization. (2021). Cardiovascular diseases (CVDs). Retrieved from: https://www.who.int/news-room/fact-sheets/detail/cardiovascular-diseases-(cvds).

Yadav, H., Jain, S., & Sinha, P. R. (2007a). Antidiabetic effect of probiotic dahi containing *Lactobacillus acidophilus* and *Lactobacillus casei* in high fructose fed rats. *Nutrition, 23*(1), 62–68.

Yadav, H., Jain, S., & Sinha, P. R. (2007b). Formation of oligosaccharides in skim milk fermented with mixed dahi cultures, *Lactococcus lactis* ssp diacetylactis and probiotic strains of lactobacilli. *Journal of Dairy Science, 74*(2), 154–159.

Yubero-Serrano, E. M., Alcalá-Diaz, J. F., Gutierrez-Mariscal, F. M., Arenas-de Larriva, A. P., Peña-Orihuela, P. J., Blanco-Rojo, R., Martinez-Botas, J., Torres-Peña, J. D., Perez-Martinez, P., Ordovas, J. M., & Delgado-Lista, J. (2021). Association between cholesterol efflux capacity and peripheral artery disease in coronary heart disease patients with and without type 2 diabetes: From the CORDIOPREV study. *Cardiovascular Diabetology, 20*(1), 1–10.

Zhao, D. (2021). Epidemiological features of cardiovascular disease in Asia. *JACC: Asia, 1*(1), 1–13.

CHAPTER 4

BENEFITS OF GARLIC IN CARDIOVASCULAR DISEASE

PEEUSH SINGHAL,[1] RITU VISHNOI,[2] MANISHA,[2] VIVEK SRIVASTAVA,[3] SOMESH THAPLIYAL,[4] and VIJAY JYOTI KUMAR[4]

[1]*Department of Pharmaceutical Sciences, Gurukul Kangri Deemed University, Haridwar, Uttarakhand, India*

[2]*Department of Botany, Chinmaya Degree College, Haridwar, Uttarakhand, India*

[3]*Amity Institute of Pharmacy, Amity University Lucknow Campus, Malhaur, Gomti Nagar Extension, Lucknow, Uttar Pradesh, India*

[4]*Department of Pharmaceutical Sciences, H.N.B. Garhwal Central University, Srinagar, Uttarakhand, India*

ABSTRACT

The rapidly increasing frequency of cardiovascular disease is a severe concern to both developed and emerging countries, necessitating an immediate response. Due to its safety profile and accessibility, public opinion is shifting in favor of Ayurvedic medicines. Because of its potent and extensive benefits, garlic is thought to be one of the top disease-preventive foods. The goal of this research is to find out how effective garlic is at preventing cardiovascular disease. We examined the research on the benefits of garlic supplements on hypertension, hypercholesterolemia, pulse wave velocity (PWV), and coronary artery calcium (CAC), as well as adverse effects data. The literature search was conducted using major databases such as Google, PubMed, and the MEDLINE library. Human clinical trials were conducted

Antioxidants as Nutraceuticals. Nayan A. Gujarathi, Raj K. Keservani, Rajesh K. Kesharwani, Bhushan R. Rane, Yogeeta Sameer Goyal (Eds.)

to determine the effect of garlic in the prevention of cardiovascular disease. Garlic supplementation lowered systolic and diastolic blood pressure by 7–16 mm Hg and 5–9 mm Hg, respectively (4 meta-analyses and 2 original studies). Total cholesterol was lowered by 7.4–29.8 mg/dL (8 meta-analyses). The studies with the most reliable outcomes used aged garlic extract (AGE). A few small trials using AGE found that it had positive benefits on CAC, CRP, and PWV. Despite the fact that garlic is generally safe, there have been a few reports of unusual adverse effects with little evidence of causality.

4.1 INTRODUCTION

In epidemiological research, spices have been associated with a lower incidence of cardiovascular disease. Garlic has a long history of being regarded as a powerful preventative and therapeutic medicinal element in the folklore of many civilizations. Garlic has aroused contemporary medicine's interest due to its numerous health advantages and the commonly held belief that garlic supports the maintenance of good health by warding off illnesses and enhancing vitality. A number of human disorders are significantly influenced by dietary variables, including cardiovascular disease. Garlic has been shown to have numerous experimental and therapeutic effects.

This study used an evidence-based method to determine the efficacy of garlic in preventing cardiovascular disease by analyzing clinical trials and conducting a systematic review in the above-mentioned field.

4.2 CARDIOVASCULAR DISEASE

Cardiovascular disease (Keservani et al., 2016) is a multifaceted, complex disease defined by a number of causes. Elevated serum lipids (cholesterol and triglycerides), increased plasma fibrinogen and coagulation factors, enhanced platelet activation, changes in glucose metabolism, and smoking have all been documented in epidemiologic investigations (Wood, 2001). Reactive oxygen species (ROS) oxidative modification of LDL is now recognized as a significant factor in the development of atherosclerosis, as is the etiology of hypertension (Sobenin et al., 2019; Dhawan & Jain, 2004). There is also compelling evidence that platelets have a role in the development of atherosclerosis. Smokers, as well as those suffering from vascular injury, hyperlipidemia, and hypertension, have higher platelet activity. Increased HDL levels are linked to a lower risk of heart disease. The improvement in cardiovascular disease is thought to be due to the normalization of aberrant lipids and lipoproteins, hypertension, platelet aggregation inhibition, and an increase in antioxidant status.

4.3 GARLIC: THE HISTORICAL PERSPECTIVE

Garlic (*Allium sativum*), a member of the Alliaceae family, is thought to have originated in Central Asia. It is utilized as a flavoring agent, traditional medicine, and a functional food to improve physical and mental health around the world. Garlic's helpful properties in treating a wide range of human diseases and disorders have been recognized for generations, and it has thus earned a special place in many cultures' folklore as a formidable preventative and curative medicinal agent. It is even mentioned in the Egyptian Codex Ebers, a 3,500-year-old manuscript, as a remedy for heart problems, tumors, worms, bites, and other maladies (Rahman, 2001). Garlic has also been shown to suppress the etiology of cardiovascular disease, as well as to prevent cancer and other age-related chronic disorders (Rahman, 2003). Over the past 25 years, much emphasis has been paid to the role that garlic plays in the prevention and treatment of cardiovascular disease.

Water makes up the majority of garlic (65%), and fructose-containing carbs make up the majority of the dry weight, followed by sulfur compounds, protein, fiber, and free amino acids (Lawson, 1996). It also includes a high amount of saponins, phosphorus, potassium, sulfur, and zinc, as well as moderate amounts of selenium and Vitamins A and C, as well as low amounts of calcium, magnesium, sodium, iron, manganese, and B-complex vitamins. Garlic also has a high phenolic content (Vinson et al., 2001). The majority of the chemicals found in garlic are water-soluble (97%), with tiny levels of oil-soluble compounds (0.15–0.7%) being present. Different garlic formulations have been studied *in vitro* and *in vivo* for their prevention and therapy of cardiovascular disease over the years (clinical trials). Typical formulations that have been researched include raw garlic, garlic powder tablets, oil of steam-distilled garlic, oil of oil-macerated garlic, oil of ether-extracted garlic, and aged garlic extract (AGE). The makeup of all of these preparations varies (Banerjee et al., 2003), making comparisons difficult.

4.4 PREPARATIONS MADE USING GARLIC AND THEIR CHEMICAL COMPONENTS

Because raw garlic homogenate is the most prevalent route of garlic ingestion, it has been the focus of extensive scientific research. The aqueous extract of garlic used in much scientific research is substantially the same as raw garlic homogenate. Allicin (allyl 2-propenethiosulfinate or diallyl-thiosulfinate) is thought to be the primary bioactive component of aqueous garlic extract or raw garlic homogenate. Allinase enzyme, found in garlic, is activated when it is diced or crushed, and it acts on alliin (found in intact garlic) to form allicin. Allyl methyl thiosulfonate, 1-propenyl allylthiosulfonate, and -L-glutamyl-S-alkyl-L-cysteine are other sulfur-containing compounds found in garlic homogenate. As the homogenate is incubated at room temperature, the concentration of adenosine increases several-fold. Heat inactivates the enzyme allinase, which converts alliin (S-allyl cysteine sulfoxide) to allicin. Thus, alliin is primarily present in the water extract of heat-treated garlic. Because garlic powder is essentially a dehydrated, powdered garlic clove, its composition, particularly its allinase activity, is equal to that of fresh garlic. However, the temperature of dehydration should not exceed 60°C, as this will inactivate allinase (Lawson, 1998).

Aged garlic extract is another frequently researched garlic preparation (AGE). AGE is raw garlic slices that have been kept in 15–20% ethanol for 20 months. This whole process is intended to result in a large loss of allicin and an increase in the activity of newer molecules including S-allyl cysteine (SAC), S-allylmercaptocysteine (SAM), allixin, and selenium, those that are stable, bioavailable, and antioxidants (Borek, 2001). N-alpha-(1-deoxy-D-fructos-1-yl)-L-arginine (Fru-Arg), a newly discovered antioxidant component of AGE, is not found in raw or heat-treated garlic (Ryu et al., 2001).

Steam distillation is the most common method for producing medicinal garlic oil. Diallyl (57%), allyl methyl (37%), and dimethyl (6%) mono to hexa sulfides make up steam-distilled garlic oil. $C_6H_{10}S_2$ (DADS, 26%), $C_6H_{10}S_3$ (DATS, 19%), $C_4H_8S_3$ (15%), $C_4H_8S_2$ (13%), $C_6H_{10}S_4$ (8%), $C_4H_8S_4$ (6%), $C_2H_6S_3$ (3%), penta sulfide (4%), pentasulf (1%). 3-vinyl-4H-1,2-dithiin and $C_9H_{14}OS_3$ are found in oil-macerated garlic oil. The Diels-Alder dimers of thioacrolein (5.7 mg/g) and $(CH_2{=}CHCH_2)_2S$ (1.4 mg/g) are nine times as abundant in ether-extracted garlic oil (essential oil), and the ajoenes (0.4 mg/g) are four times as abundant (Lawson, 1998).

4.5 HYPERTENSION

Antihypertensive therapy has been linked to a 20–25% reduction in the risk of IHD and a 30–40% reduction in the risk of stroke (Mulawarman et al., 2021). Up to 50% of hypertension patients are estimated to be utilizing garlic as a supplement or primarily for treatment (Stabler et al., 2012). Garlic is also often used for hypertension in developing countries like Nigeria, where complementary medicines are more economical and accessible (Osamor & Owumi, 2010). To our knowledge, the first meta-analysis of garlic's antihypertensive effects was published in 1994, and it found positive results (Silagy & Neil, 1994). However, we will concentrate on four meta-analyses and two new investigations that have been published since then. In 2008, two of the four meta-analyses were published (Reinhart et al., 2008) found 26 randomized studies with controls reporting blood pressure outcomes in the first study. Around 16 of these studies were eliminated due to their low quality (e.g., Two were not double-blinded, five were not placebo-controlled, and One had no baseline blood pressure measurements). Only three of the remaining 10 studies included hypertension patients (n = 132) at the outset, whereas the other seven included normotensive patients (n = 262). All three trials that included hypertensive individuals used Kwai garlic powder (KB GP). In the remaining 7 studies, which included subjects with normotension, administration of KB GP, Kyolic brand aged garlic extract (KB AGE), and Cardiomax brand garlic oil did not significantly lower blood pressure. Garlic decreases SBP and DBP in hypertensive individuals, but not in normotensive patients, according to Reinhart et al.

Ried et al. found 25 appropriate studies and 11 of them were used in their meta-analysis, which included 503 patients in the SBP arm and 565 in the DBP arm. This comprised 6 of the 10 studies from Reinhart et al.'s meta-analysis, as well as just 2 of the 3 trials with hypertensive patients at baseline. Nine research utilized KB GP, one used KB AGE, and one used distilled garlic oil in this meta-analysis. Overall, SBP reduced by 4.6±2.8 mm Hg. In individuals who were hypertensive at baseline, SBP decreased by 8.4±2.8 mm Hg and DBP decreased by 7.3–1.5 mm Hg, according to Ried et al. (2008, 2013)—conducted a regression analysis showing a connection between blood pressure levels at the start of the intervention and the degree of blood pressure reduction attained.

Simons et al. conducted a review of trials on the role of garlic in high blood pressure in their third study. They looked at 32 studies and assessed their quality, finding that the majority were of marginal quality. They graded each trial on a nine-point scale, with the majority of research receiving only 4–6 points. Given the "poor methodological quality," Simons et al. concluded that the use of garlic for treating hypertension was not advised.

However, Stabler et al. reviewed 72 publications for their Cochrane Review and only included two trials in their analysis. They discovered that garlic treatment lowers SBP by 10–12 mm Hg and DBP by 6–9 mm Hg.

Since Stabler et al. (2012) published their Cochrane Review, two more randomized, controlled trials have been found. First, Ried et al. conducted a randomized, double-blind, placebo-controlled experiment that met all quality standards. They enrolled 84 individuals with hypertension who were taking standard antihypertensive drugs. They showed a reduction in SBP of 11.8–5.4 mm Hg at a dose of 2 capsules when KB AGE was used at three different doses compared to placebo. This dose was "very well tolerated and acceptable." All garlic groups had high tolerance, compliance, and acceptability (93%) with the groups taking 1 or 2 capsules daily having the highest.

Second, in a 12-week randomized, placebo-controlled, double-blind trial that met the maximum quality standards, normotensive patients (SBP: 130–139 mm Hg) to moderately hypertensive patients (SBP: 140–159 mm Hg) were assessed by Nakasone et al. and given a Japanese garlic preparation by the brand Dentou-ninniku-ranwo. With no known side effects, Nakasone et al. reported a reduction in SBP of 6.6–7.5 mm Hg and DBP of 4.6–5.2 mm Hg.

According to numerous authors, based on our review of the literature, we found a few small trials with strict methodological standards that showed a positive effect on blood pressure due to the use of garlic formulations in the range of 7–16 mm Hg for SBP and 5–9 mm Hg for DBP compared to placebo. Only patients with hypertension at baseline showed this impact. This effect has been proven with the use of KB GP, KB AGE, and Dentou-ninniku-ranwo formulations in addition to conventional antihypertensive medications (Nakasone et al., 2013). The majority of studies have used KB AGE. There have been no trials that indicate impacts on endpoints like death, myocardial infarction, or stroke, but it's worth noting that lowering blood pressure with other therapies has been proven to reduce IHD occurrences by up to 40% (Mulawarman et al., 2021).

4.6 HYPERCHOLESTEROLEMIA

Several large-scale randomized trials have found a graded relationship between hypercholesterolemia and IHD. In a meta-analysis of 61 trials with over 100 participants, lowering TC by 38.7 mg/dL was linked to approximately 56% [HR 0.44 (95% CI: 0.42, 0.48)], 34% [0.66 (95% CI: 0.65, 0.68)], and 17% [0.83 (95% CI: 0.81, 0.85)] lower IHD mortality in both sexes at ages 40–49, 50–69, and 70–89 years, respectively (Lewington et al., 2007).

Despite the fact that *in vitro* and animal research have consistently and nearly universally proved that garlic consumption reduces hypercholesterolemia and its repercussions, clinical trials have produced mixed outcomes

(Krivskaya, 2022). We found 8 meta-analyses examining the influence of garlic consumption on TC between 1993 and 2011. Each had its own set of inclusion and exclusion criteria, resulting in a wide range of outcomes.

The most current meta-analysis by Zeng et al. looked at 26 randomized, double-blind, placebo-controlled trials with a total of 1295 participants. It also rejected nine further studies that fulfilled the inclusion criteria but lacked data that could be pooled. Furthermore, 6 trials were removed because they included diabetic patients, 2 because they employed lipid-lowering medications concurrently, 2 because they co-administered garlic with other therapies, and 1 because the garlic and placebo groups were significantly different in gender. Only four of the 26 trials examined included participants with normal lipid levels. The most popular products were garlic powder, KB AGE, and garlic oil. Overall, it was discovered that garlic reduced serum TC by 10.8 mg/dL more than the placebo did (95% confidence interval: 17.4, 4.3, P = 0.001). Lowering TC concentrations was more successful with KB AGE and KB GP. The scientists concluded that while the reduction was considerable, it was not as striking as reductions from prescription medications like statins, but that it was equivalent to diet change alone.

Two of the remaining seven meta-analyses were published in 2009 and produced contradictory results. Reinhart et al. examined 2,958 papers and assessed 29 studies from November 2007 to November 2008. They discovered a 7.35 mg/dL drop in TC (95% CI: 12.8, 2.3). Khoo and Aziz examined only 1,230 studies published till March 2008, including 12 trials with 1,056 patients, and established no change in TC through garlic use compared to placebo in the same year.

Alder et al. (2003) and Stevinson et al. (2000), all published before 2008, found that garlic had beneficial effects on TC of 24.7, 17.0, 15.9, 29.8, and 22.8 mg/dL, respectively. We discovered three randomized, controlled trials that are not applicable since the publication of the latest meta-analysis because they featured the coadministration of therapies other than garlic (Higashikawa et al., 2012; Seo et al., 2012) and open labeling (Kumar et al., 2013).

TC levels were reduced by 7.4–29.8 mg/dL in several garlic preparations. The no-effect experiment by Khoo and Aziz was published simultaneously by Reinhart et al., but it only screened and included half as many papers. This could be a sign of bias. When combined with statins or for people who cannot tolerate statins, this mild to moderate drop in TC should help lower cholesterol levels.

4.7 CAC AND EPICARDIAL ADIPOSE TISSUE

The amount of calcification identified in coronary arteries by a non-contrast computed tomography (CT) scan is used to calculate the CAC. According to the 2010 American College of Cardiology Foundation/American Heart Association parameter for assessing cardiovascular disease risk in asymptomatic adults (Greenland, 2010), CAC is not only a well-validated prognostic marker of IHD, but it can also assist in categorizing patients' risks as low or high, influencing treatment decisions. Among patients who, according to the Framingham risk factors, are at intermediate risk (10–20% 10-year risk). Furthermore, serial assessments of CAC can help further prognosticate patients, and it is increasingly being used as a surrogate endpoint in studies evaluating the efficiency of therapies rather than myocardial infarction or cardiac disease mortality (Waters & Craven, 1993). Furthermore, statin therapy has been demonstrated to slow the advancement of CAC (Achenbach et al., 2002; Callister et al., 1998). A CAC score progression of more than 15% every year has been demonstrated to significantly increase mortality (Budoff et al., 2010; Raggi et al., 2004).

There are three small randomized, double-blind, placebo-controlled studies (Budoff et al., 2004, 2009; Zeb et al., 2012) that show garlic has a positive effect on CAC advancement as a proxy measure for clinical outcomes. The standardized KB AGE formulation was used in all three experiments at recommended dosages.

Budoff et al., Relative to placebo over a year, it was discovered that KB AGE slowed the progression of CAC in 23 patients with established coronary artery disease (CAD) or high-risk patients (Framingham risk >20% over 10 years) (7.5 9.4% vs. 22.2 18.5%, respectively). Budoff et al. reported substantial outcomes in 65 intermediate-risk patients (age 60–90 years) with a Framingham risk of 10–20% and a baseline CAC of >30. KB AGE was given along with vitamin B-12, folic acid, vitamin B-6, and L-arginine in that study. CAC advancement was considerably lower in the therapy group than in the placebo group over a one-year period (6.8% vs. 26.5%, P = 0.005). Finally, Zeb et al. examined the effects of KB AGE with coenzyme Q10 on 65 asymptomatic, moderate-risk level (baseline CAC >10) males aged 55 to 65 years. At one year, mean CAC advancement in the therapy group was considerably lower than in the placebo group (32.6 versus 58.8, P = 0.01).

Due to the fact that CAC development is associated with a higher risk of IHD, and because treatment with garlic appears to slow the progression of CAC in these three small studies, it's possible that garlic could lower

IHD rates. Although all three trials employed KB AGE, two of them used additional therapies in addition to KB AGE, which could have influenced the outcomes.

CT scans can also classify the adipose tissue around the coronary arteries as white or brown epicardial adipose tissue, in addition to CAC (EAT). Because EAT is a biologically active tissue that regulates rates of inflammation and atherosclerosis progression as well as overall plaque stability via a variety of hormones and cytokines, its composition is significant (Canon & Nedergaard, 2004; Farmer, 2008). Whereas the biochemical method is complicated and not entirely understood, it has been demonstrated that a greater brown-to-white EAT ratio is beneficial and linked to a lower incidence of IHD (Iacobellis & Barbaro, 2008; Jeong et al., 2007).

With the development of precise methods for assessing brown-to-white EAT ratios using CT scan technology, over time, positive improvements in the brown-to-white EAT ratio can be shown. When compared to placebo, KB AGE plus supplements considerably raised the brown-to-white EAT ratio (125 38% vs. 11 20%) (Ahmadi et al., 2013).

4.8 PWV (ARTERIAL STIFFNESS)

PWV is an effective predictor of IHD that is simple to assess, noninvasive, operator-independent, and highly reliable, yet it is not extensively used clinically in North America (Vlachopoulos et al., 2010). This test, which is similar to the ankle-brachial index, could help the clinician determine risk levels. PWV evaluates the speed of blood flow in the aorta by measuring the time cycle between the carotid and distal pulses (e.g., radial or femoral). A meta-analysis of 17 studies including over 15,000 patients found that having a high PWV is associated with a higher risk of IHD (2.26), heart disease death (2.02), and all-cause death (1.90). PWV is included as a risk assessment measure for hypertensive patients who are not already at high risk in the 2007 European Societies of Hypertension and Cardiology Recommendation for the Control of High Blood Pressure (Mancia et al., 2007).

In a randomized, double-blind, placebo-controlled study of 65 males at medium risk, the Fire-fighter Aged Garlic Extract Research as a therapy for coronary heart disease experiment looked at the effect of garlic on PWV (Larijani et al., 2013). The intervention group (KB AGE with coenzyme Q10) had a mean decrease in PWV of 1.21 m/s after 1 year compared to the placebo group ($P = 0.005$). While a moderate PWV is preferable to a high

PWV, there is no evidence that lowering PWV leads to improved outcomes. PWV, on the other hand, is a promising clinical measure for risk stratification in primary prevention and a simple objective to achieve if it can be proven that improvement leads to better outcomes.

4.9 BIOMARKERS OF INFLAMMATION

Several biomarkers are showing promise in terms of IHD event prediction and risk stratification, regardless of the processes involved. CRP is the most researched biomarker for IHD as a clinical predictor, and it is a part of the 2009 Canadian Cardiovascular Society program for the treatment of dyslipidemia and the prevention of cardiovascular disease (McPherson et al., 2006). Men over 50 and women over 60 who are at moderate risk of IHD (as indicated by the Framingham risk) and have LDL cholesterol of less than 3.5 mmol/L should be screened. If the CRP levels in these patients are high, statin medication should be started because statins lower CRP and help prevent IHD.

There is no meta-analysis on the effects of garlic on CRP that we are aware of. We found six studies (Kumar et al., 2013; Budoff et al., 2009; Zeb et al., 2012; Warshafsky et al., 1993; Higashikawa et al., 2012; Seo et al., 2012) that looked at the effects of garlic on CRP. Zeb et al. published the only high-quality study that found a link between garlic administration and reduced CRP levels (Zeb et al., 2012). In that study, 65 intermediate-risk individuals were given KB AGE with coenzyme Q10 for a year. When compared to placebo (0.91 ± 0.56 mg/L), CRP was significantly lower (–0.12 ± 0.24 mg/L). The other five studies were either poorly designed or had no effect.

4.10 AVOIDABLE SITUATIONS AND DRUG INTERACTIONS

Garlic is extremely safe (Williams et al., 2005). However, some common side effects and uncommon case reports have been reported. Despite the fact that not all studies and meta-analyses cover side effects, body odor, and halitosis are the only statistically significant negative effects of garlic medication (Williams et al., 2005; McPherson et al., 2006; Kumar et al., 2013). These adverse effects are most noticeable when using raw garlic, although they can be mitigated by using odor-free garlic preparations such as KB AGE (Williams et al., 2005).

Gastrointestinal intolerances such as stomach pain, bloating, and flatulence are also common self-reported minor side effects (McPherson et al., 2006). However, dysphagia and garlic-induced esophagitis with hematemesis or hematochezia, as well as small-bowel blockage without a clear cause, have been reported (Williams et al., 2005; Borelli et al., 2007).

Allergic responses, including anaphylaxis, have been reported as major side effects in some cases. Eczema, acute viral nasopharyngitis, emphysematous, nettle-rash, photosensitivity, angioneurotic edema, and pemphigus are among the allergic symptoms that some individuals experience (Williams et al., 2005; McPherson et al., 2006).

Excessive use of garlic products has been linked to coagulation malfunction and bleeding in rare cases (Williams et al., 2005). This includes epidural hematoma in the spine, a longer clotting time, postoperative hemorrhage, and extraconal hematoma with no known cause. There have been two cases of warfarin interaction. Macan et al. discovered that using aged garlic extract along with warfarin medication could be acceptable.

4.11 THE WAY FORWARD: FUTURE RESEARCH

It is critical to employ standardized garlic formulations in clinical trials and to determine the bioavailability of the active components. It's also crucial to ask the correct questions: are we looking at garlic for cardiovascular disease prevention or treatment? In addition, well-designed randomized trials with sufficient duration are required to investigate morbidity and mortality outcomes, as well as lipid and thrombotic outcomes. It's also worth looking into whether garlic taken as a dietary supplement can help people avoid or delay cardiovascular disease in healthy people. It's possible that the outcome will be different if garlic is consumed before the development of cardiovascular disease. Some epidemiologic evidence backs this up (Ergül & Çakal, 2012). Finally, new biomarkers and techniques for cardiovascular disease must be included in clinical trials, and if a beneficial effect is seen, the mechanism of action on disease parameters must be determined. Because cardiovascular illness is complicated and complex and garlic contains several qualities that may lower cardiovascular disease, clinical trials must address a variety of problems.

4.12 DISCUSSION

Garlic has been demonstrated to have beneficial effects on various clinically important risk factors in the present literature; this can alter treatment options for individuals in the foremost prevention of IHD in addition to helping prognosticate. The standardization of the preparation or active ingredient is one of the obstacles in studying the effects of garlic. Because the product is calibrated to a set quantity of N-acetyl cysteine before packing, results from KB AGE have been the most reliable. Nonetheless, multiple trials and meta-analyses have demonstrated that garlic has beneficial effects on well-known risk factors like hypertension and hypercholesterolemia. When compared to placebo, SBP and DBP were reduced by 7–16 mm Hg and 5–9 mm Hg, respectively. The amount of TC in the blood is lowered by 7.4–29.8 mg/dL. Garlic has demonstrated favorable effects for surrogate endpoints like CAC development rates in a few small studies, despite the lack of bigger studies for clinical endpoints such as morbidity and death. Garlic has also been found in small studies to improve practical clinical prognosticators like PWV and CRP. Garlic is typically safe, with moderate stomach discomfort being the most prevalent intolerance, which can be alleviated by using an odorless preparation such as KB AGE. Given that it is one of the most traditional medicines ever used and may reduce the chance of developing cardiovascular disease, additional research is necessary.

4.13 CONCLUSION

We draw the conclusion that garlic supplementation has the capacity to defend the cardiovascular system in terms of risk factor reduction (hypertension and total cholesterol) and surrogate markers of atherosclerosis (CRP, PWV, and CAC). Larger studies are needed to fully assess these impacts.

KEYWORDS

- **aged garlic extract**
- **ayurvedic medicine**
- **benefits of garlic**
- **cardiovascular disease**
- **computed tomography**
- **coronary artery calcium**
- **coronary artery disease**
- **pulse wave velocity**
- **reactive oxygen species**

REFERENCES

Achenbach, S., Ropers, D., Pohle, K., Leber, A., Thilo, C., Knez, A., Menendez, T., Maeffert, R., Kusus, M., Regenfus, M., et al. (2002). Influence of lipid-lowering therapy on the progression of coronary artery calcification: A prospective evaluation. *Circulation, 106*, 1077–1082.

Ahmadi, N., Nabavi, V., Hajsadeghi, F., Zeb, I., Flores, F., Ebrahimi, R., & Budoff, M. (2013). Aged garlic extract with supplement is associated with increase in brown adipose, decrease in white adipose tissue and predict lack of progression in coronary atherosclerosis. *International Journal of Cardiology, 168*, 2310–2314.

Alder, R., Lookinland, S., Berry, J. A., & Williams, M. A. (2003). Systematic review of the effectiveness of garlic as an anti-hyperlipidemic agent. *Journal of the American Academy of Nurse Practitioners, 15*, 120.

Banerjee, S. K., Mukherjee, P. K., & Maulik, S. K. (2003). Garlic as an antioxidant: The good, the bad and the ugly. *Phytotherapy Research, 17*, 97–106.

Borek, C. (2001). Antioxidant health effect of aged garlic extract. *The Journal of Nutrition, 131*, 1010S–1015S.

Borrelli, F., Capasso, R., & Izzo, A. A. (2007). Garlic (Allium sativum L.): Adverse effects and drug interactions in humans. *Molecular Nutrition & Food Research, 51*, 1386–1397.

Budoff, M. J., Ahmadi, N., Gul, K. M., Liu, S. T., Flores, F. R., Tiano, J., Takasu, J., Miller, E., & Tsimikas, S. (2009). Aged garlic extract supplemented with B vitamins, folic acid and L-arginine retards the progression of subclinical atherosclerosis: A randomized clinical trial. *Preventive Medicine, 49*, 101–107.

Budoff, M. J., Hokanson, J. E., Nasir, K., Shaw, L. J., Kinney, G. L., Chow, D., Demoss, D., Nuguri, V., Nabavi, V., Ratakonda, R., et al. (2010). Progression of coronary artery calcium predicts all-cause mortality. *JACC Cardiovascular Imaging, 3*, 1229–1236.

Budoff, M. J., Takasu, J., Flores, F. R., Niihara, Y., Lu, B., Lau, B. H., Rosen, R. T., & Amagase, H. (2004). Inhibiting progression of coronary calcification using aged garlic extract in patients receiving statin therapy: A preliminary study. *Preventive Medicine, 39*, 985–991.

Callister, T. Q., Raggi, P., Cooil, B., Lippolis, N. J., & Russo, D. J. (1998). Effect of HMG-CoA reductase inhibitors on coronary artery disease as assessed by electron-beam computed tomography. *The New England Journal of Medicine, 339*, 1972–1978.

Cannon, B., & Nedergaard, J. (2004). Brown adipose tissue: Function and physiological significance. *Physiological Reviews, 84*, 277–359.

Dhawan, V., & Jain, S. (2004). Effect of garlic supplementation on oxidized low-density lipoproteins and lipid peroxidation in patients of essential hypertension. *Molecular and Cellular Biochemistry, 266*, 109–115. https://doi.org/10.1097/01.hjh.0000752400.24367.fa.

Ergül, B., & Çakal, B. (2012). Dysphagia caused by garlic induced esophagitis. *Clinics and Research in Hepatology and Gastroenterology, 36*(6), e134.

Farmer, S. R. (2008). Molecular determinants of brown adipocyte formation and function. *Genes & Development, 22*, 1269–1275.

Greenland, P., Alpert, J. S., Beller, G. A., Benjamin, E. J., Budoff, M. J., Fayad, Z. A., Foster, E., Hlatky, M. A., Hodgson, J. M., Kushner, F. G., et al. (2010). ACCF/AHA guideline for assessment of cardiovascular risk in asymptomatic adults: A report of the American College of Cardiology Foundation/American Heart Association Task Force on Practice Guidelines. *Journal of the American College of Cardiology, 56*, e50–103.

Higashikawa, F., Noda, M., Awaya, T., Ushijima, M., & Sugiyama, M. (2012). Reduction of serum lipids by the intake of the extract of garlic fermented with *Monascus pilosus*: A randomized, double-blind, placebo-controlled clinical trial. *Clinical Nutrition, 31*, 261–266.

Iacobellis, G., & Barbaro, G. (2008). The double role of epicardial adipose tissue as pro- and anti-inflammatory organ. *Hormone and Metabolic Research, 40*, 442–445.

Jeong, J. W., Jeong, M. H., Yun, K. H., Oh, S. K., Park, E. M., Kim, Y. K., Rhee, S. J., Lee, E. M., Lee, J., Yoo, N. J., et al. (2007). Echocardiographic epicardial fat thickness and coronary artery disease. *Circulation Journal, 71*, 536–539.

Kantor, E. D., Lampe, J. W., Vaughan, T. L., Peters, U., Rehm, C. D., & White, E. (2012). Association between use of specialty dietary supplements and C-reactive protein concentrations. *American Journal of Epidemiology, 176*, 1002–1013.

Keservani, R. K., Sharma, A. K., & Kesharwani, R. K. (2016). Nutraceutical and functional foods for cardiovascular health. In *Food Process Engineering* (pp. 291–312). Apple Academic Press, CRC Press.

Khoo, Y. S., & Aziz, Z. (2009). Garlic supplementation and serum cholesterol: A meta-analysis. *Journal of Clinical Pharmacy and Therapeutics, 34*, 133–145.

Krivskaya, T. (2022). How good is garlic for your health? *Zoe*. https://joinzoe.com/learn/is-garlic-good-for-the-heart (accessed on 12 June 2024).

Kumar, R., Chhatwal, S., Arora, S., Sharma, S., Singh, J., Singh, N., Bhandari, V., & Khurana, A. (2013). Antihyperglycemic, antihyperlipidemic, anti-inflammatory and adenosine deaminase-lowering effects of garlic in patients with type 2 diabetes mellitus with obesity. *Diabetes, Metabolic Syndrome and Obesity: Targets and Therapy, 6*, 49–56.

Larijani, V. N., Ahmadi, N., Zeb, I., Khan, F., Flores, F., & Budoff, M. (2013). Beneficial effects of aged garlic extract and coenzyme Q10 on vascular elasticity and endothelial function: The FAITH randomized clinical trial. *Nutrition, 29*, 71–75.

Lawson, L. D. (1996). The composition and chemistry of garlic cloves and processed garlic. In H. P. Koch & L. D. Lawson (Eds.), *Garlic: The Science and Therapeutic Application of Allium sativum L and Related Species* (pp. 37–107). Baltimore: Williams & Wilkins.

Lawson, L. D. (1998). Garlic: A review of its medicinal effects and indicated active compounds. In L. D. Lawson & R. Bauer (Eds.), *Phytomedicines of Europe: Chemistry and biological activity. Series 691.* (pp. 176–209). American Chemical Society.

Lewington, S., Whitlock, G., Clarke, R., Sherliker, P., Emberson, J., Halsey, J., Qizilbash, N., Peto, R., & Collins, R. (2007). Blood cholesterol and vascular mortality by age, sex, and blood pressure: A meta-analysis of individual data from 61 prospective studies with 55,000 vascular deaths. *The Lancet, 370*, 1829–1839.

Lopez, A. D., Mathers, C. D., Ezzati, M., Jamison, D. T., & Murray, C. J. (2006). Global and regional burden of disease and risk factors, 2001: Systematic analysis of population health data. *The Lancet, 367*, 1747–1757.

Ma, S., & Yin, J. (2012). Anaphylaxis induced by ingestion of raw garlic. *Foodborne Pathogens and Disease, 9*, 773–775.

Macan, H., Uykimpang, R., Alconcel, M., Takasu, J., Razon, R., Amagase, H., & Niihara, Y. (2006). Aged garlic extract may be safe for patients on warfarin therapy. *The Journal of Nutrition, 136*(3), 793S–795S.

Mancia, G., De Backer, G., Dominiczak, A., Cifkova, R., Fagard, R., Germano, G., Grassi, G., Heagerty, A. M., Kjeldsen, S. E., Laurent, S., et al. (2007). Guidelines for the management of arterial hypertension: The task force for the management of arterial hypertension of

the European Society of Hypertension (ESH) and of the European Society of Cardiology (ESC). *Journal of Hypertension, 25*, 1105–1187.
McPherson, R., Frohlich, J., Fodor, G., & Genest, J.; Canadian Cardiovascular Society. (2006). Canadian Cardiovascular Society position statement—Recommendations for the diagnosis and treatment of dyslipidemia and prevention of cardiovascular disease. *Canadian Journal of Cardiology, 22*, 913–927.
Mulawarman, R., Trifitriana, M., Felani, M. R., & Tondas, A. E. (2021). Garlic effect on reducing blood pressure and cholesterol in patients with and without hypertension: A systematic review and meta-analysis of randomized controlled trials. *Journal of Hypertension, 39*, e4.
Nakasone, Y., Nakamura, Y., Yamamoto, T., & Yamaguchi, H. (2013). Effect of traditional Japanese garlic preparation on blood pressure in prehypertensive and mildly hypertensive adults. *Experimental and Therapeutic Medicine, 5*, 399–405.
Osamor, P. E., & Owumi, B. E. (2010). Complementary and alternative medicine in the management of hypertension in an urban Nigerian community. *BMC Complementary and Alternative Medicine, 10*, 36–40.
Pekkanen, J., Linn, S., Heiss, G., Suchindran, C. M., Leon, A., Rifkind, B. M., & Tyroler, H. A. (1990). Ten-year mortality from cardiovascular disease in relation to cholesterol level among men with and without pre-existing cardiovascular disease. *The New England Journal of Medicine, 322*, 1700–1707.
Raggi, P., Callister, T. Q., & Shaw, L. J. (2004). Progression of coronary artery calcium and risk of first myocardial infarction in patients receiving cholesterol-lowering therapy. *Arteriosclerosis, Thrombosis, and Vascular Biology, 24*, 1272–1277.
Rahman, K. (2001). Historical perspective on garlic and cardiovascular disease. *The Journal of Nutrition, 131*, 977S–979S.
Rahman, K. (2003). Garlic and aging: New insights into an old remedy. *Ageing Research Reviews, 2*, 39–56.
Reinhart, K. M., Coleman, C. I., Teevan, C., Vachhani, P., & White, M. (2008). Effects of garlic on blood pressure in patients with and without systolic hypertension: A meta-analysis. *Annals of Pharmacotherapy, 42*, 1766–1771.
Reinhart, K. M., Talati, R., White, C. M., & Coleman, C. I. (2009). The impact of garlic on lipid parameters: A systematic review and meta-analysis. *Nutrition Research Reviews, 22*, 39–48.
Ried, K., Frank, O. R., & Stocks, N. P. (2013). Aged garlic extract reduces blood pressure in hypertensives: A dose-response trial. *European Journal of Clinical Nutrition, 67*, 64–70.
Ried, K., Frank, O. R., Stocks, N. P., Fakler, P., & Sullivan, T. (2008). Effects of garlic on blood pressure: A systematic review and meta-analysis. *BMC Cardiovascular Disorders, 8*, 13.
Ryu, K., Ide, N., Matsuura, H., & Itakura, Y. (2001). N alpha-(1-deoxy-D-fructos-1-yl)-L-arginine, an antioxidant compound identified in aged garlic extract. *The Journal of Nutrition, 131*, 972S–976S.
Seo, D. Y., Lee, S., Figueroa, A., Kwak, Y. S., Kim, N., Rhee, B. D., Ko, K. S., Bang, H. S., Baek, Y. H., & Han, J. (2012). Independent beneficial effects of aged garlic extract intake with regular exercise on cardiovascular risk in postmenopausal women. *Nutrition Research and Practice, 6*, 226–231.
Silagy, C. A., & Neil, H. A. (1994). A meta-analysis of the effect of garlic on blood pressure. *Journal of Hypertension, 12*, 463–468.

Silagy, C., & Neil, A. (1994). Garlic as a lipid lowering agent—A meta-analysis. *Journal of the Royal College of Physicians of London, 28*, 39–45.

Simons, S., Wollersheim, H., & Thien, T. (2009). A systematic review on the influence of trial quality on the effect of garlic on blood pressure. *Netherlands Journal of Medicine, 67*, 212–219.

Sobenin, I. A., Myasoedova, V. A., Iltchuk, M. I., Zhang, D. W., & Orekhov, A. N. (2019). Therapeutic effects of garlic in cardiovascular atherosclerotic disease. *Chinese Journal of Natural Medicines, 17*(10), 721–728.

Stabler, S. N., Tejani, A. M., Huynh, F., & Fowkes, C. (2012). Garlic for the prevention of cardiovascular morbidity and mortality in hypertensive patients. *Cochrane Database of Systematic Reviews, 8*, CD007653.

Stamler, J., Wentworth, D., & Neaton, J. D. (1986). Is relationship between serum cholesterol and risk of premature death from coronary heart disease continuous and graded: Findings in 356,222 primary screenees of the Multiple Risk Factor Intervention Trial (MRFIT). *JAMA, 256*(20), 2823–2828.

Stevinson, C., Pittler, M., & Ernst, E. (2000). Garlic for treating hypercholesterolemia: A meta-analysis of randomized clinical trials. *Annals of Internal Medicine, 133*, 420–429.

Three reasons a heart loves garlic. (2020). Providence. https://blog.providence.org/toyourhealthblogs/three-reasons-a-heart-loves-garlic (accessed on 12 June 2024).

Van Doorn, M. B., Espirito Santo, S. M., Meijer, P., Kamerling, I. M., Schoemaker, R. C., Dirsch, V., Vollmar, A., Haffner, T., & Gebhardt, R. (2006). Effect of garlic powder on C-reactive protein and plasma lipids in overweight and smoking subjects. *American Journal of Clinical Nutrition, 84*, 1324–1329.

Vinson, J. A., Su, X., Zubik, L., & Bose, P. (2001). Phenol antioxidant quantity and quality in foods: Fruits. *Journal of Agricultural and Food Chemistry, 49*, 5315–5321.

Vlachopoulos, C., Aznaouridis, K., & Stefanadis, C. (2010). Prediction of cardiovascular events and all-cause mortality with arterial stiffness: A systematic review and meta-analysis. *Journal of the American College of Cardiology, 55*, 1318–1327.

Warshafsky, S., Kamer, R. S., & Sivak, S. L. (1993). Effect of garlic on total serum cholesterol: A meta-analysis. *Annals of Internal Medicine, 119*, 599–605.

Waters, D., Craven, T. E., & Lespérance, J. (1993). Prognostic significance of progression of coronary atherosclerosis. *Circulation, 87*, 1067–1075.

Williams, M. J., Sutherland, W. H., McCormick, M. P., Yeoman, D. J., & de Jong, S. A. (2005). Aged garlic extract improves endothelial function in men with coronary artery disease. *Phytotherapy Research, 19*, 314–319.

Wood, D. (2001). Established and emerging cardiovascular risk factors. *American Heart Journal, 141*, S49–S57.

Zeb, I., Ahmadi, N., Nasir, K., Kadakia, J., Larijani, V. N., Flores, F., Li, D., & Budoff, M. J. (2012). Aged garlic extract and coenzyme Q10 have favorable effects on inflammatory markers and coronary atherosclerosis progression: A randomized clinical trial. *Journal of Cardiovascular Disease Research, 3*, 185–190.

Zeng, T., Guo, F. F., Zhang, C. L., Song, F. Y., Zhao, X. L., & Xie, K. Q. (2012). A meta-analysis of randomized, double-blind, placebo-controlled trials for the effects of garlic on serum lipid profiles. *Journal of the Science of Food and Agriculture, 92*, 1892–1902.

CHAPTER 5

HEALTH BENEFITS OF GREEN TEA: A REVIEW

NIHARIKA DEWANGAN

Shri Shankaracharya Professional University, Bhilai, Chhattisgarh, India

ABSTRACT

"Where there's tea, there's hope" is a well-known quotation about a cup of tea seen on the internet. As a tea lover, of course, the quote is very true for me. In ancient times, green tea was recommended for the treatment of headaches and body aches. It also aids in better digestion and detoxification. Green tea acts to boost energy. Green tea makes up to 20–22% of the total tea production. Tea plants are small evergreen shrubs with white flowers and are native to the mountainous regions of China, Japan, and India. The plant can grow up to a height of 30 feet, but its leaves are usually pruned at a height of 2 to 3 feet. Green tea is mainly consumed in China, Japan, Korea, and Morocco. Green tea, or non-fermented tea, contains the highest amount of flavonoids compared to its partially fermented (oolong tea) and fermented (black tea) counterparts. After water, tea is the most widely consumed beverage in the world. The Chinese have a ritual tea-drinking ceremony that originated during the Sung Dynasty. Recently, there has been a growing interest in the cardiovascular benefits of green tea due to the increasing interest in the health properties of tea and a significant rise in scientific investigation.

5.1 INTRODUCTION

Beverages are consumed by humans due to their refreshing and stimulating properties. Tea is one of the beverages that is consumed worldwide. Along

Antioxidants as Nutraceuticals. Nayan A. Gujarathi, Raj K. Keservani, Rajesh K. Kesharwani, Bhushan R. Rane, Yogeeta Sameer Goyal (Eds.)

with its refreshing properties, it also provides pleasure and has many health benefits. *Camellia sinensis* L., commonly known as the tea plant, is an evergreen shrub belonging to the family *Theaceae* (Naheed et al., 2007). The leaves of the tea plant are used to produce tea. China was the first country in the world where the production and consumption of tea began. Due to its antioxidant and anti-inflammatory properties, China considered the green tea plant as a medicinally beneficial plant. In the 19th century, in 1823 A.D., the cultivation of the tea plant was started for the first time in India in the Assam region (Nagalakshmi, 2003). Green tea (Kesharwani et al., 2016) is considered one of the most popular drinks consumed by millions of people every day all over the world (Monirul et al., 2012). In Indian homes, tea is a traditional welcome drink for guests and is also used as an energy booster. In recent decades, scientists all over the world have been investigating the potential health benefits of green tea and its most abundant catechin, epigallocatechin gallate (EGCG). Various researchers are presently investigating the effects of green tea and its constituents, especially catechins, on cardiovascular and metabolic health (Wolfram, 2007). In a survey, it is found that oxidized catechins, known as theaflavins in black tea, reduce blood cholesterol. Green tea extracts, along with other polyphenolic constituents, show synergistic properties, and thus these compounds are potentially important to the medicinal benefits of black and green teas. Also, due to presumed antioxidant and anti-aging properties, tea is now finding its way into topical preparations (Morre et al., 2005) (Figures 5.1–5.3).

The most commonly used tea in Asian countries is green tea and Oolong Tea, and in Western countries Black tea is more popular among those mentioned in Table 5.1.

Apart from the green tea obtained from the Camellia plant, a tea prepared from the combination of water extract of *Cymbopogon citratus* plant, commonly known as lemongrass; *Ocimum sanctum* plant commonly known as Tulsi in India, and *Zingiber officinale* plant commonly called Ginger can also be a healthy green tea with various health benefits. Lemongrass leaves contain flavonoids such as luteolin, and isoorientin 2′O rhamnoside (Guanasingh et al., 1981; Matouscheck et al., 1991). Quercetin, apigenin, kaempferol, etc., and flavonoids were also investigated in leaves of the lemongrass plant (Miean et al., 2001). Phenolic compounds such as elemicin, catechol, chlorogenic acid, caffeic acid, and hydroquinone are found in the plant (Faruq et al., 1994). Thus, the lemongrass plant has antibacterial, antifungal, antimalarial, anti-inflammatory, antidiarrheal, etc., activities (Shah et al., 2011). The extract of lemongrass possesses a hypocholesterolemic

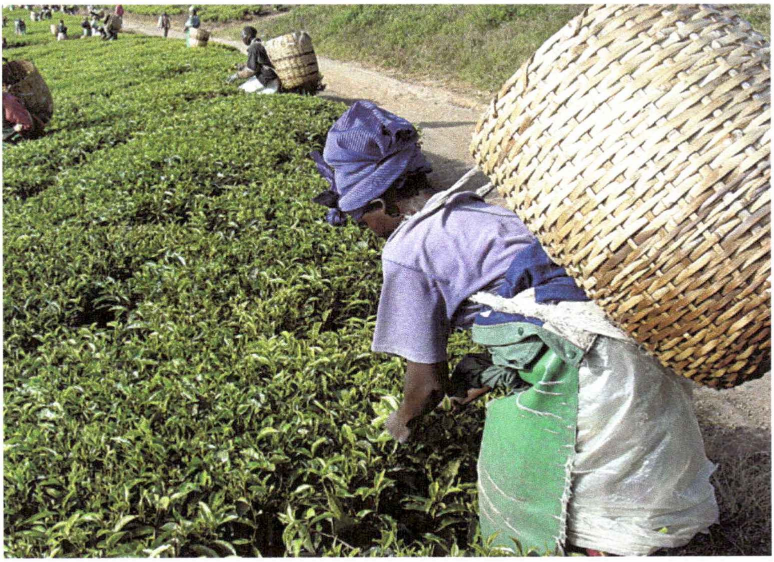

FIGURE 5.1 *Camellia sinensis* plant plantation.

Image credit: By Martin Benjamin. https://creativecommons.org/licenses/by-sa/3.0/

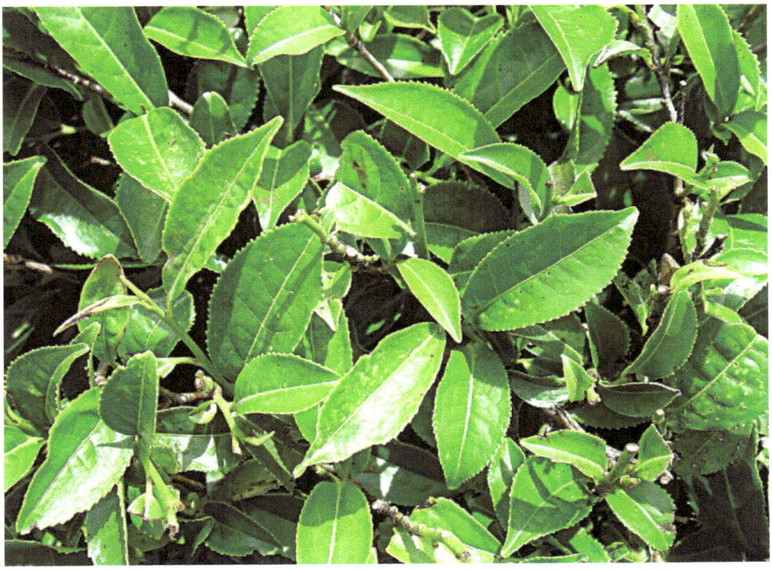

FIGURE 5.2 *Camellia sinensis* leaves.

Source: Public domain

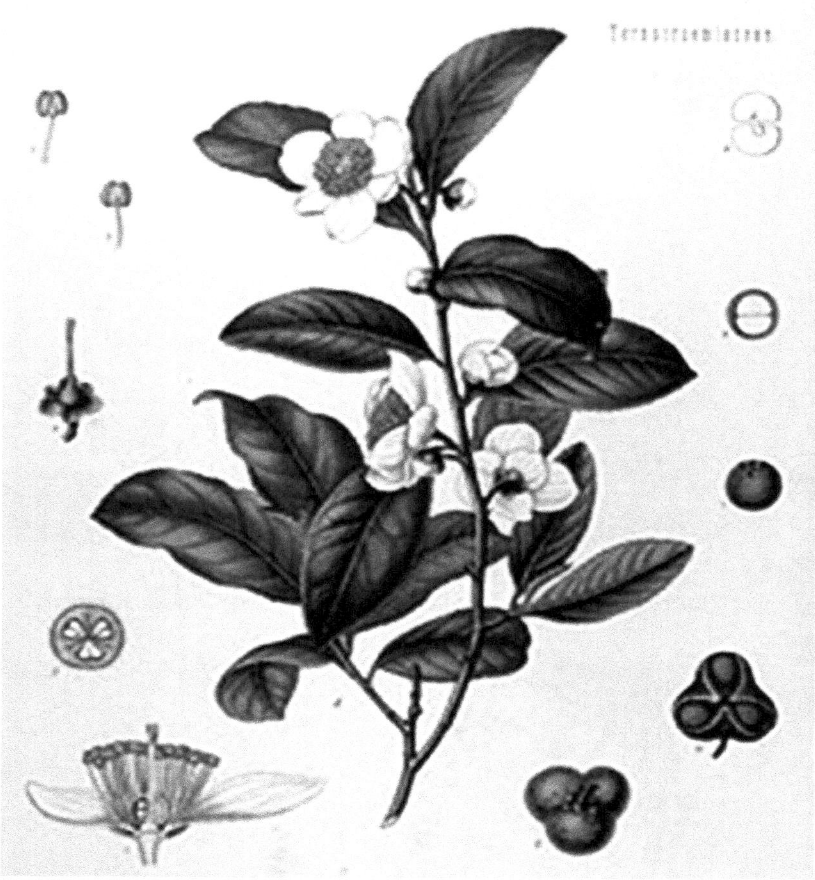

FIGURE 5.3 *C. sinensis* diagrammatic representation.

Source: Public domain

potential that can reduce cholesterol concentration (Agbafor et al., 2007). Tulsi and Ginger plants are well-known medicinally important plants with antibiotic activities, used in cough, cold, and fever. Leaves of the Tulsi plant are used while the rhizome of the ginger plant is used as a supplement in making green tea from the lemongrass plant.

The combination of these three plants supplemented with different flavors of cardamom, clove, mint, turmeric, etc., is used as a healthier tea nowadays. Along with the flavor, the supplemented plants were also equally important in providing medicinal value to a cup of tea (Figures 5.4–5.8).

TABLE 5.1 Types of Tea with Their Health Characters

Sl. No.	Types	Processing/ Preparation	Chemical Characters	Health Characters	References
1.	Green Tea	Prepared from unfermented leaves	Antioxidant polyphenol Catechins present	Refreshing and stimulating properties	Vishnoi et al. (2018)
2.	Black Tea	Prepared by fermenting process. It accounts for 72% of the world's total tea production.	Most EGCG oxidized during fermentation, and flavonoids present	Help in removing harmful toxins from the body	
3.	White Tea	Buds were picked before they were fully opened, also young leaves were plucked. They were steamed and dried.	It retains a maximum level of antioxidants and less caffeine.	Refreshing and stimulating properties	
4.	Oolong Tea	Prepared by partial fermentation	A high level of antioxidants is present	It keeps skin cells healthy and slows down the aging process.	
5.	Pu'erh Tea	Leaves were picked any time of the year	Various antioxidants are present	Refreshing and stimulating properties	
6.	Red Tea	Comes from a shrub of South Africa.	Naturally caffeine-free.	Various health benefits especially for pregnant women	
7.	Matcha Green Tea	Japanese powdered green-type tea	theanine, caffeine, catechins, phenolic acids, rutin, Quercetin vitamin c	Antioxidant and anti-inflammatory properties for health.	Kochman et al. (2020)

5.2 COMBINATION OF CYMBOPOGON GREEN TEA

The blend of three plants, enhanced with cardamom, clove, mint, turmeric, etc., is now popular as a healthier tea. These supplemented plants not only add flavor but also contribute medicinal value to the tea. TRhnis tea is an instant tea.

Lemongrass leaves contain flavonoids like luteolin and isoorientin 2′O rhamnoside. Quercetin, apigenin, kaempferol, and other flavonoids have been studied in lemongrass leaves. Phenolic compounds such as elimicin, catechol, chlorogenic acid, caffeic acid, and hydroquinone are present in the plant.

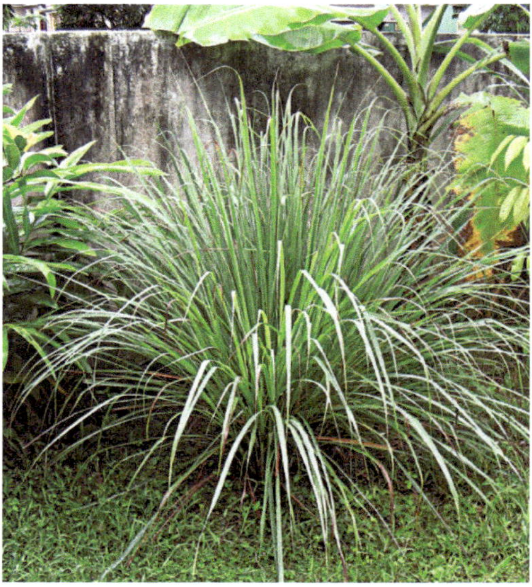

FIGURE 5.4 Cymbopogon citrus plan.

Image credit: By Hakcipta Yosri - Dibebaskan di bawah. https://creativecommons.org/licenses/by/2.0

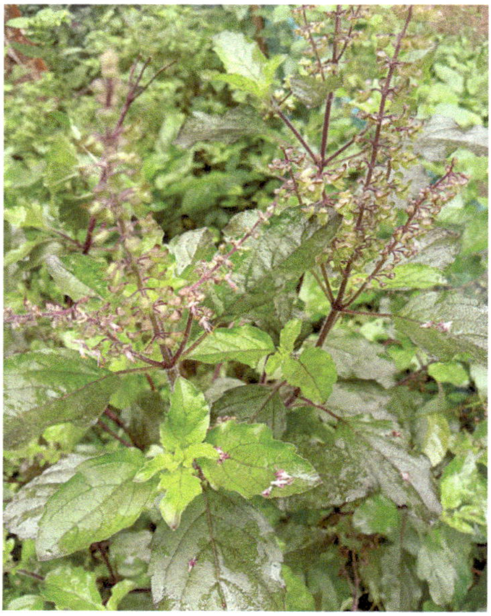

FIGURE 5.5 *Ocimum sanctum* plant.

Image Credit: By LINAVARGHESE. https://creativecommons.org/licenses/by/4.0/

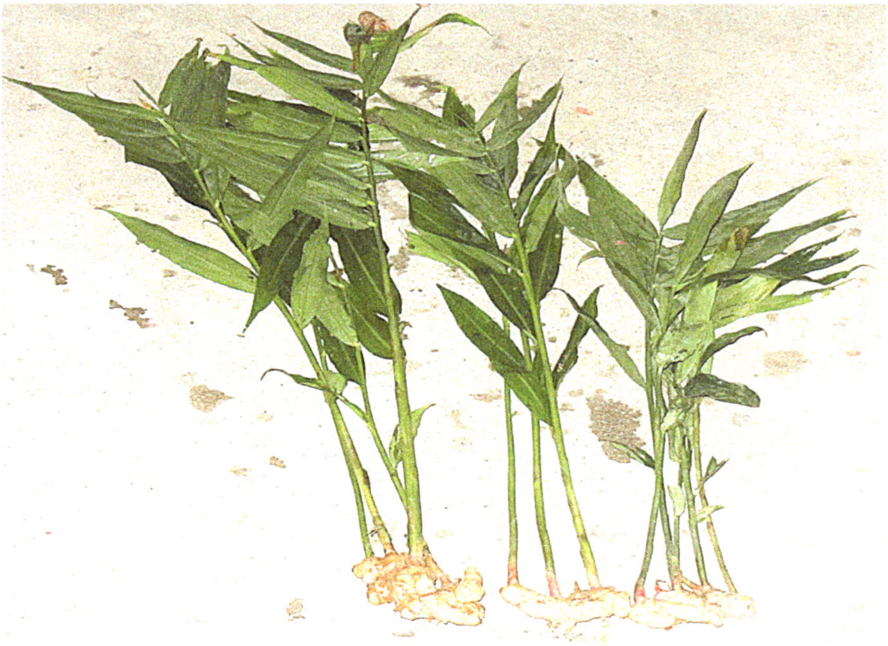

FIGURE 5.6 *Zingiber officinalis* plant.

Image credit: By Sengai Podhuvan. https://creativecommons.org/licenses/by-sa/3.0/

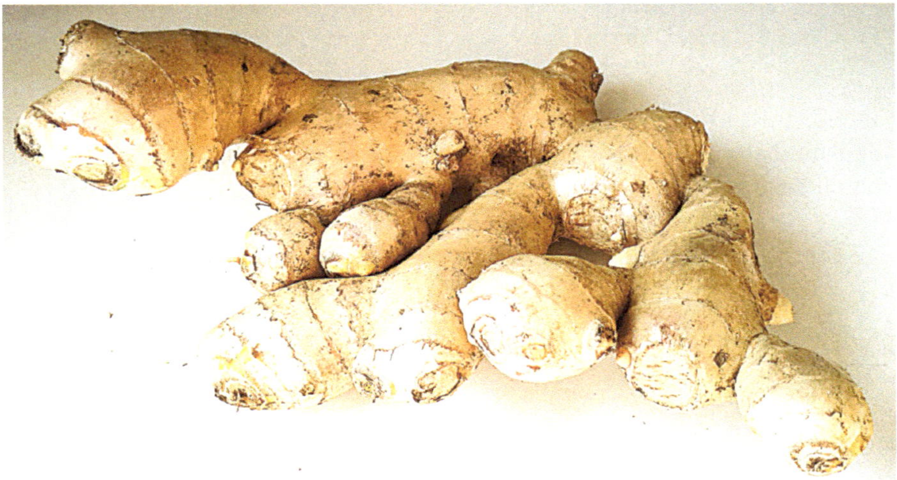

FIGURE 5.7 Rhizome of *Zingiber officinalis*.

Image credit: By Mk2010. https://creativecommons.org/licenses/by-sa/4.0/

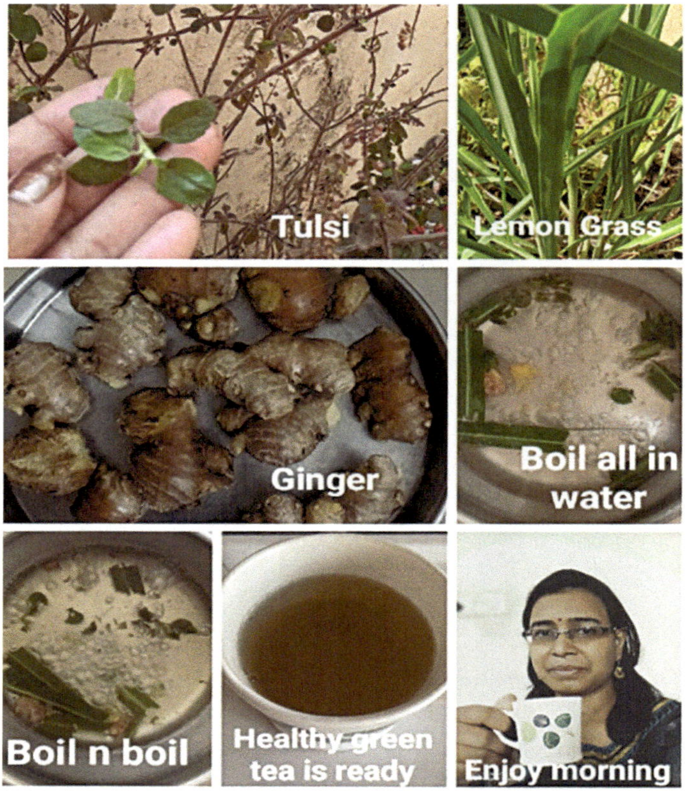
Tulsi
Lemon Grass
Ginger
Boil all in water
Boil n boil
Healthy green tea is ready
Enjoy morning

FIGURE 5.8 Easy method of preparation of *Cymbopogon* green tea.

Lemongrass exhibits antibacterial, antifungal, antimalarial, anti-inflammatory, and antidiarrheal activities. Lemongrass extract shows the potential to reduce cholesterol levels. Tulsi and ginger plants are known for their medicinal properties, including antibiotic effects for cough, cold, and fever. Tulsi leaves and ginger rhizome are used along with lemongrass in making green tea.

5.3 CLIMATIC CONDITION FOR CULTIVATION OF GREEN TEA (*CAMELLIA SINENSIS*)

Green tea and black tea are obtained from one of two major varieties of *Camellia, C. sinensis var. sinensis* and *C. sinensis* var. *assamica* (Integrated Taxonomic). The suitable climate for the cultivation of green tea is tropical and subtropical, with a temperature range between 13°C and 25°C

(Nagalakshmi, 2003). Well-drained, deep loam soil with a rich amount of organic matter and a pH range between 4.5 and 5.5 is required for tea plantation (TNAU Agritech Portal, 2021). Tea is grown in the mountainous areas of the tropics between latitudes 41°N and 16°S.

5.4 CHEMICAL CONSTITUENTS OF GREEN TEA

Some minerals, caffeine, and catechins are present in different levels of green tea. Potassium is present in large amounts followed by sodium, calcium, aluminum, manganese, and iron. A significant amount of catechin and caffeine is present in green tea. Chromium and selenium were not found (Reto et al., 2007). Green tea prepared from *Camellia sinensis* contains a high amount of polyphenols, which are disease-fighting antioxidants. Catechins are the most important compounds of green tea, accounting for 10–20% of dry tea leaves (Maruyama et al., 2017).

Catechins are of four main types:

1. Epicatechin (EC)
2. Epicatechin-3-gallate (ECG)
3. Epigallocatechin (EGC)
4. Epigallocatechin-3-gallate (EGCG).

Among these Epigallocatechin-3-gallate (EGCG) is the most dominant catechin.

Along with catechins, proteins (15%), whose enzymes contribute an important fraction of amino acids (4%) such as glutamic acid, theanine, 5-N-ethylglutamine, leucine, threonine, tryptophan, serine, arginine, aspartic acid, tyrosine, glycine, valine, and lysine; fiber (26%); other carbohydrates (7%) such as cellulose, pectins, glucose, fructose, and sucrose; lipids (7%) such as linoleic and α-linolenic acids; pigments (2%); and minerals (5%) are also included in the chemical composition of green tea (Belitz et al., 1997). Vitamins B, C, and E, and volatile compounds such as aldehydes, alcohols, esters, lactones, and hydrocarbons were also found in green tea. The fresh leaves contain, on average, 3–4% of alkaloids known as methyl-xanthines, such as caffeine, theobromine, and theophylline.

5.5 CHEMICAL STRUCTURE OF IMPORTANT COMPOUNDS OF GREEN TEA

1. Catechin, C, (+)-Catechin ($C_{15}H_{14}O_6$).

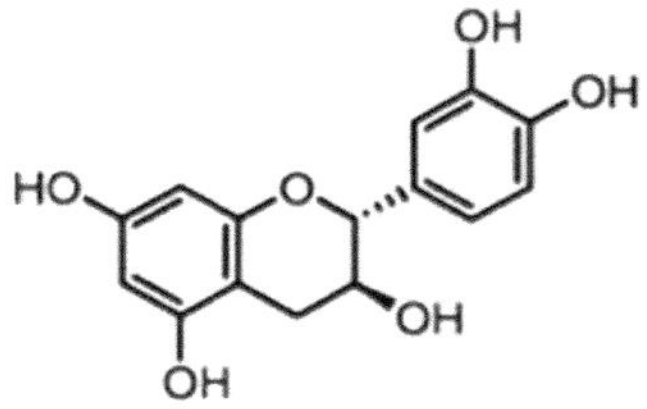

(+)-catechin

2. Epicatechin, EC, (–)-Epicatechin (cis) ($C_{15}H_{14}O_6$).

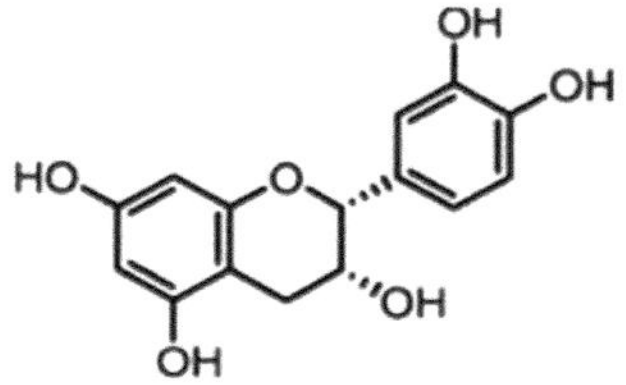

(–)-epicatechin

3. Epigallocatechin, EGC, (–)-Epigallocatechin ($C_{15}H_{14}O_7$).

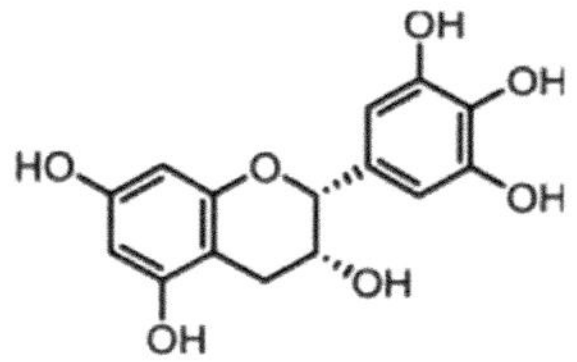

(–)-epigallocatechin

4. Gallocatechin, GC, (+) Gallocatechin ($C_{15}H_{14}O_7$).

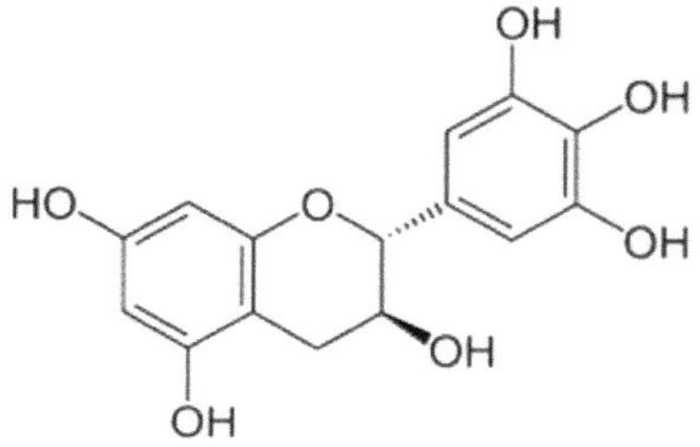

5. Epicatechin gallate, ECG, (–)-Epicatechin, Gallate ($C_{22}H_{18}O_{10}$).

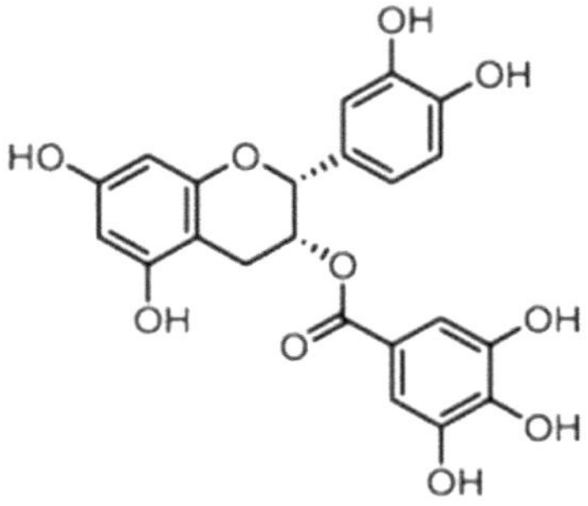

(−)-epicatechin gallate

A cup of tea, prepared in a proportion of 1 g of tea leaves to 100 ml of boiling water in a 3-minute, usually contains 250–350 mg of dry materials that are comprised of 30–42% catechins and 3–6% caffeine.

Matcha, a Japanese green tea is a powdered type of tea, in which biologically active compounds such as theanine, caffeine, catechins, phenolic acids, rutin, Quercetin vitamin C, etc., are present. Due to the presence of these, it is characterized by a high content of antioxidant and anti-inflammatory substances (Kochman et al., 2020) (Tables 5.2 and 5.3).

TABLE 5.2 Chemical Constituent of Green Tea (*Camellia Sinensis*)

Sl. No.	Compound	Elements Present	References
1.	Catechins	(+)-catechin, (–)-epicatechin, (–)-gallocatechin, (–)-epigallocatechin, (–)-catechin gallate, (–)-epicatechin gallate, (–)-gallocatechin gallate, (–)-epigallocatechin gallate	Yasin et al. (2015); Lan-Sook et al. (2014)
2.	Theaflavins	Theaflavin, theaflavin-3-O-gallate, theaflavin-3′-O-gallate, theaflavin-3-3′-O-gallate	Yasin et al. (2015)
3.	Flavanols	Quercetin, kaempferol, myricetin	Yasin et al. (2015)
4.	Alkaloids	Caffeine, theophylline, theobromine	Yasin et al. (2015)
5.	Sugars	Glucose, fructose, saccharose	Yasin et al. (2015)
6.	Amino acids	Isoleucine, leucine, methionine, threonine, phenylalanine, glutamine, asparagine, alanine, serine, proline, histidine, glutamic acid, aspartic acid, theanine	Yasin et al. (2015)
7.	Vitamins	C, α-, β-, γ-, δ-tocopherols, riboflavin	Yasin et al. (2015)
8.	Pigments	Chlorophyll and carotenoids	Yasin et al. (2015)

TABLE 5.3 Percentage of Main Chemical Constituent of Green Tea Leaves

Sl. No.	Constituent	Percentage (% of Dried Leaf)
1.	Polyphenols	37
2.	Carbohydrates	25
3.	Caffeine	3.5
4.	Protein	15
5.	Amino acids	4
6.	Lignin	6.5
7.	Organic acids	1.5
8.	Lipids	2
9.	Ash	5
10.	Chlorophyll	0.5

Source: Modified from Sinija et al. (2008).

5.6 HEALTH BENEFICIAL PROPERTIES OF GREEN TEA (*CAMELLIA SINENSIS*)

1. **Anticarcinogenic Effect:** The content of Epigallocatechin gallate is found to be tumor inhibitory (Makiuchi et al., 2016). Catechins are considered anticancer medications and can be used to support therapy as well as in cancer prevention. Vitamin C has also been associated with protective effects against cancer (Panda et al., 2013; Fujiki et al., 2015).
2. **Cardio Protective Effect:** By an experiment, it has been found that upon exposure to cigarette smoke, myocardial injury and lipid anomalies were developed. However, the oral administration of EGCG shows an inverted effect on these aberrations. EGCG is potent to exert a protective effect on the heart muscle in patients undergoing surgery (Gokulakrisnan et al., 2011).
3. **Antiviral Properties of Green Tea:** Epigallocatechin-3-gallate (EGCG) in green tea is found to be beneficial for human health. It has antiviral activities against various viral infections. The antiviral activities of EGCG show that it has antiviral molecules that act at different stages of the virus life cycle. EGCG has prophylactic activity and is found to inhibit 3CLpro, a vital enzyme found in the virus, at low concentrations and also exhibits good binding to 3CLpro, a druggable target. 3CLpro is found in SARS-CoV and SARS-CoV-2, and there is a similarity between these two viruses. So,

it is considered that green tea is a potent antiviral agent that should be explored as an alternative treatment for COVID-19 (Mhatre et al., 2020).

4. **The Immunomodulatory Properties of Green Tea:** This supports the prevention and regulation of the immune response in infectious diseases, including COVID-19 (Fan et al., 2020; Khaerunnisa et al., 2020). Many studies reveal the antiviral properties of traditional green tea. Green tea contains antiviral activity that can inactivate SARS-CoV-2. Although it is a promising report, it requires more detailed research (Fukino et al., 2005) (Table 5.4).

TABLE 5.4 Summary of Health Benefits of Consuming Green Tea

Sl. No.	Health Beneficial Properties	References
1.	Antioxidant	Soni et al. (2015); Rohdewald (1998)
2.	Antimicrobial	Hamilton-Miller (2001); Soni et al. (2015)
3.	Anticariogenic	Tsuchiya et al. (1997); Linke et al. (2003)
4.	Anti-cancerous	Jankun et al. (1997); Kanwar et al. (2012)
5.	Anti-hair fall Activity	Amin et al. (2014)
6.	Anti-diabetic Activity	Wu et al. (2004)
7.	Anti-obesity Activity	Hamao et al. (2011)
8.	In Cardiovascular disease	Hodgson et al. (2010)
9.	Smooth-muscle relaxant Activity	Hung et al. (2002)
10.	Anti-inflammatory Activity	Akhtar et al. (2011)

5.7 CONCLUSION

The content of health-promoting substances, including polyphenols, is also affected by the agro-climatic conditions during growth, such as the number and distribution of sunny and rainy days, fertilization and plant protection measures, if any, etc. Green tea is one of the most popular beverages worldwide. In the past, it was consumed for treating some diseases, and for the last 30 years, many researchers have been studying the potential health benefits of green tea. Further study and research are needed on the health-beneficial properties of green tea. Green tea is loaded with antioxidants which have a beneficial effect on health.

Tea is an important health drink proven by many scientific research studies and is consumed all over the world. Tea is a pleasant and mildly stimulating beverage and is more effective due to its therapeutic value if sugar is not added. However, further human trials are required in well-controlled conditions. Meanwhile, tea is an affordable beverage with natural medicinal value.

KEYWORDS

- **alkaloids**
- **Camellia sinensis**
- **catechins**
- **epigallocatechin gallate**
- **flavonoids**
- **Ocimum sanctum**
- **theaflavins**
- **zingiber officinale**

REFERENCES

Agbafor, K. N., & Akubugwo, E. I. (2007). Hypocholesterolaemic effect of ethanolic extract of fresh leaves of *Cymbopogon citratus* (lemon grass). *African Journal of Biotechnology, 6*, 596–598.

Akhtar, N., & Haqqi, T. M. (2011). Epigallocatechin-3-gallate suppresses the global interleukin-1beta-induced inflammatory response in human chondrocytes. *Arthritis Research & Therapy, 13*(3), 1–16.

Amin, J., Simamora, E. L. P., Anwar, E., & Djajadisastra, J. (2014). Green tea (*Camellia sinensis*, L.) ethanolic extract as hair tonic in nutraceutical: Physical stability, hair growth activity on rats and safety test. *International Journal of Pharmacy and Pharmaceutical Sciences, 6*(5), 94–99.

Basu, A., & Lucas, E. A. (2007). Mechanism and effects of green tea on cardiovascular health. *Nutrition Reviews, 65*(8), 361–375.

Belitz, D. H., & Grosch, W. (1997). Quimica de los Alimentos. Zaragoza: Acribia. xlv, 1087 p. : il. ISBN: 9788420008356.

Fan, Y., Zhang, Y., Tariq, A., Jiang, X., Ahamd, Z., Zhihao, Z., Idrees, M., Azizullah, A., Adnan, M., & Bussmann, R. W. (2020). Food as medicine: A possible preventive measure against Coronavirus Disease (COVID-19). *Phytotherapy Research, 34*(12), 3124–3136.

Faruq, M. O. (1994). TLC technique in the component characterization and quality determination of Bangladeshi lemongrass oil (*Cymbopogon citratus* (DC) Stapf.). *Bangladesh Journal of Scientific and Industrial Research, 29*, 27–38.

Fujiki, H., Sueoka, E., Watanabe, T., & Suganuma, M. (2015). Synergistic enhancement of anticancer effects on numerous human cancer cell lines treated with the combination of

EGCG, other green tea catechins, and anticancer compounds. *Journal of Cancer Research and Clinical Oncology, 141*, 1511–1522.

Fukino, Y., Shimbo, M., Aoki, N., Okubo, T., & Iso, H. (2005). Randomized controlled trial for an effect of green tea consumption on insulin resistance and inflammation markers. *Journal of Nutritional Science and Vitaminology, 51*, 335–342.

Gokulakrisnan, A., Jayachandran, D. B., & Thirunavukkarasu, C. (2011). Attenuation of the cardiac inflammatory changes and lipid anomalies by (–)-epigallocatechin-gallate in cigarette smoke-exposed rats. *Molecular and Cellular Biochemistry, 354*(1–2), 1–10.

Guanasingh, C. B., & Nagarajan, S. (1981). Flavonoids of *Cymbopogon citratus*. *Indian Journal of Pharmaceutical Sciences, 43*, 115.

Hamao, M., Matsuda, H., Nakashima, S., Semura, S., Maekubo, S., Wakasugi, S., & Yoshikawa, M. (2011). Anti-obesity effects of the methanolic extract and chakasaponins from the flower buds of *Camellia sinensis* in mice. *Bioorganic and Medicinal Chemistry, 9*, 6033–6041.

Hamilton-Miller, J. M. T. (2001). Anti-cariogenic properties of tea (*Camellia sinensis*). *Journal of Medical Microbiology, 50*, 299–302.

Hodgson, J. M., & Croft, K. D. (2010). Tea flavonoids and cardiovascular health. *Molecular Aspects of Medicine, 31*, 495–502.

Hung, Y. C., Sava, V. M., Juang, C. L., Yeh, T. C., Shen, W. C., & Huang, G. S. (2002). Gastrointestinal enhancement of MRI with melanin derived from tea leaves (*Thea sinensis* Linn.). *Journal of Ethnopharmacology, 79*, 75–79.

Jankun, J., Selman, S. H., & Swiercz, R. (1997). Why drinking green tea could prevent cancer. *Nature, 387*, 561.

Jeszka-Skowron, M., Krawczyk, M., & Zgoła-Grześkowiak, A. (2015). Determination of antioxidant activity, rutin, quercetin, phenolic acids, and trace elements in tea infusions: Influence of citric acid addition on extraction of metals. *Journal of Food Composition and Analysis, 40*, 70–77.

Kanwar, J., Taskeen, M., & Mohammad, I. (2012). Recent advances on tea polyphenols. *Frontiers in Bioscience (Elite Edition), 4*, 111–131.

Kesharwani, R. K., Singh, P., & Keservani, R. K. (2016). Green coffee bean extract and chlorogenic acids: Chemistry and novel antioxidant benefits. In D. Bagchi, H. Moriyama, & A. Swaroop (Eds.), *Green Coffee Bean Extract in Human Health* (pp. 1–17). Boca Raton: Taylor and Francis. ISBN: 9781498716376.

Khaerunnisa, S., Kurniawan, H., Awaluddin, R., Suhartati, S., & Soetjipto, S. (2020). Potential inhibitor of COVID-19 main protease (Mpro) from several medicinal plant compounds by molecular docking study. Preprints, 2020, 2020030226.

Kochman, J., Jakubczyk, K., Antoniewicz, J., Mruk, H., & Janda, K. (2020). Health benefits and chemical composition of matcha green tea: A review. *Molecules (Basel, Switzerland), 26*(1), 85.

Lee, L. S., Kim, S. H., Kim, Y. B., & Kim, Y. C. (2014). Quantitative analysis of major constituents in green tea with different plucking periods and their antioxidant activity. *Molecules, 19*, 9173–9186.

Linke, H. A. B., & LeGeros, R. Z. (2003). Black tea extract and dental caries formation in hamsters. *International Journal of Food Sciences and Nutrition, 54*, 89–95.

Makiuchi, T., Sobue, T., Kitamura, T., Ishihara, J., Sawada, N., Iwasaki, M., Sasazuki, S., Yamaji, T., Shimazu, T., & Tsugane, S. (2016). Association between green tea/coffee consumption and biliary tract cancer: A population-based cohort study in Japan. *Cancer Science, 107*, 76–83.

Maruyama, K., Kihara-Negishi, F., Ohkura, N., Nakamura, Y., Nasui, M., & Saito, M. (2017). Simultaneous determination of catechins and caffeine in green tea-based beverages and foods for specified health uses. *Food and Nutrition Sciences, 8*, 316–325.

Matouschek, B. K., & Stahl, B. E. (1991). Phytochemical study of non-volatile substances from *Cymbopogon citratus* (DC.) Stapf (Poaceae). *Pharmaceutica Acta Helvetiae, 66*, 242–245.

Mhatre, S., Srivastava, T., Naik, S., & Patravale, V. (2021). Antiviral activity of green tea and black tea polyphenols in prophylaxis and treatment of COVID-19: A review. *Phytomedicine: International Journal of Phytotherapy and Phytopharmacology, 85*, 153286.

Miean, K. H., & Mohamed, S. (2001). Flavonoid (Myricitin, Quercetin, Kaempferol, Luteolin, and Apigenin) content of edible tropical plants. *Journal of Agricultural and Food Chemistry, 49*, 3106–3112.

Naheed, Z., Barech, A. R., Sajid, M., Khan, N. A., & Hussain, R. (2007). Effect of rolling, fermentation, and drying on the quality of black tea. *Sarhad Journal of Agriculture, 23*(3), 577.

Panda, D., Sharma, A., Shukla, N. K., Jaiswal, R., Dwivedi, S., Raina, V., Mohanti, B. K., Deo, S. V., & Patra, S. (2013). Gall bladder cancer and the role of dietary and lifestyle factors: A case-control study in a North Indian population. *European Journal of Cancer Prevention, 22*, 431–437.

Reto, M., Figueira, M. E., & Filipe, H. M. (2007). Chemical composition of green tea (*Camellia sinensis*) infusions commercialized in Portugal. *Plant Foods for Human Nutrition, 62*, 139.

Rohdewald, P. (1998). Pycnogenol. In C. A. Rice-Evans & L. Packer (Eds.), *Flavonoids in health and disease* (pp. 405–419). New York: Marcel Dekker, Inc.

Shah, G., Shri, R., Panchal, V., Sharma, N., Singh, B., & Mann, A. S. (2011). Scientific basis for the therapeutic use of *Cymbopogon citratus* Stapf (lemon grass). *Journal of Advanced Pharmaceutical Technology & Research, 2*(1), 3–8.

Sinija, V. R., & Mishra, H. N. (2008). Green tea: Health benefits, review. *Journal of Nutritional and Environmental Medicine, 17*(4), 232–242.

Soni, R. P., Katoch, M., Kumar, A., Ladohiya, R., & Verma, P. (2015). Tea: Production, composition, consumption and its potential as an antioxidant and antimicrobial agent. *International Journal of Food and Fermentation Technology, 5*(2), 95–106.

TNAU Agritech Portal: Tamil Nadu Tea Plantation Corporation. http://www.agritech.tnau.ac.in/horticulture/horti_plantation%20crops_tea.html.

Tsuchiya, H., Sato, M., Kato, H., Okubo, T., Juneja, L. R., & Kim, M. (1997). Simultaneous determination of catechins in human saliva by high-performance liquid chromatography. *Journal of Chromatography B: Biomedical Sciences and Applications, 703*(1–2), 253–258.

Vishnoi, H., Bodla, R. B., & Kant, R. (2018). Green tea (*Camellia sinensis*) and its antioxidant property: A review. *International Journal of Pharmaceutical Sciences and Research, 9*(5), 1723–1736.

Wu, C. D., & Wei, G. X. (2002). Tea as a functional food for oral health. *Nutrition, 18*(5), 443–444.

Wu, L. Y., Juan, C. C., Ho, L. T., Hsu, Y. P., & Hwang, L. S. (2004). Effect of green tea supplementation on insulin sensitivity in Sprague-Dawley rats. *Journal of Agricultural and Food Chemistry, 52*(3), 643–648.

Yashin, A. Y., Nemzer, B. V., Combet, E., & Yashin, Y. I. (2015). Determination of the chemical composition of tea by chromatographic methods: A review. *Journal of Food Research, 4*(3), 56–71.

Zuo, Y., Chen, H., & Deng, Y. (2002). Simultaneous determination of catechins, caffeine, and gallic acids in green, Oolong, black and Pu-erh teas using HPLC with a photodiode array detector. *Talanta, 57*(2), 307–316.

CHAPTER 6

ROLE OF VITAMINS IN HEART DISEASE

ABABIO GRACE K.

University of Ghana Medical School, Medical Biochemistry, Ghana, Africa

ABSTRACT

The role of antioxidant vitamins has generated much interest due to the supposed inhibition of lipid peroxidation in cardiovascular events. Even though an inverse relation between vitamin E and cardiovascular events has been indicated, vitamin C and provitamin A carotenoids remain cardio-protective. In this write-up, antioxidant properties of vitamin C were reviewed and a conceptual framework for vitamin E, which seems consistent with the literature, was made.

6.1 INTRODUCTION

6.1.1 GENERAL OVERVIEW

Vitamins are organic substances needed in smaller quantities for healthy living. Normally, vitamins are not produced by the human body, hence it is needed in the diet.

All vitamins preserve the integrity of bones, heal wounds, and boost the immune system. Two main classifications exist (Figure 6.1), namely water-soluble and fat-soluble vitamins (Tables 6.2 and 6.3).

There are several food sources for vitamins (Table 6.1).

Antioxidants as Nutraceuticals. Nayan A. Gujarathi, Raj K. Keservani, Rajesh K. Kesharwani, Bhushan R. Rane, Yogeeta Sameer Goyal (Eds.)

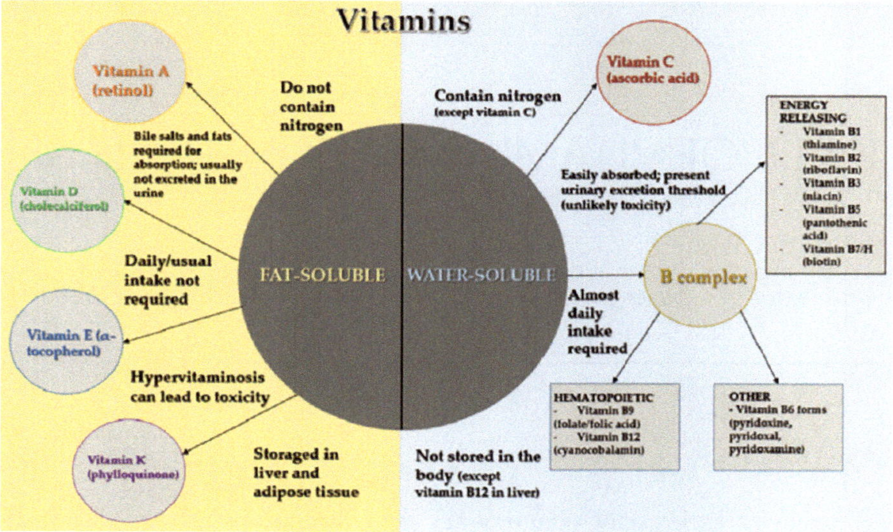

FIGURE 6.1 Classification of vitamins.

Source: Lesic et al., 2024. https://creativecommons.org/licenses/by/4.0/

TABLE 6.1 Sources of Vitamins

	Vitamin	Natural Sources
Fat Soluble	A	Spinach, pumpkin, orange, carrots, liver, leafy vegetables
	D	Liver, fish, mushroom, eggs
	E	Fruits and vegetables
	K	Spinach (green leafy vegetables), egg yolk, liver
Water Soluble Vitamin	B_1	Eggs, brown rice, potatoes, eggs, oatmeal, pork, liver
	B_2	Bananas, asparagus, dairy products, green beans
	B_3	Mushrooms, meat, eggs, tree nuts, fish, vegetables
	B_5	Avocado, broccoli, meat
	B_6	Bananas, meat, tree nuts, vegetables
	B_7	Peanuts, raw egg yolk, some vegetables
	B_9	Bread, cereal, liver, leafy vegetables
	B_{12}	Animal products
	C	Liver, fruits, and vegetables

Starvation and dietary deficiency normally cause primary vitamin deficiency, while increased loss of vitamin (lactation) or malabsorption, decreased intake, and increased requirement (pregnancy) cause secondary vitamin deficiency.

TABLE 6.2 Water Soluble Vitamins

Vitamins	Structure	Active forms	Function
Ascorbic acid	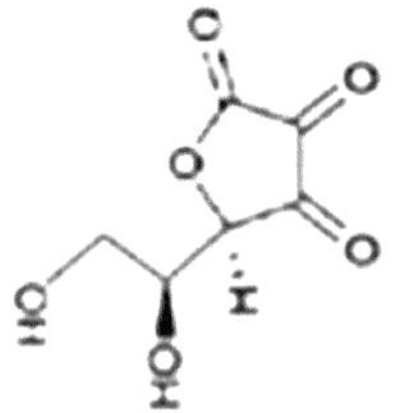	Ascorbic acid	• Antioxidant • Iron and copper metabolism • Collagen synthesis • Carnitine and tyrosine metabolism • Immune function
Biotin	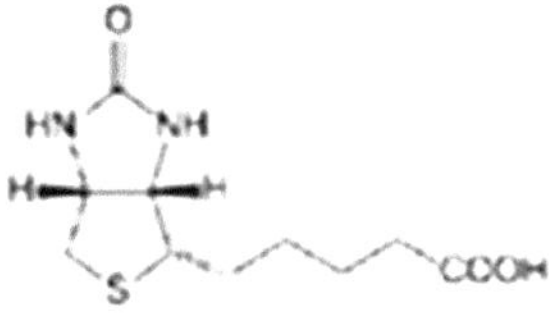	Biotin	• Metabolism of fatty acids carbohydrates,and amino acids • Energy metabolism • Regulation of cellular oxidative stress • Gene expression • Immune function • Maintenance of normal intestinal homeostasis
cobalamin	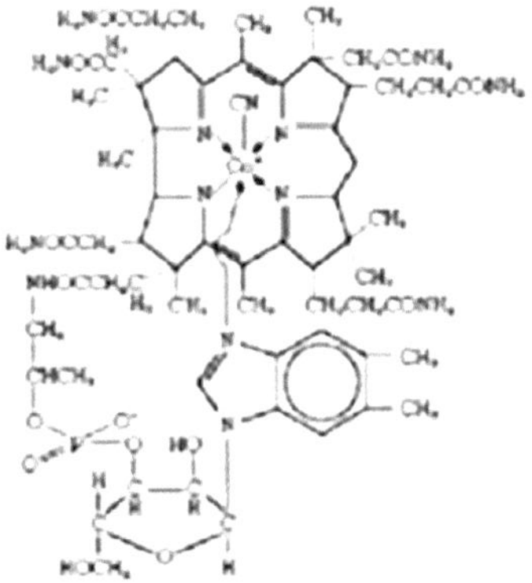	upper ligand (replacing the cyanide (CN) group: -Methyl-5'-deoxyadenosyl-	• Methyl tansfer • Metabolism of odd chain fatty acid,branched amino acids, and cholesterol

TABLE 6.2 *(Continued)*

Vitamins	Structure	Active forms	Function
Folate	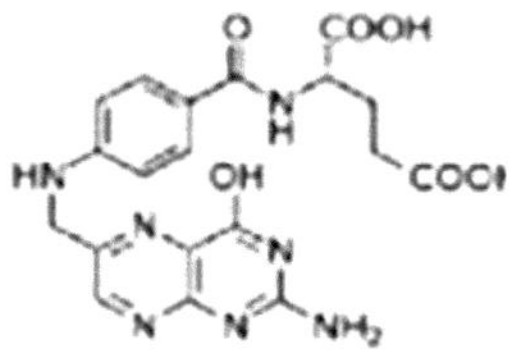	Many derivatives,e.g., tetrahydrofolate (THF) N^5-methyl-THF,N^{10}-for myl-THF	• DNA synthesis • Metabolism of amino acids
Niacin	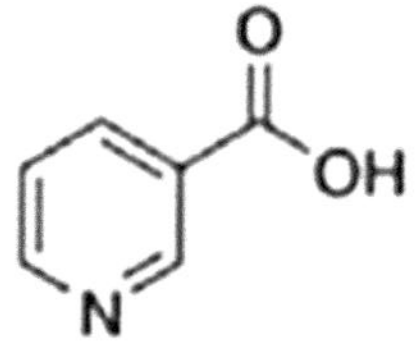	Niacin-adenine-dinucleotid (NAD), Niacin-adenine-dinucleotid-phosphate (NADP)	• Glycoysis • Maintenance of cellular redox state • Maintenance of normal intestinal homeostasis
Pantothenic acid	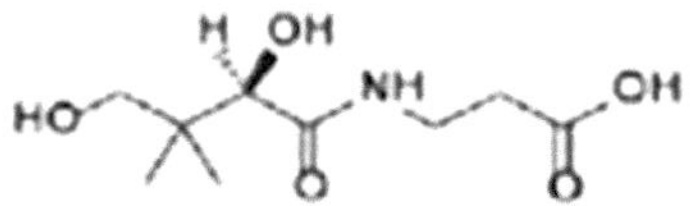	Part of coenzyme A	• Metabolism of carbohydrates,lipid and proteins
Pyridoxine	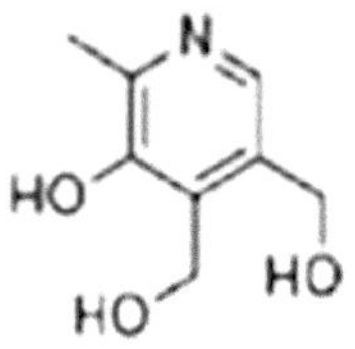	Pyridoxine,pyridoxal pyridoxamin	• Metabolism of carbohydrates,lipid and proteins • Production of neurotransmitters

TABLE 6.2 *(Continued)*

Vitamins	Structure	Active forms	Function
Riboflavin	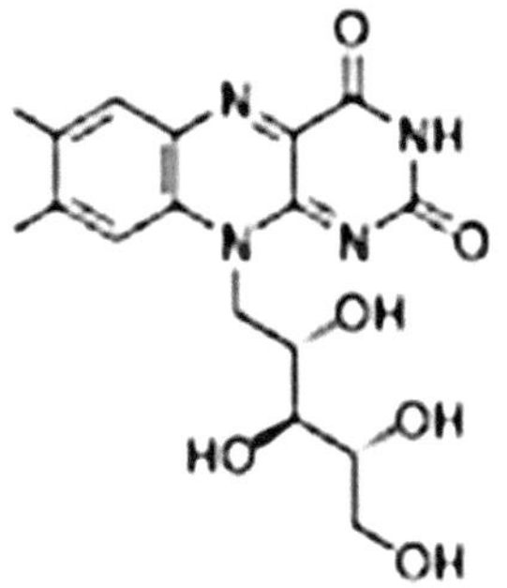	flavinmononucleotide (FMN), flavinadenindinucleotid (FAD)	• Oxidation-reduction • Protein foldings ,energy Metabolism,antioxidant, • anti- inflammatory
Thiamin	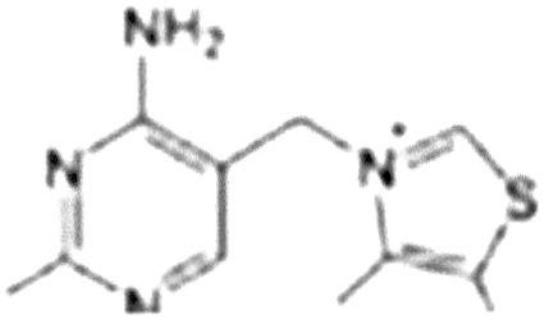	Thiamin pyrophosphate (TPP)	• Energy Metabolism • ATP production • Reduction of cellular oxidative stress

Source: Said, Hamid & Nexø, Ebba (2018).

TABLE 6.3 Fat Soluble Vitamins

Vitamin	Recommended Dietary Allowances	Dietary Sources	Function	Deficiency Symptoms
A	1000 ug (800 ug of retinol)	Green leafy vegetables, dairy products, fruits, eggs, fish oil	Maintaining mucus membrane, formation of visual pigments, and transport of nutrients across cell membranes	Increased pressure on the brain, night blindness, skin lesions, bone decalcification
D	75 ug of cholecalciferol	Liver, fish oil, provitamin activated by sunlight	Regulates phosphate and calcium metabolism	Rickets, mental retardation
E	10 mg (8 mg) of alpha-tocopherol	Wheat germ, green leafy vegetables, vegetable oil	Maintaining cell membrane	Fragile red blood cells increase
K	70–140 ug	Synthesized by bacteria in the gut, green leafy vegetables	Synthesis of blood clotting factors	Liver damage, failure of coagulation, hemolytic anemia

6.2 VITAMINS AND HEART DISEASE

Hypertension exposes patients to lipid peroxidation (Russo et al., 1998), and observational trials have indicated an inverse correlation between antioxidant vitamins (Chen et al., 2002; Salonen et al., 1988) and hypertension. Notable antioxidant vitamins have been extensively dealt with in this write-up.

6.2.1 VITAMIN A

Vitamin A (Figure 6.2) belongs to the same family as retinoids. In foods from animal origin, its major form is retinyl palmitate which can be converted to retinol. Its precursors (provitamins) remain members of the carotenoid family. Carotenoids' implication in oxidative protection seems inconsistent. Data range from neutral oxidation (Gazaino et al., 1995; Price et al., 1992; Reaven et al., 1993), antioxidant (Tsuchihashi et al., 1995; Jialal et al., 1991), and pro-oxidant (Tsuchihashi et al., 1995; Rautalahti et al., 1997; Palozza et al., 1995) properties. Carotenoids have been inversely related to cardiovascular events (Hozawa et al., 2007; D'Ortio et al., 2000; Ito et al., 2006). However, these studies established possible combination effects and not the independent assessment of beta-carotene. Increased intake of vitamin E (Knekt et al., 2004; Kushi et al., 1996; Knekt et al., 1994; Rimm et al., 1993; Stampfer et al., 1993), beta-carotene (Rimm et al., 1993; Osganian et al., 2003; Klipstein-Grobusch et al., 1999), and vitamin C (Osganian et al., 2003; Enstrom et al., 1992) has been inversely related to the incidence of coronary heart disease. Even though increased intake of beta carotene has been related to decreased cardiovascular mortality (Buijsse et al., 2008; SENECA investigators, 2005), the latter association was restricted to the aged. Many clinical trials have attempted to show a favorable safety profile (Hathcock et al., 2005; Kappus & Biplock, 1992) but clinical findings have been inconsistent (Wright et al., 2006; Hercberg et al., 2004; Lee et al., 2005; Salonen et al., 2003; Hodis et al., 2002; Christen et al., 2000; Salonen et al., 2000; Hennekens et al., 1996; Omenn et al., 1996; Alpha-Tocopherol Beta Carotene Cancer Prevention Study Group, 1994; Blot et al., 1993; Cook et al., 2007; Waters et al., 2002; Heart Protection Collaboration Group, 2002; Brown et al., 2001).

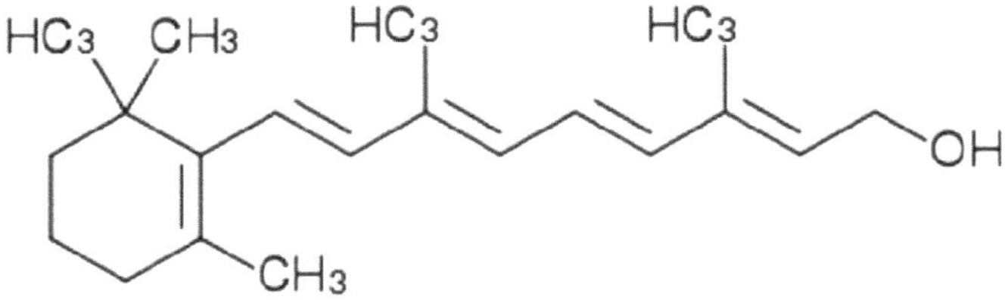

FIGURE 6.2 Vitamin A.

Notwithstanding the added input, vitamin A is involved in immune function, vision, bone metabolism, gene transcription, antioxidant activity, embryonic development and reproduction, skin health, and hematopoiesis, decreasing the risk of heart diseases and cancers.

6.2.2 *VITAMIN C*

Vitamin C (Figure 6.3) or ascorbic acid is a strong reducing agent used in redox reactions. Vitamin C utilizes the same redox properties in collagen synthesis, antioxidant reactions, stimulation of the immune system, and iron absorption. Vitamin C is available as a supplement since humans cannot synthesize their vitamin C as they lack L-gulonolactone oxidase (Harris, 1996). Vitamin C is also present as a food additive. Guinea pigs, fruit-eating bats, and simians seem to have lost the ability to synthesize vitamin C (Expert Group on Vitamins and Minerals, 2003).

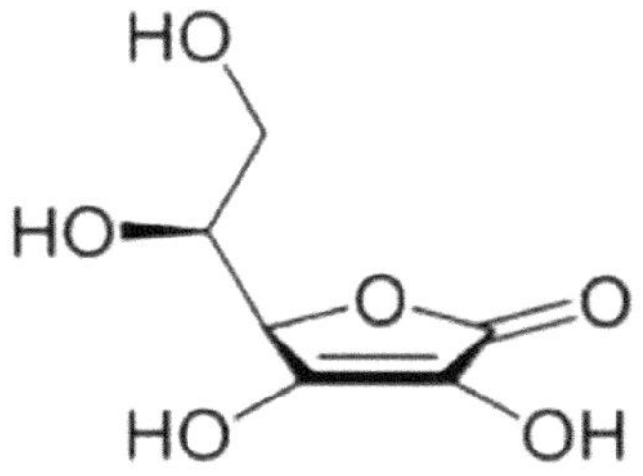

FIGURE 6.3 Vitamin C.

Regarding vitamin C's protective effects, there is an inverse relationship between vitamin C and ischemic stroke events (Del Rio et al., 2011). The Rotterdam study indicated vitamin C's protective effects through antioxidant reactions in smokers (Voko et al., 2003). It has also been suggested that the use of vitamin C as prophylaxis decreased the occurrence of postoperative atrial fibrillation in patients undergoing surgery. Surprisingly, administering beta-blockers and vitamin C together was more effective than administering beta-blockers alone (Rasoli et al., 2011).

The single role of vitamin C in heart disease has not been investigated extensively. Vitamin C still maintains antioxidant properties (Niki et al., 1991; Jialal & Grundy, 1991; Kagan et al., 1992). Vitamin C suppresses endothelial apoptosis mediated by LDL oxidation and inflammatory cytokines *in vivo* (Rossig et al., 2001) and promotes the proliferation of endothelial cells while inhibiting the growth of vascular smooth muscle (Ulrich-Merzenich et al., 2002) through the extracellular signal-regulated kinase pathway (Ulrich-Merzenich et al., 2007). Vitamin C down-regulates intercellular adhesion molecule-1 gene expression and decreases monocyte adhesion to the endothelium (Rayment et al., 2003). Vitamin C enhances nitric oxide synthesis (Heller et al., 1999) and *in vivo* sustains vasodilation (Gokce et al., 1999). Vitamin C supplementation has been suggested to prevent plaque instability in late-stage atherosclerosis (Siow et al., 1999).

6.2.3 *VITAMIN E*

Vitamin E (Figure 6.4) is made up of tocopherols that consist of various methylated phenols. Of the eight recognized forms of vitamin E (Herrera

& Barbas, 2001; Packer et al., 2001), α-tocopherol is the most widely studied and has higher bioavailability (Brigelius-Flohé & Traber, 1999). α-tocopherol is therefore mostly used as a supplement. α-tocopherol is involved in redox reactions and reacts with lipid radicals in lipid peroxidation. Oxidized α-tocopheroxyl radicals from this reaction could be recycled to an active reduced form by antioxidant reduction. Notable antioxidants that could perform this sort of reduction include retinol, ascorbate, and ubiquinol.

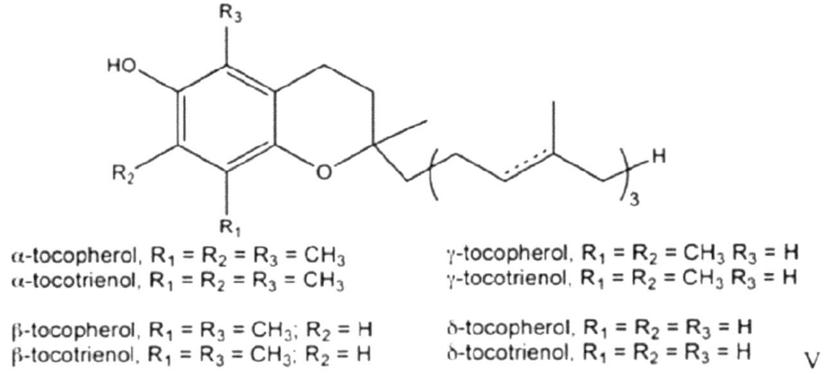

FIGURE 6.4 Vitamin E.

γ-tocopherol is a nucleophile that reacts with mutagens (Brigelius-Flohé & Traber, 1999; Sen et al., 2006; Malafa, 2008) and reduces cholesterol as well (Das et al., 2008). Notwithstanding, the significant roles of the various vitamin E forms remain unclear (Brigelius-Flohé & Davies, 2007; Atkinson et al., 2007). A recently suggested notion states that vitamin E remains a signaling molecule and has no role in antioxidant metabolism.

Experimental findings have indicated that vitamin E supplements decrease the incidence of stroke, myocardial infarction, and mortality caused by *haptoglobin 2–2* patients. As such, the *haptoglobin 2–2* genotype may identify patients who might benefit from vitamin E therapy. It has been noted that vitamin E works synergistically with other antioxidant vitamins. Vitamin E decreases foam cell formation by reducing monocytes (Devaraj & Jialal, 1996; Wu et al., 1999), chemokine (Devaraj & Jialal, 1999), and macrophage scavenger receptors (CD36) (Munteanu et al., 2006; Devaraj et al., 2001; Keaney et al., 1999). Vitamin E enhances nitric oxide availability and decreases adhesion molecule levels (Islam & Jialal, 1996; Zapolska-Downar et al., 2000) as well as inhibiting smooth muscle cell proliferation

(Keaney et al., 1999; Ozer et al., 1993) and platelet aggregation (Freedman et al., 1996; Steiner, 1991).

In this write-up, it is therefore proposed that vitamin E could stimulate the phosphatase PP2A, and Bcl_2 apoptosis forming a complex that could inhibit the oxidized-LDL-induced NF-kB product from fatty streak or foam cell formation in a typical cardiovascular event. This process decreases 1 kB as well. This notion seems to attract several supporting studies (Murohara et al., 2002; Boscoboinik et al., 1991; Sugiyama et al., 1998; Li et al., 2002; Goya et al., 2006; Keaney et al., 1996; Kuzuya et al., 1991; Uemura et al., 2002).

6.3 CLINICAL INVESTIGATIONS

As the majority of trial subjects met their recommended daily allowance of the antioxidant vitamins, none of the actual clinical trials assessed oxidative stress baseline levels hence it was possible that 'non-responders' inclusion diluted or phased out the overall benefit as seen with responders. This accounted for the disappointing overall findings (Table 6.4).

6.5 CONCLUSION

Bridging the gap between clinical trials and observational studies requires the discovery of standardized oxidative biomarkers for the assessment of antioxidant vitamins and identifying potential individuals who could benefit from supplementation and or lifestyle management.

ACKNOWLEDGMENT

The author is grateful to the University of Ghana Medical School for the online platform of varying resources.

KEYWORDS

- **antioxidant**
- **cardiovascular event**
- **heart disease**
- **oxidative stress**
- **vitamin C**

TABLE 6.4 Intervention Studies

Target Group	Trial	Study Design	Antioxidant and Dosage	Results and Conclusion
Primary prevention	Chinese study (Blot et al., 1993)	30,000 men and women at high risk of heart disease were treated for 52 years.	First factor: b-Carotene: 15 mg/d Vitamin E: 30 mg/d Se: 50 mg/d Second factor: Mo: 30 mg/d Vitamin C: 120 mg/d	First factor: supplementation caused no decrease in the incidence of heart disease Second factor: a combination of Mo and vitamin C caused no decrease in the incidence of heart disease
Primary prevention	SU.VI.MAX (Hechhberg et al., 2004)	12,800 middle-aged women and men were treated for 75 years. Primary endpoint: incidence of ischemic Heart disease, cancer and all-cause mortality	Vitamin C: 120 mg/d Vitamin E: 30 mg/d Se: 100 mg/d b-Carotene: 6 mg/d Trace elements (Zn): 20 mg/d	No difference in the incidence of cardiovascular events and all-cause mortality between the intervention and placebo group
Secondary prevention	HATS (Brown et al., 2001)	160 patients with pre-existing coronary heart disease, normal LDL, and low HDL were treated for 3 years Primary endpoint: arteriographic evidence of coronary stenosis changes and the first occurrence of a cardiovascular event (death, myocardial infarction, stroke, or revascularization)	Vitamin C: 1000 mg/d Vitamin E: 800 IU/d (d-a-tocopherol) Se: 100 mg/d b-Carotene: 25 mg/d Second treatment: Simvastatin and niacin 2 x 2 factorial design	In combination with simvastatin and niacin, antioxidants blunted their effect on the rise in HDL-2 levels (15% reduction), the reduction in the level of stenosis (0.4% regression v. 0.7% progression) and there was a 12% reduction in the number of individuals free of events

TABLE 6.4 *(Continued)*

Target Group	Trial	Study Design	Antioxidant and Dosage	Results and Conclusion
Secondary prevention	MRC/BHF Heart Protection Study (Heart Protection Collaboration Group, 2002)	20,500 individuals with pre-existing heart disease or diabetes were treated for 5 years Primary endpoint: incidence of vascular and non-vascular mortality and major morbidity	Vitamin C: 250 mg/d Vitamin E: 600 mg/d (all-rac-a-tocopherol) b-Carotene: 20 mg/d	No significant difference in all-cause and cardiovascular mortality and incidence of vascular events between the vitamin- and placebo-allocated groups. There was an increase in all-cause mortality in the supplemented group compared with the placebo group

REFERENCES

Alpha-Tocopherol Beta Carotene Cancer Prevention Study Group. (1994). The effect of vitamin E and β-carotene on the incidence of lung cancer and other cancers in male smokers. The Alpha-Tocopherol, β-Carotene Cancer Prevention Study Group. *New England Journal of Medicine, 330*, 1029–1035.

Atkinson, J., Epand, R. F., & Epand, R. M. (2007). Tocopherols and tocotrienols in membranes: A critical review. *Free Radical Biology and Medicine, 44*(5), 739–764.

Blot, W. J., Li, J. Y., Taylor, P. R., Guo, W., Dawsey, S., Wang, G. Q., Yang, C. S., Zheng, S. F., Gail, M., Li, G. Y., & Yu, Y. (1993). Nutrition intervention trials in Linxian, China: Supplementation with specific vitamin/mineral combinations, cancer incidence, and disease-specific mortality in the general population. *Journal of the National Cancer Institute, 85*, 1483–1492.

Boscoboinik, D., Szewczyk, A., Hensey, C., & Azzi, A. (1991). Inhibition of cell proliferation by α-tocopherol. Role of protein kinase C. *Journal of Biological Chemistry, 266*, 6188–6194.

Brigelius-Flohé, R., & Davies, K. J. (2007). Is vitamin E an antioxidant, a regulator of signal transduction and gene expression, or a 'junk' food? *Free Radical Biology and Medicine, 43*(1), 2–3.

Brigelius-Flohé, R., & Traber, M. G. (1999). Vitamin E: function and metabolism. *The FASEB Journal, 13*(10), 1145–1155.

Brown, B. G., Zhao, X. Q., Chait, A., Fisher, L. D., Cheung, M. C., Morse, J. S., Dowdy, A. A., Marino, E. K., Bolson, E. L., Alaupovic, P., & Frohlich, J. (2001). Simvastatin and niacin, antioxidant vitamins, or the combination for the prevention of coronary disease. *New England Journal of Medicine, 345*(22), 1583–1592.

Buijsse, B., Feskens, E. J., Kwape, L., Kok, F. J., & Kromhout, D. (2008). Both α- and β-carotene, but not tocopherols and vitamin C, are inversely related to 15-year cardiovascular mortality in Dutch elderly men. *Journal of Nutrition, 138*, 344–350.

Chen, J., He, J., Hamm, L., Batuman, V., & Whelton, P. K. (2002). Serum antioxidant vitamins and blood pressure in the United States population. *Hypertension, 40*, 810–816.

Christen, W. G., Gaziano, J. M., Hennekens, C. H., Physicians, F. T. S. C. O., & Study II, H. E. A. L. T. H. (2000). Design of Physicians' Health Study II – A randomized trial of β-carotene, vitamins E and C, and multivitamins, in prevention of cancer, cardiovascular disease, and eye disease, and review of results of completed trials. *Annals of Epidemiology, 10*, 125–134.

Cook, N. R., Albert, C. M., Gaziano, J. M., Zaharris, E., MacFadyen, J., Danielson, E., Buring, J. E., & Manson, J. E. (2007). A randomized factorial trial of vitamins C and vitamin E and β-carotene in the secondary prevention of cardiovascular events in women: results from the Women's Antioxidant Cardiovascular Study. *Archives of Internal Medicine, 167*(15), 1610–1618.

D'Odorico, A., Martines, D., Kiechl, S., Egger, G., Oberhollenzer, F., Bonvicini, P., Sturniolo, G. C., Naccarato, R., & Willeit, J. (2003). High plasma levels of α- and β-carotene are associated with a lower risk of atherosclerosis: Results from the Bruneck study. *Atherosclerosis, 153*, 231–239.

Das, S., Lekli, I., Das, M., Szabo, G., Varadi, J., Juhasz, B., Bak, I., Nesaretam, K., Tosaki, A., Powell, S. R., & Das, D. K. (2008). Cardioprotection with palm oil tocotrienols: Comparison of different isomers. *American Journal of Physiology-Heart and Circulatory Physiology, 294*(2), 970–978.

Del Rio, D., Agnoli, C., Pellegrini, N., Krogh, V., Brighenti, F., Mazzeo, T., Masala, G., Bendinelli, B., Berrino, F., Sieri, S., & Tumino, R. (2011). Total antioxidant capacity of the diet is associated with lower risk of ischemic stroke in a large Italian cohort. *The Journal of Nutrition, 141*(1), 118–123.

Devaraj, S., & Jialal, I. (1999). α-Tocopherol decreases interleukin-1 β release from activated human monocytes by inhibition of 5-lipoxygenase. *Arteriosclerosis, Thrombosis, and Vascular Biology, 19*, 1125–1133.

Devaraj, S., Hugou, I., & Jialal, I. (2001). α-Tocopherol decreases CD36 expression in human monocyte-derived macrophages. *Journal of Lipid Research, 42*, 521–527.

Devaraj, S., Li, D., & Jialal, I. J. (1996). The effects of α-tocopherol supplementation on monocyte function. Decreased lipid oxidation, interleukin 1β secretion, and monocyte adhesion to endothelium. *Journal of Clinical Investigation, 98*, 756–763.

Enstrom, J. E., Kanim, L. E., & Klein, M. A. (1992). Vitamin C intake and mortality among a sample of the United States population. *Epidemiology, 3*, 194–202.

Expert Group on Vitamins and Minerals. (2003). Vitamin C: Risk assessment. UK Food Standards Agency.

Freedman, J. E., Farhat, J. H., Loscalzo, J., & Keaney, J. F. (1996). α-Tocopherol inhibits aggregation of human platelets by a protein kinase C-dependent mechanism. *Circulation, 94*, 2434–2440.

Gaziano, J. M., Manson, J. E., Branch, L. G., Colditz, G. A., Willett, W. C., & Buring, J. E. (1995). A prospective study of consumption of carotenoids in fruits and vegetables and decreased cardiovascular mortality in the elderly. *Annals of Epidemiology, 5*, 255–260.

Gokce, N., Keaney Jr, J. F., Frei, B., Holbrook, M., Olesiak, M., Zachariah, B. J., Leeuwenburgh, C., Heinecke, J. W., & Vita, J. A. (1999). Long-term ascorbic acid administration reverses endothelial vasomotor dysfunction in patients with coronary artery disease. *Circulation, 99*(25), 3234–3240.

Goya, K., Sumitani, S., Otsuki, M., Xu, X., Yamamoto, H., Kurebayashi, S., Saito, H., Kouhara, H., & Kasayama, S. (2006). The thiazolidinedione drug troglitazone up-regulates nitric oxide synthase expression in vascular endothelial cells. *Journal of Diabetes and Its Complications, 20*, 336–342.

Harris, J. R. (1996). Ascorbic Acid: Subcellular Biochemistry. New York: Springer. Pp. 464. ISBN 0306451484.

Hathcock, J. N., Azzi, A., Blumberg, J., Bray, T., Dickinson, A., Frei, B., Jialal, I., Johnston, C. S., Kelly, F. J., Kraemer, K., Packer, L., & Traber, M. G. (2005). Vitamins E and C are safe across a broad range of intakes. *American Journal of Clinical Nutrition, 81*, 736–745.

Heart Protection Study Collaborative Group. (2002). MRC/BHF Heart Protection Study of antioxidant vitamin supplementation in 20 536 high-risk individuals: a randomized placebo-controlled trial. *The Lancet, 360*(9326), 23–33.

Heller, R., Münscher-Paulig, F., Gräbner, R., & Till, U. (1999). L-Ascorbic acid potentiates nitric oxide synthesis in endothelial cells. *Journal of Biological Chemistry, 274*(12), 8254–8260.

Hennekens, C. H., Buring, J. E., Manson, J. E., Stampfer, M., Rosner, B., Cook, N. R., Belanger, C., LaMotte, F., Gaziano, J. M., Ridker, P. M., & Willett, W. (1996). Lack of effect of long-term supplementation with β-carotene on the incidence of malignant neoplasms and cardiovascular disease. *New England Journal of Medicine, 334*, 1145–1149.

Hercberg, S., Galan, P., Preziosi, P., Bertrais, S., Mennen, L., Malvy, D., Roussel, A. M., Favier, A., & Briançon, S. (2004). The SU.VI.MAX Study: A randomized, placebo-controlled trial of the health effects of antioxidant vitamins and minerals. *Archives of Internal Medicine, 164*, 2335–2342.

Herrera, E., & Barbas, C. (2001). Vitamin E: Action, metabolism and perspectives. *Journal of Physiology and Biochemistry, 57*(2), 43–56.

Hodis, H. N., Mack, W. J., LaBree, L., Mahrer, P. R., Sevanian, A., Liu, C. R., Liu, C. H., Hwang, J., Selzer, R. H., & Azen, S. P. (2002). α-Tocopherol supplementation in healthy individuals reduces low-density lipoprotein oxidation but not atherosclerosis: The Vitamin E Atherosclerosis Prevention Study (VEAPS). *Circulation, 106*, 1453–1459.

Hozawa, A., Jacobs Jr, D. R., Steffes, M. W., Gross, M. D., Steffen, L. M., & Lee, D. H. (2007). Relationships of circulating carotenoid concentrations with several markers of inflammation, oxidative stress, and endothelial dysfunction: The Coronary Artery Risk Development in Young Adults (CARDIA)/Young Adult Longitudinal Trends in Antioxidants (YALTA) study. *Clinical Chemistry, 53*, 447–455.

Islam, K. N., Devaraj, S., & Jialal, I. (1998). α-Tocopherol enrichment of monocytes decreases agonist-induced adhesion to human endothelial cells. *Circulation, 98*, 2255–2261.

Ito, Y., Kurata, M., Suzuki, K., Hamajima, N., Hishida, H., & Aoki, K. (2006). Cardiovascular disease mortality and serum carotenoid levels: A Japanese population-based follow-up study. *Journal of Epidemiology, 16*, 154–160.

Järvinen, R., Knekt, P., Seppänen, R., Reunanen, A., Heliövaara, M., Maatela, J., & Aromaa, A. (1994). Antioxidant vitamin intake and coronary mortality in a longitudinal population study. *American Journal of Epidemiology, 139*, 1180–1189.

Jialal, I., & Grundy, S. M. (1991). Preservation of the endogenous antioxidants in low density lipoprotein by ascorbate but not probucol during oxidative modification. *Journal of Clinical Investigation, 87*(2), 597–601.

Jialal, I., Norkus, E. P., Cristol, L., & Grundy, S. M. (1991). β-Carotene inhibits the oxidative modification of low-density lipoprotein. *Biochimica et Biophysica Acta (BBA) – Lipids and Lipid Metabolism, 1086*, 134–138.

Kagan, V. E., Serbinova, E. A., Forte, T., Scita, G., & Packer, L. (1992). Recycling of vitamin E in human low-density lipoproteins. *Journal of Lipid Research, 33*(3), 385–397.

Kappus, H., & Diplock, A. T. (1992). Tolerance and safety of vitamin E: A toxicological position report. *Free Radical Biology & Medicine, 13*, 55–74.

Keaney Jr, J. F., Simon, D. I., & Freedman, J. E. (1999). Vitamin E and vascular homeostasis: implications for atherosclerosis. *The FASEB Journal, 13*, 965–975.

Keaney, J. F., Guo, Y., Cunningham, D., Shwaery, G. T., Xu, A., & Vita, J. A. (1996). Vascular incorporation of α-tocopherol prevents endothelial dysfunction due to oxidized LDL by inhibiting protein kinase C stimulation. *Journal of Clinical Investigation, 98*, 386–394.

Klipstein-Grobusch, K., Geleijnse, J. M., den Breeijen, J. H., Boeing, H., Hofman, A., Grobbee, D. E., & Witteman, J. C. (1999). Dietary antioxidants and risk of myocardial infarction in the elderly: The Rotterdam Study. *American Journal of Clinical Nutrition, 69*, 261–266.

Knekt, P., Ritz, J., Pereira, M. A., O'Reilly, E. J., Augustsson, K., Fraser, G. E., Goldbourt, U., Heitmann, B. L., Hallmans, G., Liu, S., & Pietinen, P. (2004). Antioxidant vitamins and coronary heart disease risk: A pooled analysis of 9 cohorts. *American Journal of Clinical Nutrition, 80*, 1508–1520.

Kushi, L. H., Folsom, A. R., Prineas, R. J., Mink, P. J., Wu, Y., & Bostick, R. M. (1996). Dietary antioxidant vitamins and death from coronary heart disease in postmenopausal women. *New England Journal of Medicine, 334*, 1156–1162.

Kuzuya, M., Naito, M., Funaki, C., Hayashi, T., Yamada, K., Asai, K., & Kuzuya, F. (1991). Antioxidants stimulate endothelial cell proliferation in culture. *Artery, 18*(3), 115–124.

Lee, I. M., Cook, N. R., Gaziano, J. M., Gordon, D., Ridker, P. M., Manson, J. E., Hennekens, C. H., & Buring, J. E. (2005). Vitamin E in the primary prevention of cardiovascular disease and cancer: The Women's Health Study: A randomized controlled trial. *JAMA, 294*, 56–65.

Lesic, Stjepanka & Ivanisević, Zrinka & Spiljak, Bruno & Tomas, Matej & Šoštarić, Magdalena & Vcev, Aleksandar. (2024). The Impact of Vitamin Deficiencies on Oral Manifestations in Children. Dentistry Journal. 12. 109. 10.3390/dj12040109.

Li, D., Saldeen, T., & Mehta, J. L. (2000). Effects of α-tocopherol on ox-LDL-mediated degradation of IκB and apoptosis in cultured human coronary artery endothelial cells. *Journal of Cardiovascular Pharmacology, 36*, 297–301.

Li, D., Saldeen, T., Romeo, F., et al. (2000). Oxidized LDL upregulates angiotensin II type receptor expression in cultured cells. *National Library of Medicine, 102*(16), 1970–1976.

Malafa, M. P. (2008). New insights and gains in pancreatic cancer. *Cancer Control, 15*(4), 276–277.

Munteanu, A., Taddei, M., Tamburini, I., Bergamini, E., Azzi, A., & Zingg, J. M. (2006). Antagonistic effects of oxidized low-density lipoprotein and α-tocopherol on CD36 scavenger receptor expression in monocytes: involvement of protein kinase b and peroxisome proliferator-activated receptor-γ. *Journal of Biological Chemistry, 281*, 6489–6497.

Murohara, T., Ikeda, H., Katoh, A., Takajo, Y., Otsuka, Y., Haramaki, N., & Imaizumi, T. (2002). Vitamin E inhibits lysophosphatidylcholine-induced endothelial dysfunction and platelet activation. *Antioxidants & Redox Signaling, 4*, 791–798.

Niki, E., Yamamoto, Y., Komuro, E., & Sato, K. (1991). Membrane damage due to lipid oxidation. *The American Journal of Clinical Nutrition, 53*(1), 201S–205S.

Omenn, G. S., Goodman, G. E., Thornquist, M. D., Balmes, J., Cullen, M. R., Glass, A., Keogh, J. P., Meyskens Jr, F. L., Valanis, B., Williams Jr, J. H., & Barnhart, S. (1996). Effects of a combination of β-carotene and vitamin A on lung cancer and cardiovascular disease. *New England Journal of Medicine, 334*, 1150–1155.

Osganian, S. K., Stampfer, M. J., Rimm, E., Spiegelman, D., Hu, F. B., Manson, J. E., & Willett, W. C. (2003). Vitamin C and risk of coronary heart disease in women. *Journal of the American College of Cardiology, 42*, 246–252.

Osganian, S. K., Stampfer, M. J., Rimm, E., Spiegelman, D., Manson, J. E., & Willett, W. C. (2003). Dietary carotenoids and risk of coronary artery disease in women. *American Journal of Clinical Nutrition, 77*, 1390–1399.

Özer, N. K., Palozza, P., Boscoboinik, D., & Azzi, A. (1993). d-α-Tocopherol inhibits low density lipoprotein induced proliferation and protein kinase C activity in vascular smooth muscle cells. *FEBS Letters, 322*, 307–310.

Packer, L., Weber, S. U., & Rimbach, G. (2001). Molecular aspects of alpha-tocotrienol antioxidant action and cell signaling. *The Journal of Nutrition, 131*(2), 369S–373S.

Palozza, P., Calviello, G., & Bartoli, G. M. (1995). Prooxidant activity of β-carotene under 100% oxygen pressure in rat liver microsomes. *Free Radical Biology and Medicine, 19*, 887–892.

Princen, H. M., van Poppel, G., Vogelezang, C., Buytenhek, R., & Kok, F. J. (1992). Supplementation with vitamin E but not β-carotene in vivo protects low density lipoprotein from lipid peroxidation in vitro. Effect of cigarette smoking. *Arteriosclerosis, Thrombosis, and Vascular Biology, 12*, 554–562.

Rasoli, S., Kakouros, N., Harling, L., Gukop, P., Soni, M., Athanasiou, T., & Kourliouros, A. (2011). Antioxidant vitamins in the prevention of atrial fibrillation: what is the evidence? *Cardiology Research and Practice, 2011*(1), 164078.

Rautalahti, M., Albanes, D., Virtamo, J., Taylor, P. R., Huttunen, J. K., & Heinonen, O. P. (1997). β-Carotene did not work: Aftermath of the ATBC study. *Cancer Letters, 114*, 235–236.

Rayment, S. J., Shaw, J., Woollard, K. J., Lunec, J., & Griffiths, H. R. (2003). Vitamin C supplementation in normal subjects reduces constitutive ICAM-1 expression. *Biochemical and Biophysical Research Communications, 308*(2), 339–345.

Reaven, P. D., Khouw, A., Beltz, W. F., Parthasarathy, S., & Witztum, J. L. (1993). Effect of dietary antioxidant combinations in humans. Protection of LDL by vitamin E but not by β-carotene. *Arteriosclerosis, Thrombosis, and Vascular Biology, 13*, 590–600.

Rimm, E. B., Stampfer, M. J., Ascherio, A., Giovannucci, E., Colditz, G. A., & Willett, W. C. (1993). Vitamin E consumption and the risk of coronary heart disease in men. *New England Journal of Medicine, 328*, 1450–1456.

Rössig, L., Hoffmann, J., Hugel, B., Mallat, Z., Haase, A., Freyssinet, J. M., Tedgui, A., Aicher, A., Zeiher, A. M., & Dimmeler, S. (2001). Vitamin C inhibits endothelial cell apoptosis in congestive heart failure. *Circulation, 104*(18), 2182–2187.

Russo, C., Olivieri, O., Girelli, D., Faccini, G., Zenari, M. L., Lombardi, S., & Corrocher, R. (1998). Anti-oxidant status and lipid peroxidation in patients with essential hypertension. *Journal of Hypertension, 16*, 1267–1271.

Said, H. M., & Nexo, E. (2018). Gastrointestinal handling of water-soluble vitamins. *Comprehensive Physiology, 8*(4), 1291–1311.

Salonen, J. T., Nyyssönen, K., Salonen, R., Lakka, H. M., Kaikkonen, J., Porkkala-Sarataho, E., Voutilainen, S., Lakka, T. A., Rissanen, T., Leskinen, L., & Tuomainen, T. P. (2000). Antioxidant Supplementation in Atherosclerosis Prevention (ASAP) study: A randomized trial of the effect of vitamins E and C on 3-year progression of carotid atherosclerosis. *Journal of Internal Medicine, 248*, 377–386.

Salonen, J. T., Salonen, R., Ihanainen, M., Parviainen, M., Seppänen, R., Kantola, M., Seppänen K., & Rauramaa, R. (1988). Blood pressure, dietary fats, and antioxidants. *American Journal of Clinical Nutrition, 48*, 1226–1232.

Salonen, R. M., Nyyssönen, K., Kaikkonen, J., Porkkala-Sarataho, E., Voutilainen, S., Rissanen, T. H., Tuomainen, T. P., Valkonen, V. P., Ristonmaa, U., Lakka, H. M., & Vanharanta, M. (2003). Six-year effect of combined vitamin C and E supplementation on atherosclerotic progression: The Antioxidant Supplementation in Atherosclerosis Prevention (ASAP) Study. *Circulation, 107*, 947–953.

Sen, C., Khanna, S., & Roy, S. (2006). Tocotrienols: Vitamin E beyond tocopherols. *Life Sciences, 78*(18), 2088–2098.

SENECA investigators. (2005). Plasma carotene and α-tocopherol in relation to 10-y all-cause and cause-specific mortality in European elderly: The Survey in Europe on Nutrition and the Elderly, a Concerted Action (SENECA). *American Journal of Clinical Nutrition, 82*, 879–886.

Siow, R. C., Richards, J. P., Pedley, K. C., Leake, D. S., & Mann, G. E. (1999). Vitamin C protects human vascular smooth muscle cells against apoptosis induced by moderately oxidized LDL containing high levels of lipid hydroperoxides. *Arteriosclerosis, Thrombosis, and Vascular Biology, 19*(10), 2387–2394.

Stampfer, M. J., Hennekens, C. H., Manson, J. E., Colditz, G. A., Rosner, B., & Willett, W. C. (1993). Vitamin E consumption and the risk of coronary disease in women. *New England Journal of Medicine, 328*, 1444–1449.

Steiner, M. (1991). Influence of vitamin E on platelet function in humans. *Journal of the American College of Nutrition, 10*, 466–473.

Sugiyama, S., Kugiyama, K., Ogata, N., Doi, H., Ota, Y., Ohgushi, M., Matsumura, T., Oka, H., & Yasue, H. (1998). Biphasic regulation of transcription factor nuclear factor-κB activity in human endothelial cells by lysophosphatidylcholine through protein kinase C-mediated pathway. *Arteriosclerosis, Thrombosis, and Vascular Biology, 18*(4), 568–576.

Tsuchihashi, H., Kigoshi, M., Iwatsuki, M., & Niki, E. (1995). Action of β-carotene as an antioxidant against lipid peroxidation. *Archives of Biochemistry and Biophysics, 323*, 137–147.

Uemura, M., Manabe, H., Yoshida, N., Fujita, N., Ochiai, J., Matsumoto, N., Takagi, T., Naito, Y., & Yoshikawa, T. (2002). α-Tocopherol prevents apoptosis of vascular endothelial cells via a mechanism exceeding that of mere antioxidation. *European Journal of Pharmacology, 456*(1–2), 29–37.

Ulrich-Merzenich, G., Metzner, C., Schiermeyer, B., & Vetter, H. (2002). Vitamin C and vitamin E antagonistically modulate human vascular endothelial and smooth muscle cell DNA synthesis and proliferation. *European Journal of Nutrition, 41*(1), 27–34.

Ulrich-Merzenich, G., Zeitler, H., Panek, D., Bokemeyer, D., & Vetter, H. (2007). Vitamin C promotes human endothelial cell growth via the ERK-signaling pathway. *European Journal of Nutrition, 46*(2), 87–94.

Voko, Z., Hollander, M., Hofman, A., Koudstaal, P. J., Breteler, M. M. (2003). Dietary antioxidants and the risk of ischemic stroke: the Rotterdam Study. *Neurology, 61*(9), 1273–1275.

Waters, D. D., Alderman, E. L., Hsia, J., Howard, B. V., Cobb, F. R., Rogers, W. J., Ouyang, P., Thompson, P., Tardif, J. C., Higginson, L., & Bittner, V. (2002). Effects of hormone replacement therapy and antioxidant vitamin supplements on coronary atherosclerosis in postmenopausal women: a randomized controlled trial. *JAMA, 288*(19), 2432–2440.

Wright, M. E., Lawson, K. A., Weinstein, S. J., Pietinen, P., Taylor, P. R., Virtamo, J., & Albanes, D. (2006). Higher baseline serum concentrations of vitamin E are associated with lower total and cause-specific mortality in the Alpha-Tocopherol, Beta-Carotene Cancer Prevention Study. *American Journal of Clinical Nutrition, 84*, 1200–1207.

Wu, D., Koga, T., Martin, K. R., & Meydani, M. E. (1999). Effect of vitamin E on human aortic endothelial cell production of chemokines and adhesion to monocytes. *Atherosclerosis, 147*, 297–307.

Zapolska-Downar, D., Zapolski-Downar, A., Markiewski, M., Ciechanowicz, A., Kaczmarczyk, M., & Naruszewicz, M. (2000). Selective inhibition by α-tocopherol of vascular cell adhesion molecule-1 expression in human vascular endothelial cells. *Biochemical and Biophysical Research Communications, 274*, 609–615.

CHAPTER 7

NUTRACEUTICAL INTERVENTION OF TOMATO AND LYCOPENE IN HEART DISEASE

TARKESHWAR,[1] PRADIP KUMAR SAINI,[2] VIKASH KUMAR SINGH,[3] SUBASH CHAND VIMAL,[1] and JITENDER BHATI[4]

[1]*Department of Genetics and Plant Breeding, Acharya Narendra Deva University of Agriculture and Technology, Ayodhya, Uttar Pradesh, India*

[2]*Research Scholar, Crop Physiology, Acharya Narendra Deva University of Agriculture and Technology, Ayodhya, Uttar Pradesh, India*

[3]*Research Scholar, Vegetable Science, Acharya Narendra Deva University of Agriculture and Technology, Ayodhya, Uttar Pradesh, India*

[4]*Assistant Professor, Department of Genetics and Plant Breeding, Chandra Shekhar Azad University of Agriculture and Technology, Kanpur, Uttar Pradesh, India*

ABSTRACT

Heart diseases are the main cause of death in humans around the world. Cardiovascular disorders are caused by pathophysiological mechanisms such as oxidative stress and inflammation. That is why bioactive food elements such as lycopene, which appears to be a compound increasingly encouraged in the diet of persons with cardiovascular problems, are so crucial in

Antioxidants as Nutraceuticals. Nayan A. Gujarathi, Raj K. Keservani, Rajesh K. Kesharwani, Bhushan R. Rane, Yogeeta Sameer Goyal (Eds.)

their prevention. The health-promoting properties of tomatoes are also due to lycopene, a red pigment present in tomatoes and tomato-based products. It is distinguished by its high antioxidant potential, which is the highest of all carotenoid pigments. For this reason, epidemiological studies suggest a number of positive associations between dietary lycopene consumption and a lower risk of cardiovascular disease. While studies into its preventive effects on the cardiovascular system are still controversial, rising evidence supports its positive significance for the endothelium layer of internal organs, heart, blood vessels of the body, and overall health. Lycopene's methods of action are currently being identified, which may explain some of the discrepancies in the literature. This chapter attempts to summarize the knowledge that has recently been gained regarding the function of lycopene in the prevention of cardiovascular diseases.

7.1 INTRODUCTION

Nutraceuticals are foods or food derivatives that have medicinal or health benefits, such as illness prevention, management, or therapy (Keservani et al., 2017, 2010a, b, 2020). They include isolated nutrients, encapsulated nutritional supplements, herbal items, and processed foods including cereals, soups, and beverages (Roberfroi, 2002; Hugenholtz et al., 2002; Andlauer et al., 2002; Kwak et al., 2001). Before their usage in cardiovascular prophylaxis and treatment, most nutraceuticals still require substantial clinical trials to verify their efficacy and safety profile (Zuchi et al., 2010). Much research has found that diet and blood pressure reduction promote cardiovascular health (Heiss et al., 2010; Taubert et al., 2007; Chen et al., 2009), but the link between different nutraceuticals and hypertension remains unknown. Most of this is due to biases and inconclusive, inconsistent research, which has resulted in limited recommendations for the safe and effective use of nutraceuticals for hypertension treatment when compared to a prescribed diet and medicine (Turner et al., 2016). The purpose of this chapter is to outline the effects and mechanisms of action of a number of well-known nutraceuticals used to treat cardiovascular disorders (Keservani et al., 2016), particularly hypertension. Heart disease is a major social issue around the world. The result is, that not only is the annual frequency of these diseases high, but the fatality rate is as well. According to statistics, there were 17.8 million deaths from CVD in 2019, and 23 million are predicted to occur by 2030 (Roth et al., 2018; Amini et al., 2021). It's also worth noting that young people are becoming more susceptible to cardiovascular disease, with one-third of deaths occurring in persons under the age of 70. Myocardial infarction and stroke are the most common causes (Zhang et al., 2020). According to the WHO, cardiovascular diseases comprise both heart and blood vessel disorders, including hypertension, coronary artery disease, peripheral arterial disease, and heart failure (CVDs, 2021). Regardless of where you live on the planet, the primary cause of death from cardiovascular disease is atherosclerosis-related issues. This is thought to be an artery-wall degenerative process brought on by oxidative stress and expressed as persistent inflammation (Pham et al., 2021).

There is a complex relationship between metabolic and molecular changes in inflammation, oxidative stress, endothelium, myocardial dysfunction, lipid metabolism, and other cardiovascular diseases, such as heart failure (Steven et al., 2019). Lycopene is believed to have anti-cancer properties in addition to its anti-inflammatory properties. In the treatment of prostate, stomach, lung, and breast cancer, it has a high percentage of effectiveness. Moreover, this substance, in addition to inhibiting neoplastic cell proliferation, causes their programmed death and inhibits metastasis. The skeletal system benefits greatly from lycopene as well. It promotes bone mineralization and prevents osteoporosis from developing. It also has neuroprotective properties, it is advantageous for both the prevention and treatment of neurodegenerative illnesses like Alzheimer's, Parkinson's, and Huntington's disease (Przybylska et al., 2020). More than 80% of the dietary lycopene consumed in the developed world comes from processed tomato products including ketchup, tomato juice, spaghetti sauce, and pizza sauce (Maiani et al., 2009). Tomato products are a dietary source of lycopene with improved bioavailability due to thermal processing, but also due to the processing's release of lycopene from the cellular structure's fibrous matrix (Burton-Freeman et al., 2014).

Regardless of the individual circumstances of the European population, the average daily lycopene consumption ranges between 5 and 7 mg (Petyaev, 2016). In the United States, men consume between 6.6 and 10.5 mg per day, while women consume between 5.7 and 10.4 mg per day (Story et al., 2010). Lycopene is now being studied in a growing number of clinical trials for a variety of health advantages, including its ability to protect against cardiovascular disease (Puah et al., 2021). The all-trans lycopene isoform dominates in fresh, ripe tomatoes, representing about 90% of the total. As a result, the forms of cis-lycopene dominate their processed goods, such as ketchup, tomato concentrates, and juices. Because of its cis form, lycopene is believed to be extremely accessible in human diets (Honda et al., 2018; Saini et al., 2020).

7.2 LYCOPENE AND TOMATOES

Papayas, tomatoes, red peppers, watermelons, and other red fruits and vegetables contain lycopene, a carotenoid (Cruz et al., 2013). Tomatoes are well-known for their culinary flexibility, as well as their nutritious importance in the diet (Burton-Freeman et al., 2014). Lycopene accounts for over 90% of the total carotenoids in tomatoes (Hsu et al., 2008), while they also contain carotene, folate, phenolic compounds, and vitamins C and E (Raiola et al., 2014). The link between tomato and lycopene consumption and a lower risk of cardiovascular disease has piqued researchers' interest (Burton-Freeman et al., 2014). The consumption of lycopene has a strong inverse relationship with the risk of myocardial infarction, coronary insufficiency, and angina pectoris, according to the Framingham Heart Offspring Study (Jacques et al., 2013). Furthermore, lycopene plasma levels were identified as low in hypertension, acute myocardial infarction, stroke, and atherosclerosis (Wolak et al., 2013; Riccioni et al., 2009). Lycopene is the most effective antioxidant of the main carotenoids, and it plays a significant role in preventing cardiovascular disease in humans (Agarwal et al., 2000). The bioavailability of lycopene in supplements has not been investigated as thoroughly, and it remains a promising subject for future research (Burton-Freeman et al., 2014). Tomato supplementation for three months promoted changes in miRNA expression and reduced oxidative stress in Wistar rats, according to an experimental investigation. Furthermore, these modifications appear to be responsible for a decrease in the cross-sectional area of left ventricular myocytes as well as improved diastolic performance. Regardless, further research is needed to determine the possible targets of tomato and lycopene in the prevention and treatment of cardiovascular illnesses, as well as to define their beneficial cardiac effects, which have yet to be investigated (Pereira et al., 2015). Endothelial function is widely known to represent vascular health (CITE). Endothelial dysfunction is also linked to the development of atherosclerosis, and endothelial dysfunction in the coronary or peripheral arteries appears to be an independent predictor of cardiovascular events (Bonetti et al., 2003). Endothelial dysfunction could be exacerbated by increased oxidative stress (Widlansky et al., 2003). Interestingly, 8-week lycopene supplementation was demonstrated to induce positive effects on oxidative stress biomarkers in a randomized, double-blind, placebo-controlled research (through the reduction of oxidative DNA damage and increased plasma superoxide dismutase enzymatic activity). Furthermore, their antioxidant properties may have a significant role in enhancing endothelial function, which is closely linked to inflammatory indicators. These findings indicate the health benefits of consuming lycopene on a daily basis (Kim et al., 2011). Although the effect of lycopene supplementation is still unknown, many studies have linked tomatoes and lycopene to a lower risk of cardiovascular disease (Wolak et al., 2013; Riccioni et al., 2009; Chen et al., 2013). Although lycopene accounts for about 90% of the total carotenoids found in tomatoes (Hsu et al., 2008), the other bioactive chemicals found in tomatoes should also be investigated to better understand their beneficial effects. Furthermore, it is recommended to consume fruits and vegetables high in natural carotenoids until further research clarifies and verifies the major benefits of lycopene supplementation in humans (Chen et al., 2013). In addition, until new research clarifies and confirms the significant benefits of lycopene supplementation in humans, it is recommended to consume fruits and vegetables rich in natural carotenoids (Chen et al., 2013).

7.3 LYCOPENE CHEMISTRY

Copene is a pigment that belongs to the non-oxygenated carotenoid group and has 11 conjugated double bonds. Its chemical formula is $C_{40}H_{56}$, and its molecular weight is 536.88. Lycopene is a symmetrical molecule made up of eight C5 isoprenoid units connected head-to-tail, except at the center, where the order is reversed by a tail-to-tail connection. The linear, all-trans conformation of carotenoids is present in most food sources, whereas cis-isomers are found in most human tissues (Figure 7.1).

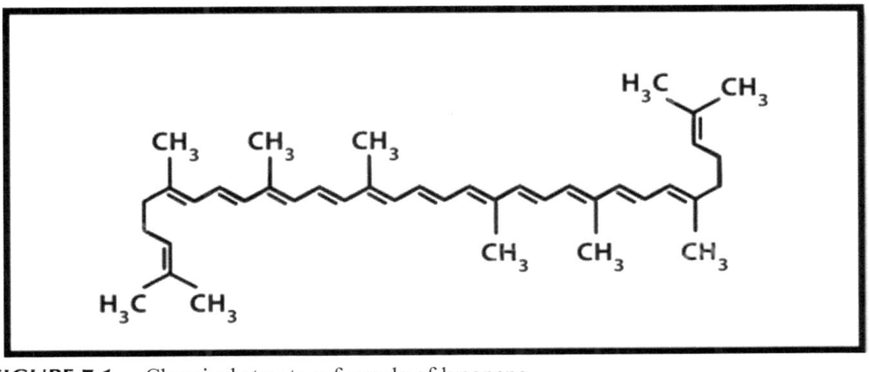

FIGURE 7.1 Chemical structure formula of lycopene.

Several research teams have claimed that cis-isomers of lycopene are more readily absorbed than the all-transform due to the shorter length of the cis-isomer, the greater solubility of cis-isomers in mixed micelles, and/or the decreased propensity of cis-isomers to collect.

7.4 LYCOPENE'S BIOLOGICAL ACTIVITY

Several research studies looked at the link between antioxidant intake and lipid peroxidation in the hopes of figuring out which antioxidants would help prevent cardiovascular disease. The hydrocarbon carotenoids, including beta-carotene and lycopene, are largely carried in LDL, putting them in an advantageous position to protect LDL against oxidation (Goulinet et al., 1997). Steinberg et al. (1998) discovered that supplementing smokers' meals with an antioxidant-rich tomato-based juice for 4 weeks resulted in considerably increased CD lag time, for conjugated dienes (CD), lower CD propagation rate, and decreased breath pentane excretion compared to individuals given a placebo juice. Although it is impossible to distinguish the effects of lycopene from those of the other antioxidants added to the juice, the authors speculated that lycopene doses were more closely linked to LDL oxidation inhibition. In a separate intervention study, 22 people (11 smokers and 11 nonsmokers) ate a diet rich in fruits and vegetables for two weeks, receiving 10 mg beta-carotene, 10 mg lycopene, and 10 mg lutein daily (Hininger et al., 1997). After the supplementation, the researchers noticed a 14% increase in CD lag time in smokers and a 28% increase in nonsmokers. These findings cannot be attributed only to lycopene, but they add to the growing body of data that carotenoids may protect against diseases caused by oxidative stress. Romanchik et al. (1997) took LDL samples from five people and enriched them with beta-carotene, lycopene, and lutein to see if it would affect LDL oxidation.

The carotenoids were destroyed before significant amounts of lipid peroxidation products were generated during copper-mediated oxidation of LDL, indicating that these pigments may act as antioxidants. Despite the fact that lycopene was the carotenoid analyzed that was degraded the fastest, only the LDL enhanced with β-carotene had a longer lag time. The same researchers found enhanced oxidation of LDL (as evaluated by the ferrous oxidation–xylenol orange assay) following enrichment with lycopene and lutein in a second analysis of LDL from 11 different people, demonstrating that the relationship between lycopene and LDL oxidation is complex (Dugas et al., 1998). *In vitro* and people, lycopene has an intriguing nonantioxidant effect. The addition of lycopene to macrophage cell lines reduced cholesterol production while increasing LDL receptors (Fuhrman et al., 1997). *In vitro,* incubation with lycopene resulted in a 73% reduction in cholesterol production, which was higher than β-carotene. Lycopene also caused a 34% rise in LDL breakdown in the cells and a 110% increase in LDL elimination from the circulation. The researchers gave 6 males 60 mg lycopene/d for 3 months to test their findings in humans (about similar to the amount of lycopene in 1 kilogram of tomatoes). They discovered a 14% decrease in plasma LDL cholesterol with no change in HDL cholesterol. We would predict a 30–40% reduction in risk in people who consume this amount of lycopene on a regular basis, based on the calculations of (Peto et al., 1995) that there is a 3:1 ratio between lowering cholesterol and lowering the risk of myocardial infarction.

7.5 ANTIOXIDANT AND ANTI-INFLAMMATORY STRATEGIES OF LYCOPENE IN THE CARDIOVASCULAR SYSTEM

7.5.1 ANTIOXIDANT EFFECTS OF LYCOPENE

Cardiovascular disease is thought to be caused by an increase in oxidative stress. It causes myocardial infarction, ischemia/reperfusion, and heart failure, among other things (Dubois-Deruy et al., 2020). Excess ROS generation causes a decrease in nitric oxide availability and vasoconstriction, resulting in arterial hypertension. ROS also has a deleterious impact on calcium management in the myocardium, resulting in arrhythmia and accelerating cardiac remodeling by triggering signal hypertrophy and apoptosis. ROS is also responsible for the production of atherosclerotic plaques (Senoner et al., 2019). As a result, bioactive food components like lycopene may play a role in reversing these alterations. Lycopene is a carotenoid pigment with the chemical formula $C_{40}H_{56}$ (Maoka, 2020; ChemSpider, 2021). Due to the high reactivity of the long polyene chain with free radicals, lycopene is a highly potent antioxidant that allows for the removal of singlet oxygen and the decrease of reactive oxygen species (ROS) (Caseiro et al., 2020). In biological systems, the reactivity of lycopene is determined by its molecular and physical structure, position or site of action inside the cells, ability to interact with other antioxidants, concentration, and oxygen partial pressure (Young et al., 2001). Due to its antioxidant properties, lycopene is also essential in the defense of DNA, lipids, and other macromolecules involved in the healthy functioning of the body (Li et al., 2021).

7.5.2 LYCOPENE'S ANTI-INFLAMMATORY ACTIVITY

According to scientific evidence, inflammation is linked to and causes a variety of disorders affecting the cardiovascular system, in addition to many others, such as hypercholesterolemia, diabetes (type 2), and obesity (Sorriento et al., 2019). Based on atherosclerotic alterations, inflammation is thought to be the primary cause of coronary heart disease (CHD). Epidemiological studies, on the other hand, suggest that chronic and severe systemic inflammation may be a result of cardiovascular disease. Lycopene plays a critical role in limiting the inflammatory response, and its ability to do so is mostly due to the reduction of inflammatory basic mediators such as reactive oxygen species (ROS). Lycopene at this concentration reduces cardiac hypertrophy and fibrosis, as well as lowered arterial hypertension (Ferreira-Santos et al., 2018). Increased HO-1 expression in atherosclerotic plaques with lycopene participation slows the course of atherosclerosis, confirming its preventive effect. Furthermore, the anti-inflammatory effects of lycopene-induced HO-1 were studied (Sahin et al., 2014).

7.5.3 EFFECTIVENESS OF LYCOPENE IN LOWERING CARDIOVASCULAR DISEASE RISK

Tierney et al. published a study in 2020 that included 43 research studies that looked at the impact of lycopene from food and supplements on the possibility of developing heart disease. The amount of lycopene in the respondents' diets varied depending on how it was given (supplements with or without food, tomato juice/paste/raw product, or in conjunction with olive oil), and the daily dose was 1.44 to 75 mg. Lycopene did not diminish risk factors for cardiovascular disease in 11 of the 43 investigations (Tierney et al., 2020). Lycopene has the ability to bind to plasma LDL cholesterol, which protects against atherosclerosis by inhibiting lipid peroxidation.

7.5.4 THE ROLE OF LYCOPENE IN ATHEROSCLEROSIS

High blood lipids are the main risk factor for cardiovascular disease (ASCVD), which includes cholesterol and triglycerides (TG) (Benjamin et al., 2019). Atherosclerosis is regarded as the primary cause of the majority of heart disease types, including acute coronary syndromes. Atherosclerosis is more prone to occur in those over the age of 45, often known as ischemic heart disease. A poor diet high in stimulants, obesity, animal fats, and diabetes are the most common causes. Controlling cardiovascular risk factors such as a healthy diet, treating obesity, and lowering high blood sugar levels is thought to greatly minimize mitochondrial stress and damage (Suárez-Rivero et al., 2021). Lycopene does not increase HDL cholesterol, but it has been demonstrated to enhance the LDL/HDL ratio, and HDL functionality, and minimize cholesterol accumulation in the rabbit aorta, highlighting lycopene's therapeutic benefits during the early stages of atherosclerosis (Thies et al., 2017). Lycopene also aids in the prevention of cardiovascular problems, such as blood clots caused by atherosclerotic alterations. Lycopene's anti-atherosclerotic activity is primarily brought on by its ability to prevent endothelial damage, suppress cholesterol synthesis by blocking 3-hydroxy-3-methylglutaryl-coenzyme A reductase, prevent LDL oxidation and restore HDL functionality, lower TG and LDL cholesterol, and inhibit pro-inflammatory activity elicited by macrophages, T lymphocytes, and macrophages (Thies et al., 2017; Palozza et al., 2010).

7.5.5 THE EFFECT OF LYCOPENE ON HYPERTENSION

Hypertension is one of the primary risk factors for cardiovascular disorders such as coronary heart disease, atrial fibrillation, and stroke. The existence of this disease entity is the most significant contributor to heart failure (Whelton et al., 2018; Al Ghorani et al., 2021). Around 1 billion individuals, or 26.4% of the world's population, have hypertension, although only one in five people have it under control. Despite the availability of effective antihypertensive medications, global blood pressure (BP) target achievement remains low (Mills et al., 2020). As a result, bioactive dietary elements, such as lycopene, are crucial in the treatment of arterial hypertension in this scenario. Lycopene reduces oxidative stress caused by angiotensin II and indirectly increases nitric oxide synthesis in the endothelium by decreasing the angiotensin-converting enzyme (ACE) and raising nitric oxide production in the endothelium due to its antioxidant impact (Han et al., 2017). Most epidemiological studies emphasize the importance of tomatoes and tomato products in improving vascular function, which is mostly due to their strong antioxidant activity, helping to lower arterial hypertension (Belovic et al., 2016). Lycopene's antihypertensive mechanism is thought to involve inhibition of the ACE, which reduces oxidative stress caused by angiotensin II while indirectly enhancing NO generation (Cheng et al., 2019).

7.5.6 SUPPLEMENTING WITH LYCOPENE AND THE RISK OF CARDIOVASCULAR DISEASE

It should be noted that this shortage may not be remedied by even carefully planned food strategies that try to give people's bodies more lycopene. Integrating lycopene into lipoprotein carriers, results in poor intestinal absorption, low bioavailability, and diminished liver capacity (Honda et al., 2020). As a result, in light of current nutritional science, the development of novel lycopene supplements with higher bioavailability is critical. Improved bioavailability of lycopene in the form of a lycosome, on the other hand, increased its antioxidant and anti-inflammatory capabilities, as well as having a favorable effect on the cardiovascular system of the study participants. The reduction of C-reactive protein, improvement of lipid profiles, lowering of blood pressure, and suppression of pro-inflammatory mediators were found to be the most efficient ways for lycopene to protect the cardiovascular system (Thies et al., 2017). Consuming one or more servings of lycopene-rich tomato products each day lowers the risk of cardiovascular disease by more than 30%, as is widely known (Costa-Rodrigues et al., 2018). Consumption of tomato products in amounts (70–400 g/day) for 1–180 days provides significant cardioprotective protection, according to (Cheng et al., 2017).

7.5.7 OTHER ILLNESSES

Male infertility has been linked to oxidative stress as a contributing factor (Zini et al., 1993). Antioxidants for male infertility could have a significant impact on the treatment of infertile couples. A modest number of studies have looked at the impact of vitamins and antioxidants in male infertility (mainly as single agents), but further research is needed (Rao et al., 2006). The action of vitamin C on semen quality was demonstrated by Dawson et al. (1993), while the activity of vitamin E on semen quality was demonstrated by Geva et al. (1996) and Suleiman et al. (1996). Semen lycopene levels were observed to be lower in men with antibody-mediated infertility than in fertile controls (Palan et al., 1996). Low lycopene levels in the blood have also been linked to an increased risk of psychiatric illnesses (Li et al., 2007). A study of 17 persons with asthma who were given a placebo, tomato extract (Lyc-o-Mato®, 45 mg/day lycopene), or tomato juice (45 mg/day lycopene) for 7 days found that the tomato extract and tomato juice treatments reduced airway neutrophil inflow and sputum neutrophil elastase activity. Plasma lycopene concentrations fell, neutrophil percentages increased, and neutrophil elastase levels increased during placebo treatment (Wood et al., 2008).

7.6 CONCLUSIONS AND PROSPECTS FOR THE FUTURE

The importance of lycopene in improving vascular function and preventing cardiovascular diseases is supported in this chapter. Lycopene is a carotenoid molecule that has been studied extensively, not only in neoplastic illnesses but also in cardiovascular ailments. We covered the most essential features of lycopene in the prevention of cardiovascular illnesses, with a focus on atherosclerosis and hypertension, in our chapter. According to epidemiological data, their occurrence is the leading cause of cardiovascular illnesses and mortality worldwide. To avoid this, it is vital to begin cultivating a healthy lifestyle, particularly good food, at a young age. It is critical that you consume as many veggies and fruits as possible. Tomatoes high in bioactive compounds, such as lycopene, may be especially important in this case. Consumption of lycopene in the form of fresh tomatoes and their products, as well as in supplements, has been shown to lower the risk of cardiovascular disease. A great number of epidemiological studies have concluded that a daily dose of 2–20 mg lycopene provides considerable anti-CVD benefits. The high antioxidant and anti-inflammatory properties of lycopene play a key role in incorporating it into the diet and boosting cardiovascular health. The trials showed that lycopene is an excellent antioxidant and that including it in one's diet can enhance blood pressure, endothelial function, metabolic profile, and atherosclerotic plaque size. Despite some conflicting research on the effects of lycopene on CVD disorders, a growing body of evidence demonstrates that it is beneficial in improving the health of patients with atherosclerosis and hypertension, among others. The way lycopene is consumed, as well as the frequency with which it is consumed in the form of fresh tomatoes or processed goods such as sauces, juices, concentrates, ketchup, and as a supplement, appears to be important. The bioavailability of dietary lycopene is another key consideration. Processed tomato products appear to absorb lycopene more effectively than raw tomatoes. Another crucial consideration is lycopene bioavailability in the diet. Many factors, including absorption, metabolism, isomerization, and interactions with other carotenoids, determine the level of its bioactive characteristics. Despite its cardioprotective properties, lycopene has limited biological applications due to poor bioavailability, which can be addressed through modern technologies such as nanotechnology or frequent ingestion of processed or fresh tomatoes with the addition of olive oil. While many elements of lycopene's metabolism, activity, and clinical implications in humans are yet unknown, tomato-based products can be considered an effective cardiovascular disease prevention strategy.

KEYWORDS

- **triglycerides**
- **cardiovascular disease**
- **angiotensin-converting enzyme**
- **conjugated dienes**
- **reactive oxygen species**

REFERENCES

Agarwal, S., & Rao, A. V. (2000). Tomato lycopene and its role in human health and chronic diseases. *CMAJ, 163*(6), 739–744.

Al Ghorani, H., Götzinger, F., Böhm, M., & Mahfoud, F. (2021). Arterial hypertension clinical trials update. *Nutrition, Metabolism and Cardiovascular Diseases, 32*, 21–31.

Amini, M., Zayeri, F., & Salehi, M. (2021). Trend analysis of cardiovascular disease mortality, incidence, and mortality-to-incidence ratio: Results from global burden of disease study 2017. *BMC Public Health, 21*(1), 1–2.

Andlauer, W., & Fürst, P. (2002). Nutraceuticals: A piece of history, present status and outlook. *Food Research International, 35*(2–3), 171–176.

Belović, M. M., Gironés-Vilaplana, A., Moreno, D. A., Milovanović, I. L., Novaković, A. R., Karaman, M. A., & Ilić, N. M. (2016). Tomato (*Solanum Lycopersicum* L.) processing main product (juice) and by-product (pomace) bioactivity potential measured as antioxidant activity and angiotensin-converting enzyme inhibition. *Journal of Food Processing and Preservation, 40*(6), 1229–1237.

Benjamin, E. J., Muntner, P., Alonso, A., Bittencourt, M. S., Callaway, C. W., Carson, A. P., Chamberlain, A. M., Chang, A. R., Cheng, S., Das, S. R., et al. (2019). Heart disease and stroke statistics-2019 update: A report from the American Heart Association. *Circulation, 139*, e56–e528.

Bonetti, P. O., Lerman, L. O., & Lerman, A. (2003). Endothelial dysfunction: A marker of atherosclerotic risk. *Arteriosclerosis, Thrombosis, and Vascular Biology, 23*(2), 168–175.

Burton-Freeman, B. M., & Sesso, H. D. (2014). Whole food versus supplement: Comparing the clinical evidence of tomato intake and lycopene supplementation on cardiovascular risk factors. *Advances in Nutrition, 5*(5), 457–485.

Cardiovascular Diseases (CVDs)—World Health Organization. (2021). Definition of cardiovascular diseases. Available online: https://www.who.int/news-room/fact-sheets/detail/cardiovascular-diseases-(cvds).

Caseiro, M., Ascenso, A., Costa, A., Creagh-Flynn, J., Johnson, M., & Simões, S. (2020). Lycopene in human health. *LWT, 127*, 109323.

ChemSpider. (2021). Search and share chemistry. Available online: http://www.chemspider.com/ (accessed on 12 June 2024).

Chen, J., Song, Y., & Zhang, L. (2013). Effect of lycopene supplementation on oxidative stress: An exploratory systematic review and meta-analysis of randomized controlled trials. *Journal of Medicinal Food, 16*(5), 361–374.

Chen, Z. Y., Peng, C., Jiao, R., Wong, Y. M., Yang, N., & Huang, Y. (2009). Anti-hypertensive nutraceuticals and functional foods. *Journal of Agricultural and Food Chemistry, 57*(11), 4485–4499.

Cheng, H. M., Koutsidis, G., Lodge, J. K., Ashor, A. W., Siervo, M., & Lara, J. (2019). Lycopene and tomato and risk of cardiovascular diseases: A systematic review and meta-analysis of epidemiological evidence. *Critical Reviews in Food Science and Nutrition, 59*(1), 141–158.

Cheng, H. M., Koutsidis, G., Lodge, J. K., Ashor, A., Siervo, M., & Lara, J. (2017). Tomato and lycopene supplementation and cardiovascular risk factors: A systematic review and meta-analysis. *Atherosclerosis, 257*, 100–108.

Costa-Rodrigues, J., Pinho, O., & Monteiro, P. R. (2018). Can lycopene be considered an effective protection against cardiovascular disease? *Food Chemistry, 245*, 1148–1153.

Dawson, V. L., Dawson, T. M., Bartley, D. A., Uhl, G. R., & Snyder, S. H. (1993). Mechanisms of nitric oxide-mediated neurotoxicity in primary brain cultures. *Journal of Neuroscience, 13*(6), 2651–2661.

Dubois-Deruy, E., Peugnet, V., Turkieh, A., & Pinet, F. (2020). Oxidative stress in cardiovascular diseases. *Antioxidants, 9*(9), 864.

Dugas, T. R., Morel, D. W., & Harrison, E. H. (1998). Impact of LDL carotenoid and α-tocopherol content on LDL oxidation by endothelial cells in culture. *Journal of Lipid Research, 39*(5), 999–1007.

Emami, M. R., Safabakhsh, M., Alizadeh, S., Asbaghi, O., & Khosroshahi, M. Z. (2019). Effect of vitamin E supplementation on blood pressure: A systematic review and meta-analysis. *Journal of Human Hypertension, 33*, 499–507.

Ferreira-Santos, P., Aparicio, R., Carrón, R., Sevilla, M. Á., Monroy-Ruiz, J., & Montero, M. J. (2018). Lycopene-supplemented diet ameliorates cardiovascular remodeling and oxidative stress in rats with hypertension induced by Angiotensin II. *Journal of Functional Foods, 47*, 279–287.

Fuhrman, B., Elis, A., & Aviram, M. (1997). Hypocholesterolemic effect of lycopene and β-carotene is related to suppression of cholesterol synthesis and augmentation of LDL receptor activity in macrophages. *Biochemical and Biophysical Research Communications, 233*(3), 658–662.

Geva, E., Bartoov, B., Zabludovsky, N., Lessing, J. B., Lerner-Geva, L., & Amit, A. (1996). The effect of antioxidant treatment on human spermatozoa and fertilization rate in an in vitro fertilization program. *Fertility and Sterility, 66*(3), 430–434.

Goulinet, S., & Chapman, M. J. (1997). Plasma LDL and HDL subspecies are heterogeneous in particle content of tocopherols and oxygenated and hydrocarbon carotenoids: Relevance to oxidative resistance and atherogenesis. *Arteriosclerosis, Thrombosis, and Vascular Biology, 17*(4), 786–796.

Han, G. M., & Liu, P. (2017). Higher serum lycopene is associated with reduced prevalence of hypertension in overweight or obese adults. *European Journal of Integrative Medicine, 13*, 34–40.

Heiss, C., & Kelm, M. (2010). Chocolate consumption, blood pressure, and cardiovascular risk. *European Heart Journal, 31*(13), 1554–1556.

Hininger, I., Chopra, M., Thurnham, D. I., Laporte, F., Richard, M. J., Favier, A., & Roussel, A. M. (1997). Effect of increased fruit and vegetable intake on the susceptibility of lipoprotein to oxidation in smokers. *European Journal of Clinical Nutrition, 51*(9), 601–606.

Honda, M., Kageyama, H., Hibino, T., Ichihashi, K., Takada, W., & Goto, M. (2020). Synergistic effects of food ingredients and vegetable oils on thermal isomerization of lycopene. *Journal of Oleo Science, 69*(12), 1529–1540.

Honda, M., Maeda, H., Fukaya, T., & Goto, M. (2018). Effects of Z-isomerization on the bioavailability and functionality of carotenoids: A review. *Progress in Carotenoid Research*, 139–159.

Hsu, Y. M., Lai, C. H., Chang, C. Y., Fan, C. T., Chen, C. T., & Wu, C. H. (2008). Characterizing the lipid-lowering effects and antioxidant mechanisms of tomato paste. *Bioscience, Biotechnology, and Biochemistry, 72*(3), 677–685.

Hugenholtz, J., & Smid, E. J. (2002). Nutraceutical production with food-grade microorganisms. *Current Opinion in Biotechnology, 13*(5), 497–507.

Jacques, P. F., Lyass, A., Massaro, J. M., Vasan, R. S., & D'Agostino, R. B. (2013). Relationship of lycopene intake and consumption of tomato products to incident CVD. *British Journal of Nutrition, 110*(3), 545–551.

Keservani, R. K., Kesharwani, R. K., Sharma, A. K., Vyas, N., & Chadoker, A. (2010). Nutritional supplements: An overview. *International Journal of Current Pharmaceutical Review and Research, 1*(1), 59–75.

Keservani, R. K., Kesharwani, R. K., Vyas, N., Jain, S., Raghuvanshi, R., & Sharma, A. K. (2010). Nutraceutical and functional food as future food: A review. *Der Pharmacia Lettre, 2*(1), 106–116.

Keservani, R. K., Sharma, A. K., & Kesharwani, R. K. (2016). Nutraceutical and Functional Foods for Cardiovascular Health. In *Food Process Engineering* (pp. 291–312). Apple Academic Press, CRC Press.

Keservani, R. K., Sharma, A. K., & Kesharwani, R. K. (2017). An overview and therapeutic applications of nutraceutical and functional foods. In *Recent Advances in Drug Delivery Technology* (pp. 160–201). ISBN: 9781522507543.

Keservani, R. K., Sharma, A. K., & Kesharwani, R. K. (Eds.). (2020). Nutraceuticals and Dietary Supplements: Applications in Health Improvement and Disease Management, Apple Academic Press, CRC Press. Pp. 1–344. ISBN: 9781771888738..

Kim, E. C., Ou, W., Dai Phung, C., Nguyen, T. T., Pham, T. T., Poudel, K., Gautam, M., Nguyen, H. T., Jeong, J. H., Yong, C. S., & Park, S. Y. (2021). Targeting and clearance of senescent foamy macrophages and senescent endothelial cells by antibody-functionalized mesoporous silica nanoparticles for alleviating aorta atherosclerosis. *Biomaterials, 269*, 120677.

Kim, J. Y., Paik, J. K., Kim, O. Y., Park, H. W., Lee, J. H., Jang, Y., & Lee, J. H. (2011). Effects of lycopene supplementation on oxidative stress and markers of endothelial function in healthy men. *Atherosclerosis, 215*(1), 189–195.

Kwak, N. S., & Jukes, D. J. (2001). Functional foods. Part 1: The development of a regulatory concept. *Food Control, 12*(2), 99–107.

Li, N., Wu, X., Zhuang, W., Xia, L., Chen, Y., Wu, C., Rao, Z., Du, L., Zhao, R., Yi, M., & Wan, Q. (2021). Tomato and lycopene and multiple health outcomes: Umbrella review. *Food Chemistry, 343*, 128396.

Li, Y., & Zhang, J. (2007). Serum concentrations of antioxidant vitamins and carotenoids are low in individuals with a history of attempted suicide. *Nutritional Neuroscience, 10*(1–2), 51–58.

Maiani, G., Periago Castón, M. J., Catasta, G., Toti, E., Cambrodón, I. G., Bysted, A., Granado-Lorencio, F., Olmedilla-Alonso, B., Knuthsen, P., Valoti, M., & Böhm, V. (2009). Carotenoids: Actual knowledge on food sources, intakes, stability and bioavailability and their protective role in humans. *Molecular Nutrition & Food Research, 53*(S2), S194–218.

Maoka, T. (2020). Carotenoids as natural functional pigments. *Journal of Natural Medicines, 74*(1), 1–6.

Mills, K. T., Stefanescu, A., & He, J. (2020). The global epidemiology of hypertension. *Nature Reviews Nephrology, 16*, 223–237.

Palan, P., & Naz, R. (1996). Changes in various antioxidant levels in human seminal plasma related to immunoinfertility. *Archives of Andrology, 36*(2), 139–143.

Palozza, P., Parrone, N., Simone, R. E., & Catalano, A. (2010). Lycopene in atherosclerosis prevention: An integrated scheme of the potential mechanisms of action from cell culture studies. *Archives of Biochemistry and Biophysics, 504*(1), 26–33.

Pereira, B. L., Arruda, F. C., Reis, P. P., Felix, T. F., Santos, P. P., Rafacho, B. P., Gonçalves, A. F., Claro, R. T., Azevedo, P. S., Polegato, B. F., & Okoshi, K. (2015). Tomato (*Lycopersicon esculentum*) supplementation induces changes in cardiac miRNA expression, reduces oxidative stress and left ventricular mass, and improves diastolic function. *Nutrients, 7*(11), 9640–9649.

Peto, R., Collins, R., & Gray, R. (1995). Large-scale randomized evidence: Large, simple trials and overviews of trials. *Journal of Clinical Epidemiology, 48*, 23–40.

Petyaev, I. M. (2016). Lycopene deficiency in ageing and cardiovascular disease. *Oxidative Medicine and Cellular Longevity, 2016*, 2016.

Przybylska, S. (2020). Lycopene–a bioactive carotenoid offering multiple health benefits: A review. *International Journal of Food Science & Technology, 55*(1), 11–32.

Puah, B. P., Jalil, J., Attiq, A., & Kamisah, Y. (2021). New Insights into Molecular Mechanism behind Anti-Cancer Activities of Lycopene. *Molecules, 26*(13), 3888.

Raiola, A., Rigano, M. M., Calafiore, R., Frusciante, L., & Barone, A. (2014). Enhancing the health-promoting effects of tomato fruit for biofortified food. *Mediators of Inflammation, 2014*, 2014.

Rao, A. V., Ray, M. R., & Rao, L. G. (2006). Lycopene. *Advances in Food and Nutrition Research, 51*, 99–164.

Riccioni, G., D'Orazio, N., Palumbo, N., Bucciarelli, V., & Di Ilio, E. (2009). Relationship between plasma antioxidant concentrations and carotid intima-media thickness: The asymptomatic carotid atherosclerotic disease in Manfredonia study. *European Journal of Cardiovascular Prevention & Rehabilitation, 16*, 351–357.

RM CB. (2013). Functional properties and health benefits of lycopene. *Nutrición Hospitalaria, 28*(1), 6–15.

Roberfroid, M. (2002). Functional food concept and its application to prebiotics. *Digestive and Liver Disease, 34*(Suppl 2), S105–S110.

Romanchik, J. E., Harrison, E. H., & Morel, D. W. (1997). Addition of lutein, lycopene, or β-carotene to LDL or serum in vitro: Effects on carotenoid distribution, LDL composition, and LDL oxidation. *The Journal of Nutritional Biochemistry, 8*(12), 681–688.
Roth, G. A., Abate, D., Abate, K. H., Abay, S. M., Abbafati, C., Abbasi, N., & Abdela, J. (2018). Global, regional, and national age-sex-specific mortality for 282 causes of death in 195 countries and territories, 1980–2017: A systematic analysis for the Global Burden of Disease Study 2017. *The Lancet, 392*, 1736–1788.
Sahin, K., Orhan, C., Tuzcu, M., Sahin, N., Ali, S., Bahcecioglu, I. H., & Kucuk, O. (2014). Orally administered lycopene attenuates diethylnitrosamine-induced hepatocarcinogenesis in rats by modulating Nrf-2/HO-1 and Akt/mTOR pathways. *Nutrition and Cancer, 66*(4), 590–598.
Saini, R. K., Bekhit, A. E., Roohinejad, S., Rengasamy, K. R., & Keum, Y. S. (2019). Chemical stability of lycopene in processed products: A review of the effects of processing methods and modern preservation strategies. *Journal of Agricultural and Food Chemistry, 68*(3), 712–726.
Senoner, T., & Dichtl, W. (2019). Oxidative stress in cardiovascular diseases: Still a therapeutic target? *Nutrients, 11*(9), 2090.
Sorriento, D., & Iaccarino, G. (2019). Inflammation and cardiovascular diseases: The most recent findings. *International Journal of Molecular Sciences, 20*(16), 3879.
Steinberg, F. M., & Chait, A. (1998). Antioxidant vitamin supplementation and lipid peroxidation in smokers. *The American Journal of Clinical Nutrition, 68*(2), 319–327.
Steven, S., Frenis, K., Oelze, M., Kalinovic, S., Kuntic, M., Bayo Jimenez, M. T., & Daiber, A. (2019). Vascular inflammation and oxidative stress: Major triggers for cardiovascular disease. *Oxidative Medicine and Cellular Longevity, 2019*, 2019.
Story, E. N., Kopec, R. E., Schwartz, S. J., & Harris, G. K. (2010). An update on the health effects of tomato lycopene. *Annual Review of Food Science and Technology, 1*, 189–210.
Suárez-Rivero, J. M., Pastor-Maldonado, C. J., Povea-Cabello, S., Álvarez-Córdoba, M., Villalón-García, I., Talaverón-Rey, M., & Sánchez-Alcázar, J. A. (2021). From mitochondria to atherosclerosis: The inflammation path. *Biomedicines, 9*(3), 258.
Suleiman, S. A., Ali, M. E., Zaki, Z. M., El-Malik, E. M., & Nasr, M. A. (1996). Lipid peroxidation and human sperm motility: Protective role of vitamin E. *Journal of Andrology, 17*(5), 530–537.
Taubert, D., Roesen, R., & Schömig, E. (2007). Effect of cocoa and tea intake on blood pressure: A meta-analysis. *Archives of Internal Medicine, 167*(7), 626–634.
Thies, F., Mills, L. M., Moir, S., & Masson, L. F. (2017). Cardiovascular benefits of lycopene: Fantasy or reality? *Proceedings of the Nutrition Society, 76*(2), 122–129.
Tierney, A. C., Rumble, C. E., Billings, L. M., & George, E. S. (2020). Effect of dietary and supplemental lycopene on cardiovascular risk factors: A systematic review and meta-analysis. *Advances in Nutrition, 11*(6), 1453–1488.
Turner, J. M., & Spatz, E. S. (2016). Nutritional supplements for the treatment of hypertension: A practical guide for clinicians. *Current Cardiology Reports, 18*(12), 1–9.
Whelton, P. K., Carey, R. M., Aronow, W. S., Casey, D. E., Jr., Collins, K. J., Dennison Himmelfarb, C., & Jamerson, K. A. (2018). 2017 ACC/AHA/AAPA/ABC/ACPM/AGS/APhA/ASH/ASPC/NMA/PCNA guideline for the prevention, detection, evaluation, and management of high blood pressure in adults: Executive summary: A report of the American College of Cardiology/American Heart Association Task Force 2 on Clinical Practice Guidelines. *Journal of the American College of Cardiology, 71*(19), 2199–2269.

Widlansky, M. E., Gokce, N., Keaney, J. F., & Vita, J. A. (2003). The clinical implications of endothelial dysfunction. *Journal of the American College of Cardiology, 42*(7), 1149–1160.
Willcox, J. K., Catignani, G. L., & Lazarus, S. (2003). Tomatoes and cardiovascular health. *Critical Reviews in Food Science and Nutrition, 43*, 1–18.
Wolak, T., & Paran, E. (2013). Can carotenoids attenuate vascular aging? *Vascular Pharmacology, 59*(3–4), 63–66.
Wood, L. G., Garg, M. L., Powell, H., & Gibson, P. G. (2008). Lycopene-rich treatments modify noneosinophilic airway inflammation in asthma: Proof of concept. *Free Radical Research, 42*(1), 94–102.
Young, A. J., & Lowe, G. M. (2001). Antioxidant and prooxidant properties of carotenoids. *Archives of Biochemistry and Biophysics, 385*(1), 20–27.
Zhang, J., Xu, J. H., Qu, Q. Q., & Zhong, G. Q. (2020). Risk of cardiovascular and cerebrovascular events in polycystic ovarian syndrome women: A meta-analysis of cohort studies. *Frontiers in Cardiovascular Medicine, 2020*, 184.
Zini, A., De Lamirande, E., & Gagnon, C. (1993). Reactive oxygen species in semen of infertile patients: Levels of superoxide dismutase-and catalase-like activities in seminal plasma and spermatozoa. *International Journal of Andrology, 16*(3), 183–188.
Zuchi, C., Ambrosio, G., Lüscher, T. F., & Landmesser, U. (2010). Nutraceuticals in cardiovascular prevention: Lessons from studies on endothelial function. *Cardiovascular Therapeutics, 28*(4), 187–201.

CHAPTER 8

NUTRACEUTICAL POTENTIAL OF LYCOPENE AND TOMATOES

NEHA SAINI, ITTISHREE BHARDWAJ, and RITU KATARIA

G.V.M. College of Pharmacy, Sonipat, Haryana, India

ABSTRACT

Nutraceuticals are the nutritional pharmaceutical products which are used to maintain good human health. There are various products used as nutraceuticals such as dietary fibers, prebiotics, probiotics, herbal products, etc. Nowadays, nutraceuticals are more acceptable by people because of their numerous advantages like keeping a human body full of nutrition and nutrients and hydrated as required by an individual. Tomatoes and tomato-based products are a rich source of Lycopene. Lycopene is a carotenoid that is mainly used to treat various diseases like cardiovascular disease, cancer, skin diseases, neurobehavioral disorders, hypertension, obesity, coronary artery disease, and infertility. Recent studies have shown that the use of lycopene reduces the risk of heart disease and also oxidative stress in an individual. Lycopene acts in various mechanisms to treat diseases such as an antioxidant, photoprotection, anti-angiogenesis, immunomodulation, anti-inflammatory, induction, and apoptosis. There are various marketed formulations available worldwide to treat such kind of fatal diseases. Lycopene has already gained popularity due to numerous successful studies conducted on it. It is also available in different types of nano-formulations like solid lipid nanoparticles, nano-emulsions, nano-dispersions, nanostructured lipid carriers, etc.

Antioxidants as Nutraceuticals. Nayan A. Gujarathi, Raj K. Keservani, Rajesh K. Kesharwani, Bhushan R. Rane, Yogeeta Sameer Goyal (Eds.)

8.1 INTRODUCTION

Nutraceutical is a combination of the words "nutrition" and "pharmaceutical." Nutraceuticals are a type of Food that plays an important role in adjusting and preserving normal physiological function to maintain human health balance. The current population and health trends are the primary drivers of the global nutraceutical market. Probiotics, Omega-3 fatty acids, flavonoids, Polyphenols, vitamins, essential nutrient-rich diet, and herbal/natural foods are examples of food products used as nutraceuticals (Das et al., 2010; Keservani et al., 2010a, b, 2017, 2020; Sharma et al., 2020). The ingestion of an adequate number of nutrients from a variety of meals is essential for the body's optimal functioning. As a result, medical experts and individuals have paid close attention to health-promoting foods and associated sectors. To tackle the problem, fresh innovative techniques such as nutraceuticals, nutritional treatment, phytonutrients, and physiotherapy have been found (Bland et al., 1996; Berger et al., 2006).

In the Western world, coronary heart disease (CHD) is one of the leading causes of mortality. The increased focus so far has been on the correlation between serum cholesterol levels and the hazard of CHD. Recent research has indicated that oxidative stress caused by reactive oxygen species (ROS) has a role in the pathophysiology of this disease (Clinton, 2010). The oxidation of circulatory low-density lipoprotein (LDL (ox) is hypothesized to have a role in atherosclerosis and CHD etiology. According to this theory, macrophages within the artery wall take up LDL (ox) and start the plaque formation process. *In vitro* studies have reported that dietary antioxidants like vitamin E and beta-carotene reduce the development of LDL (ox) and their absorption by macrophages. Lycopene is an unsaturated lipid-soluble carotene observed in red fruits and veggies such as tomatoes, papaya, watermelon, red grapefruits, and guava. It is a lipophilic, unsaturated carotenoid. Lycopene may contribute to enhancing vascular function and preventing cardiovascular disease in both the primary and secondary preventative stages (Mozos et al., 2018; Alves et al., 2019). The link between tomato and lycopene consumption and a lower risk of cardiovascular disease has piqued researchers' interest. Lycopene is the most potent antioxidant and aids in the treatment of heart disease in human beings. The bioavailability of lycopene in supplements has not been investigated as thoroughly, and it remains a promising subject for future research (Arab et al., 2000).

Tomato-based products including tomato sauce, tomato soup, and pizza marinara are the most abundant sources of lycopene in the American diet, accounting for more than 80% of total lycopene consumption. Unlike many other carotenoids, lycopene levels do not consistently decrease in smokers compared to nonsmokers, demonstrating that any potential anti-cancer properties are not attributable to antioxidant action (Thies et al., 2017) (Figure 8.1).

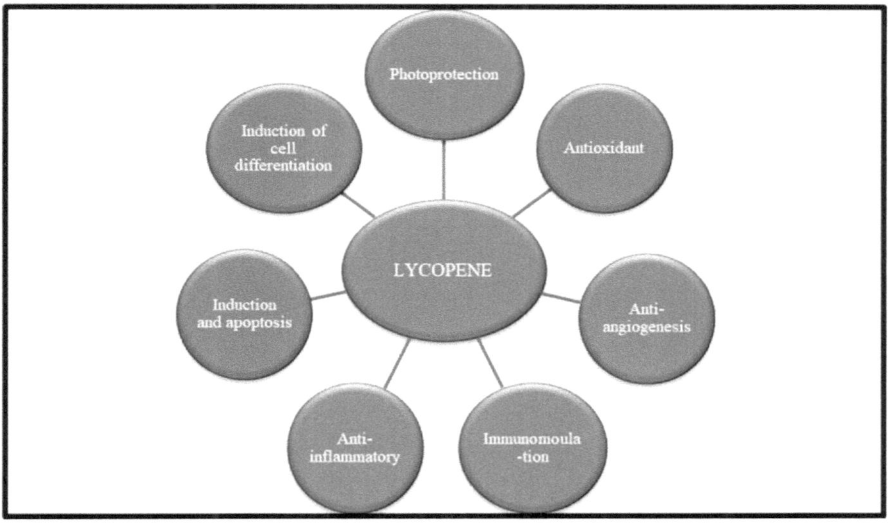

FIGURE 8.1 Lycopene's ability to alter cellular activity could be due to a variety of mechanisms.

Source: Adapted from Chen et al., 2013.

8.2 BIOAVAILABILITY OF LYCOPENE

Lycopene has a low bioavailability rate and is integrated into the lipoproteins as well as apo-B proteins carrying lipoproteins in the circulation to enhance the bioavailability. The bioavailability of lycopene and other carotenoids is poorly understood and explored. Chloroplasts are impervious to stomach and intestinal digestion. The structural specialization of lycopene in the chloroplasts of fruits and vegetables has recently been proven to be a crucial factor limiting lycopene bioavailability from dietary sources. The distribution of lycopene in various tissues seems to be quite selective. The largest concentrations of lycopene are identified in the testicles, adrenal glands, liver, and prostate, while other organs have relatively low levels. In the human body, plasma lipoproteins are the primary transporters of carotenoids and lycopene. Lycopene is extremely bioavailable when in an oily phase, primarily in monounsaturated oils, fats, proteins, and other tomato-based products (Shi et al., 2000; Bin et al., 2022) (Figure 8.2).

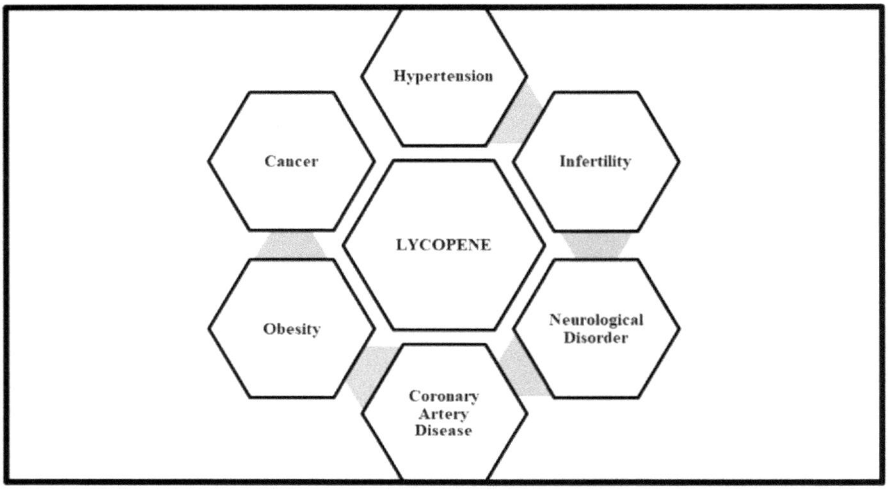

FIGURE 8.2 Nutraceutical compound. Applications of lycopene to treat a variety of diseases.
Source: Reprinted from Basuny, 2012. https://creativecommons.org/licenses/by/3.0/

8.3 CHEMICAL NATURE OF LYCOPENE

Lycopene is an acyclic carotenoid with conjugated double bonds, usually in the all-trans form, according to its chemical definition. Lycopene is a 40-carbon-atom lipophilic straight-chain hydrocarbon with 11 conjugated and 2 non-conjugated double bonds. Isomerization of the double bonds occurs, and several cis isomers (mostly 5, 9, 13, or 15) can be identified in plants and blood plasma. Because the human body is unable to manufacture carotenoids from endogenously produced biochemicals, it is completely reliant on carotenoids obtained from food. Tomato fruit and tomato-based food products contribute at least 85% of dietary lycopene to humans. Watermelon, guava, pink grapefruit, and papaya—all fruits that contain lycopene but at considerably lower levels than tomatoes—provide the remaining 15%. It is a lipophilic, bioactive, unsaturated, acyclic carotenoid having the chemical formula $C_{40}H_{56}$. Even though it is an essential phase in carotenoid synthesis in plants, lycopene has no role as a provitamin A precursor in the human diet due to the lack of suitable enzymes.

Lycopene accounts for over 90% of the total carotenoids found in tomatoes, while it is also present in plenty of other foods. Carotene, folate, phenolic compounds, and vitamins C and E are also present in tomatoes. The link between tomato and lycopene consumption and a lower risk of cardiovascular disease has piqued researchers' interest (Hsu et al., 2008; Alves et al., 2019). Much research has linked tomatoes and lycopene to lower rates of heart disease prevalence rate; however, the impact of lycopene intake is currently unclear and unconfirmed (García-Fernández et al., 2016) (Figure 8.3).

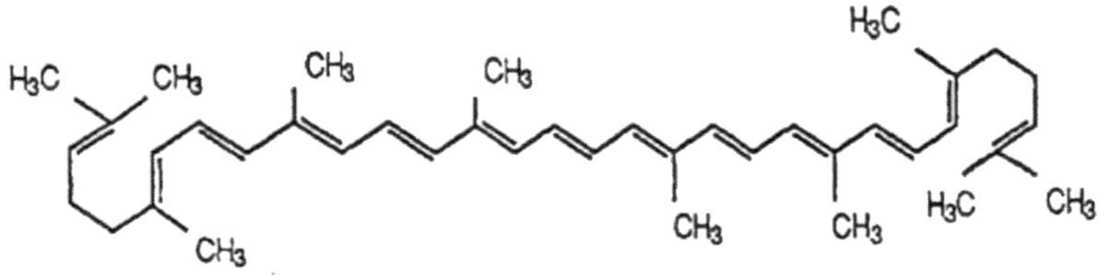

FIGURE 8.3 Chemical structure of lycopene.

Source: Reprinted from Kumar et al., 2017. https://creativecommons.org/licenses/by/4.0/

8.4 ROLE OF LYCOPENE IN CARDIOVASCULAR DISEASE

Cardiovascular disease (CVD) is still the major cause of death and disability worldwide. When evaluated by comparing to certain other West European and American territories, epidemiological evidence suggests that Middle Eastern countries have a reduced rate of mortality risk (Ivan, 2016). In various reports, it has been seen that patients treated with lycopene have reduced levels of LDL cholesterol and an upgrade in HDL cholesterol levels, as well as a decrease in carotid artery thickness and protection from oxidative damage (Przybylska & Tokarczyk, 2022).

Lycopene is essential in preventing exacerbations, such as blood clots caused by atherosclerotic changes. High blood lipid levels, such as bad cholesterol and triglycerides, are the leading cause of heart disease. Lycopene has the ability to adhere to plasma LDL cholesterol and, by doing so, it protects against atherosclerosis by inhibiting lipid oxidation. Ischemic heart disease is the primary cause of cardiovascular disease, as in this disease mainly accumulation of the lipids takes place in the arterial walls which causes plaques and an increase in the level of ROS, which ultimately causes inflammation, dysfunction, and vasculitis in the heart. The risk factors of heart disease can be controlled by maintaining lipid levels (Saini et al.,

2020). Cardiovascular diseases (CVD) are chiefly linked with systemic and low-grade chronic inflammation caused by oxidative stress (Thies et al., 2017; Przybylska, &Tokarczyk, 2022).

People with metabolic syndrome, a group of health problems that can lead to heart disease, may live longer if their blood levels of lycopene are high. Lycopene's antioxidant properties appear to be especially advantageous to people who have low blood antioxidant levels or are under a lot of oxidative stress. This includes seniors, smokers, and persons with diabetes or heart problems (Lenore & Steck, 2020).

According to findings, lycopene without provitamin A activity is present in higher levels in a few plant-based products with substantial antioxidant effects in treating various heart diseases and cancers in human beings. There is no evidence to show lycopene absorption; however, studies have shown that lycopene enters the bloodstream more freely if the tomato is subjected to heat and a source of fat is added to the diet. In a group of subjects that received 180 g of tomato juice, which contains around 12 mg of lycopene daily for 6 weeks, it was shown that plasma lycopene levels increased slightly. Other studies have discovered a relatively insignificant rise in lycopene concentrations in plasma after consuming unheated tomato products (Stahl & Sies, 1992).

Smoking cigarettes has long been recognized as a risk factor for coronary atherosclerosis. According to theory, smoke exposes a source of harmful radicals into the bloodstream, causing lipid oxidation and associated complications. According to research, the magnitude of coronary artery disease is linked to bad cholesterol oxidation vulnerability. Antioxidants that defend LDL from oxidative stress may thus protect living beings from cardiovascular disease (Salonen et al., 1992; Kim et al., 2017).

According to the Rotterdam Study, smoking is a powerful oxidative stress that can impede arterial elastic properties and endothelial dysfunction, and lycopene is the only significant serum beta-carotene that can lessen atherosclerotic danger in former and present smokers (Rao & Agarwal, 1998).

8.5 REPORTED NANO-FORMULATIONS OF LYCOPENE

Nano-formulations are prepared for better efficacy and results of the drug or phytoconstituents. There are so many available nano-formulations in the market which have promising results for the patients. Nowadays, these types of formulations are more acceptable due to their numerous advantages.

Lycopene is also used to prepare various nano-formulations such as solid lipid nanoparticles, nano-emulsions, nano-dispersion, and nanostructured lipid particles by various methods as given in Table 8.1.

TABLE 8.1 Types of Nano-Formulation with Lycopene and Its Method of Preparation

Sl. No.	Nano-Formulation of Lycopene	Method
1.	Lycopene loaded Solid lipid Nanoparticles	Hot Homogenization method. Rao & Agarwal (1998)
2.	Nano-emulsion	Emulsification-Evaporation method (https://www.healthline.com/nutrition/lycopene)
3.	Nano-Dispersion	Ultrasound Assisted Nano precipitation. Nazemiyeh et al. (2016)
4.	Nanostructured Lipid carriers	High-pressure homogenization
5.	Lycopene in emulsions	Emulsion preparation method (https://doi.org/10.3389/fphar.2018.00521)

8.6 MECHANISM OF ACTION

Lycopene has been shown to enhance cardiovascular health and make a significant contribution to the primary and subsequent prevention of cardiovascular disease. Lycopene's primary activity profile includes anti-atherosclerotic, antioxidant, anti-inflammatory, antihypertensive, antiplatelet, anti-apoptotic, and protective endothelial effects, as well as the capacity to enhance metabolism and decrease arterial stiffness. A large Japanese cohort study discovered a negative correlation between plasma lycopene accumulation and cardiovascular disease mortality (Song et al., 2017).

In a recent meta-analysis study published in 2017, the relationship between lycopene intake, plasma levels, and cardiovascular disease was evaluated. Analysis of the data showed that lycopene was associated with a 17% reduction in the risk of cardiovascular disease when the results of the higher intake were compared to the lowest one. Numerous theories have been suggested to describe lycopene's cardiac preventive properties, such as the lowering of LDL cholesterol and immune response, the significant decrease of biosynthetic pathway oxidation, the advancement of junctional connectivity and apoptosis stimulation, and eventually, the antiproliferative effects (Bohm, 2012; Fuhrman et al., 1997).

So many studies have concluded that a nutritious rich diet reduces the risk of cardiovascular diseases. Carotene carotene-rich diet is primarily responsible for the positive effects of preventing coronary heart disease (Waqas et al., 2020; Meroni & Raikos, 2018; https://www.chemeurope.com/en/encyclopedia/Lycopene.html).

8.7 MARKETED FORMULATIONS AVAILABLE TO DECREASE THE RISK OF CVS

Lycopene is sold in the market in combination with other carotenoids and antioxidants. It is marketed under various brand names by a number of pharmaceutical companies (https://www.dawabazar.in/lycopene/0/1964/generic). Some commonly used Dosage forms containing Lycopene, which is used in heart diseases are:

TABLE 8.2 Available Marketed Formulations of Lycopene to Decrease CVS Disease

Sl. No.	Brand Name	Dosage Form	Manufacturer
1.	Athax	Capsule	Athens Labs Ltd.
2.	Lycodev Plus	Capsule	Zee laboratories
3.	Lycofol Plus	Syrup	Alkem Laboratories Ltd.
4.	Lyconext	Capsule	Bionext Pharma Private Ltd.
5.	Lycoral	Syrup	Cubit Healthcare
6.	Lycoral-Z	Tablet	Cubit Healthcare
7.	Lycotek Plus	Capsule	Grentek Healthcare
8.	Lygem	Soft Gel Capsules	Zota Health Care Ltd.
9.	MCM-XL	Capsule	Zee laboratories
10.	Propep	Tablet	Biosciences Pharmakon
11.	Vaglyco	Tablet	Dr. John's Labs
12.	Pinelex plus	Capsule	Axygen Life sciences

8.8 CONCLUSION

Multiple non-alimentary illnesses and pathological conditions linked to micronutrient deficiencies have been recognized due to recent innovations in medical and analytical chemistry. Significant variations in plasma and tissue levels of numerous key nutrients, including lycopene and other carotenoids, have been connected with health disorders associated with oxidative stress such as population aging, heart disease, and type 2 diabetes mellitus. A new enzymatic pathway for lycopene breakdown has been discovered, which results in the creation of various end products excreted from the human body. As a result, health disorders associated with long-term oxidative stress may lead to lycopene depletion, necessitating continuous and effective restoration of carotene in the form of antioxidants in living organisms. New carotenoids and lycopene nutraceutical compositions with improved bioavailability are definitely needed. Using micro-emulsifying methods and/or nano-delivery techniques, novel preparations of antioxidants, carotenoids, and lycopene with enhanced bioavailability have been developed in recent years.

KEYWORDS

- **cardiovascular disease**
- **coronary heart disease**
- **low-density lipoprotein**
- **lycopene**
- **reactive oxygen species**

REFERENCES

Agarwal, S., & Rao, A. V. (1998). Tomato lycopene and low-density lipoprotein oxidation: a human dietary intervention study. *Lipids*, *33*(10), 981–984.

Alves, Q. L., Camargo, S. B., & Silva, D. F. (2019). Role of Nutraceuticals in the Prevention and Treatment of Hypertension and Cardiovascular Diseases. *Journal of Hypertension Management*, *5*, 037. https://doi.org/10.23937/2474-3690/1510037.

Arab, L., & Steck, S. (2000). Lycopene and cardiovascular disease. *The American Journal of Clinical Nutrition*, *71*(6), 1691S–1695S.

Arab, L., & Steck, S. (2020). Lycopene and cardiovascular disease. *The American Journal of Clinical Nutrition*, *71*(6), 1691S–1695S. https://doi.org/10.1093/ajcn/71.6.1691.

Available from: https://www.chemeurope.com/en/encyclopedia/Lycopene.html.

Available from: https://www.dawabazar.in/lycopene/0/1964/generic.

Basuny, A. M. (2012). The Anti-Atherogenic Effects of Lycopene. InTech. doi: 10.5772/48134.

Berger, M. M., & Shenkin, A. (2006). Vitamins and trace elements: Practical aspects of supplementation. *Nutrition*, *22*(9), 952–955.

Bin-Jumah, M. N., Nadeem, M. S., Gilani, S. J., Mubeen, B., Ullah, I., Alzarea, S. I., Ghoneim, M. M., Alshehri, S., Al-Abbasi, F. A., & Kazmi, I. (2022). Lycopene: A Natural Arsenal in the War against Oxidative Stress and Cardiovascular Diseases. *Antioxidants (Basel, Switzerland)*, *11*(2), 232. https://doi.org/10.3390/antiox11020232.

Bland, J. S. (1996). Phytonutrition, phytotherapy and phytopharmacology. *Alternative Therapies in Health and Medicine*, *2*(3), 73–76.

Böhm, V. (2012). Lycopene and heart health. *Molecular Nutrition & Food Research*, *56*(2), 296–303.

Burton-Freeman, B., & Sesso, H. D. (2014). Whole food versus supplement: comparing the clinical evidence of tomato intake and lycopene supplementation on cardiovascular risk factors. *Advances in Nutrition*, *5*(5), 457–485.

Chen, J., Song, Y., & Zhang, L. (2013). Effect of lycopene supplementation on oxidative stress: An exploratory systematic review and meta-analysis of randomized controlled trials. *Journal of Medicinal Food*, *16*(4), 361–374.

Clinton, S. K. (1998). Lycopene: chemistry, biology, and implications for human health and disease. *Nutrition Reviews*, *56*(2), 35–51.

Das, L., Bhaumik, E., Raychaudhuri, U., & Chakraborty, R. (2012). Role of nutraceuticals in human health. *Journal of Food Science and Technology*, *49*(2), 173–183. https://doi.org/10.1007/s13197-011-0269-4.

Fuhrman, B., Elis, A., & Aviram, M. (1997). Hypocholesterolemic effect of lycopene and β-carotene is related to suppression of cholesterol synthesis and augmentation of LDL receptor activity in macrophage. *Biochemical and Biophysical Research Communications*, *233*(3), 658–662.

García-Fernández, E., Rico-Cabañas, L., Estruch, R., & Bach-Faig, A. (2014). Mediterranean diet and cardio diabesity: a review. *Nutrients*, *6*(9), 3474–3500.

Hsu, Y. M., Lai, C. H., Chang, C. Y., Fan, C. T., Chen, C. T., et al. (2008). Characterizing the lipid-lowering effects and antioxidant mechanisms of tomato paste. *Bioscience, Biotechnology, and Biochemistry*, *72*(3), 677–685.

Joseph Levy, Yoav Sharoni (2018). The Functions of Tomato Lycopene and Its Role in Human Health, 62, 49–56. https://www.herbalgram.org/resources/herbalgram/issues/62/table-of-contents/article2696.

Keservani, R. K., Kesharwani, R. K., Sharma, A. K., Vyas, N., & Chadoker, A. (2010b). Nutritional Supplements: An Overview. *International Journal of Current Pharmaceutical Review and Research*, *1*(1), 59–75.

Keservani, R. K., Kesharwani, R. K., Vyas, N., Jain, S., Raghuvanshi, R., & Sharma, A. K. (2010a). Nutraceutical and functional food as future food: a review. *Der Pharmacia Lettre*, *2*(1), 106–116.

Keservani, R. K., Sharma, A. K., & Kesharwani, R. K. (2017). An overview and therapeutic applications of nutraceutical and functional foods. In *Recent Advances in Drug Delivery Technology* (pp. 160–201). ISBN:9781522507543.

Kim, G. H., & Youn, H. J. (2017). Is carotid artery ultrasound still useful method for evaluation of atherosclerosis? *Korean Circulation Journal*, *47*, 1–8. https://doi.org/10.4070/kcj.2016.0232.

Kong, K. W., Khoo, H. E., Prasad, K. N., Ismail, A., Tan, C. P., & Rajab, N. F. (2010). Revealing the power of the natural red pigment lycopene. *Molecules*, *15*, 959–987. https://doi.org/10.3390/molecules15020959.

Kumar, Venkata & Pa, Elango & S., Asmathulla & Kavimani, S.. (2017). A Systematic Review on Lycopene and its Beneficial Effects". Biomedical and Pharmacology Journal. 10. 2113-2120. 10.13005/bpj/1335.

Lycopene uses and side effect https://www.dawabazar.in/lycopene/0/1964/generic.

Lycopene: Health Benefits and Top Food Sources, https://www.healthline.com/nutrition/lycopene#antioxidant.

Meroni, E., & Raikos, V. (2018). Lycopene in Beverage Emulsions: Optimizing Formulation Design and Processing Effects for Enhanced Delivery. *Beverages*, *4*(1), 14. https://doi.org/10.3390/beverages4010014.

Mozos I, Stoian D, Caraba A, Malainer C, Horbańczuk JO and Atanasov AG (2018) Lycopene and Vascular Health. *Front. Pharmacol. 9,* 521. doi: 10.3389/fphar.2018.00521.

Mozos, I., Stoian, D., Caraba, A., Malainer, C., Horbańczuk, J. O., & Atanasov, A. G. (2018). Lycopene and Vascular Health. *Frontiers in Pharmacology*, *9*, 521. https://doi.org/10.3389/fphar.2018.00521.

Nazemi, Y., et al. (2016). Formulation and Physicochemical Characterization of Lycopene-Loaded Solid Lipid Nanoparticles. *Advanced Pharmaceutical Bulletin*, *6*(2), In press. DOI:10.15171/apb.2016.032.

Petyaev, I. M. (2016). Lycopene Deficiency in Ageing and Cardiovascular Disease. *Oxidative Medicine and Cellular Longevity*, 1–344. Article ID 3218605. https://doi.org/10.1155/2016/3218605.

Przybylska, S., & Tokarczyk, G. (2022). Lycopene in the Prevention of Cardiovascular Diseases. *International Journal of Molecular Sciences*, *23*, 1997. DOI:10.3390/ijms23041957.

Rao, A. V., & Agarwal, S. (1998). Bioavailability and in vivo antioxidant properties of lycopene from tomato products and their possible role in the prevention of cancer. *Nutrition and Cancer*, *31*(4), 199–203.

Saini, R. K., Kannan, R. R., Rengasamy, F. M., & Keum, Y. -S. (2020). Protective effects of lycopene in cancer, cardiovascular, and neurodegenerative diseases: An update on epidemiological and mechanistic perspectives. *Pharmacological Research*, *155*, 104730. https://doi.org/10.1016/j.phrs.2020.104730.

Salonen, J. T., Yla-Herttuala, S., Yamamoto, R., et al. (1992). Autoantibody against oxidised LDL and progression of carotid atherosclerosis. *Lancet*, *339*, 883–887.

Sharma, A. K., Keservani, R. K., & Gautam Surya, P. (2020). *Herbal Product Development*. Apple Academic Press, CRC Press, Taylor & Francis Group. ISBN: 9781771888776.

Shi, J., & Le Maguer, M. (2000). Lycopene in tomatoes: chemical and physical properties affected by food processing. *Critical Reviews in Biotechnology*, *20*(4), 293–334.

Song, B., Liu, K., Gao, Y., Zhao, L., Fang, H., & Li, Y., et al. (2017). Lycopene and risk of cardiovascular diseases: A meta-analysis of observational studies. *Molecular Nutrition & Food Research*, *61*(9), 1–4.

Stahl, W., & Sies, H. (1992). Uptake of lycopene and its geometrical isomers is greater from heat-processed than from unprocessed tomato juice in humans. *Journal of Nutrition*, *122*(11), 2161–2166.

Thies, F., Mills, L., Moir, S., & Masson, L. (2017). Cardiovascular benefits of lycopene: Fantasy or reality? *Proceedings of the Nutrition Society*, *76*(2), 122–129. doi:10.1017/S0029665116000744.

Venkata, N. K., Elango, P., Asmathulla, S., & Kavimani, S., (2017). A Systematic Review on Lycopene and Its Beneficial Effects. *Biomedical & Pharmacology Journal, 10*(4), 2113–2120.

Waqas, A., Anam, L., Zhang, L., Zhang, J., Wang, C., Abdur, R., Hussain, A., Siddiquy, M., & Karim, A. (2020). Technological Advancement in the Processing of Lycopene: A Review. *Food Reviews International*, *38,* 857. DOI: 10.1080/87559129.2020.1749653.

CHAPTER 9

ROLE OF NUTRACEUTICALS IN DYSLIPIDEMIA

VIPIN NAUTIYAL[1] and DEEPANSHU RANA[2]

[1]*Assistant Professor, Department of Paramedical Sciences, Uttaranchal (P.G.) College of Biomedical Sciences and Hospital, Dehradun, Uttarakhand, India*

[2]*Assistant Professor, Department of Microbiology, Sardar Bhagwan Singh University, Balawala, Dehradun, Uttarakhand, India*

ABSTRACT

In the current scenario, the major population across the world is emphasizing the modulation of diet to get positive health effects and eliminate the risk of cardiovascular and several other diseases. Nutraceuticals are simply food or part of food that are capable of providing health benefits to individuals. Nutraceuticals could be classified in several ways, depending on their beneficial effects like prevention of CVD, and maintenance of bowel and endothelial dysfunction. These food additives could be a good alternative to synthetic drugs, particularly in patients having diseases associated with the accumulation of lipid molecules.

9.1 INTRODUCTION

A healthy diet plan is essential for good health. However, the new lifestyle has changed the diet as well as the basic food habits of the major population of the world. The consumption of junk food is continuously increasing, resulting in the depletion of nutrients which leads to the emergence of various diseases (Das et al., 2012). Heart disorders, obesity, arthritis, and cancer are

Antioxidants as Nutraceuticals. Nayan A. Gujarathi, Raj K. Keservani, Rajesh K. Kesharwani, Bhushan R. Rane, Yogeeta Sameer Goyal (Eds.)

some well-known diseases related to malnutrition, particularly in developing countries. The treatment of such diseases by modern medicines and therapies is very expensive, and therefore, alternative medicines are seeking attention from researchers as well as industries in order to exploit their biological and therapeutical potential. In this quest, nutraceuticals have emerged as a potential class of natural products that can meet the requirements of the major population (Adelaja & Schiling, 1999). Animal-originated and plant-based nutraceuticals provide tremendous opportunities for the food industries to come up with novel food products of wider therapeutic value.

The term "nutraceutical" is the combination of two words, "nutrition" and "pharmaceutical," which was first coined by Stephen De Felice in 1989 (Brower, 1998; Maddi et al., 2007). De Felice defined nutraceutical as a food that gives positive health benefits by preventing and treating disease. Nutraceuticals may also be defined as food-derived products sold in different medical forms like pills and powder (Wildman, 2001; Bull, 2000). These products could be from isolated nutrients, dietary supplements, processed products, herbal products, and genetically modified foods (Malik, 2008; Dureja et al., 2003).

Nutraceuticals show a wide range of therapeutic activities that include anti-arthritic, anti-cancer, and antidiabetic activities (Keservani et al., 2010a, b, 2017, 2020; Pandey et al., 2010).

9.2 CLASSIFICATION OF NUTRACEUTICALS

Nutraceuticals can be categorized based on food sources, action, and chemical nature. The natural food sources used as nutraceuticals can be categorized as shown in Figure 9.1 (Kalia, 2005; Kokate et al., 2002; Pandey et al., 2010). The health benefits of nutraceutical food sources are depicted in Figure 9.1.

Dyslipidemia (increased fat levels in the blood) is considered one of the major risk factors associated with cardiovascular disease (CVD) (Kannel et al., 1971). Such elevated lipid concentrations are responsible for vascular damage due to the generation of oxidative stress, inflammation, and autoimmune disorders (Tian et al., 2010; Ungvari et al., 2010) (Table 9.1). The involvement of reactive oxygen species (ROS) in various pathological conditions is shown in Figure 9.2.

9.2.1 *NIACIN (VITAMIN B3)*

Niacin acts as a potent antioxidant compound. In addition to this, it inhibits LDL oxidation, catabolic rate of HDL-Apo A1, platelet function, decreases cytokines and cell adhesion molecules, lowers lipoprotein (a), while it increases lipolysis of triglycerides in adipose tissues, Apo B degradation,

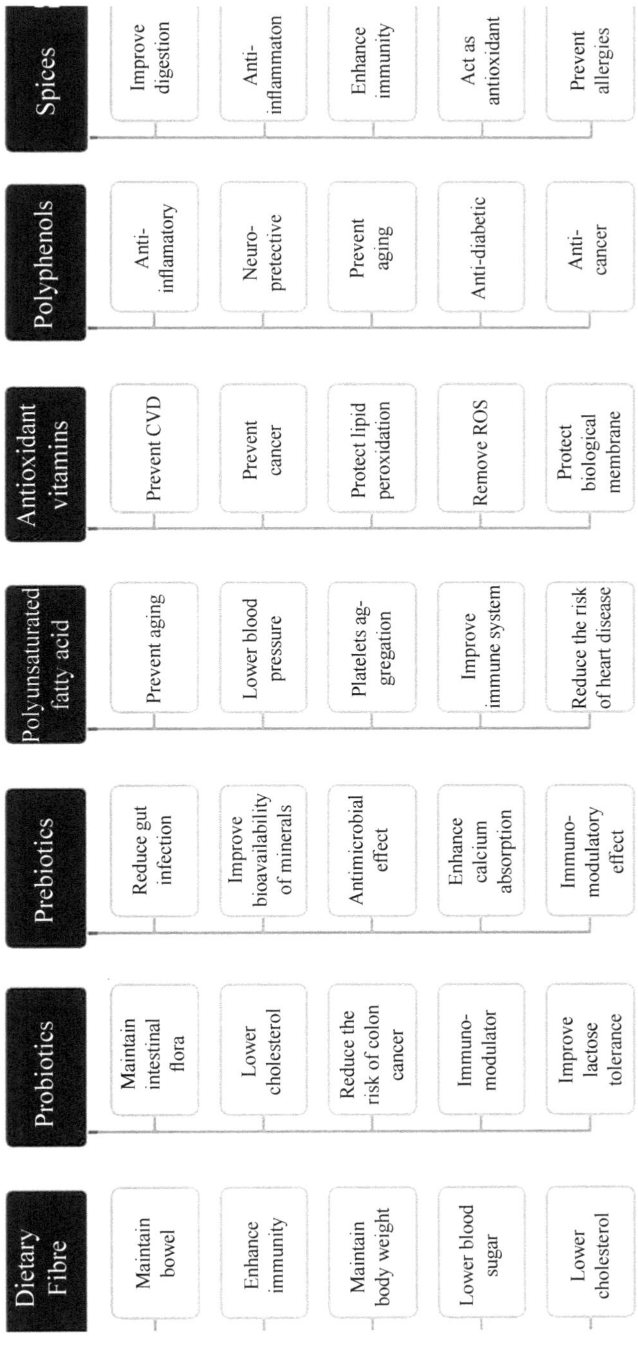

FIGURE 9.1 Health benefits of nutraceutical food sources.

TABLE 9.1 Recommended Dose of Nutraceutical for Dyslipidemia

Sl. No.	Supplement	Daily Dose
1.	Vitamin B3	500–4,000 mg in divided doses
2.	Phytosterols	2.15 g
3.	Fermented soy	30–50 g
4.	Green tea or extract	500–700 mg
5.	Omega 3 fatty acid	3,000–5,000 mg
6.	Flax seed	40 g
7.	Monounsaturated fats	20–40 g
8.	Sesame	40 g
9.	Gamma/delta tocotrienols	200 mg
10.	Pantethine	900 mg in divided doses
11.	Resveratrol (trans form)	250 mg
12.	N acetyl cysteine	2,000 mg in divided doses
13.	Curcumin	2,000 mg in divided doses
14.	Pomegranate juice	8 ounces
15.	Citrus bergamot	1,000 mg
16.	Vitamin C	500 mg

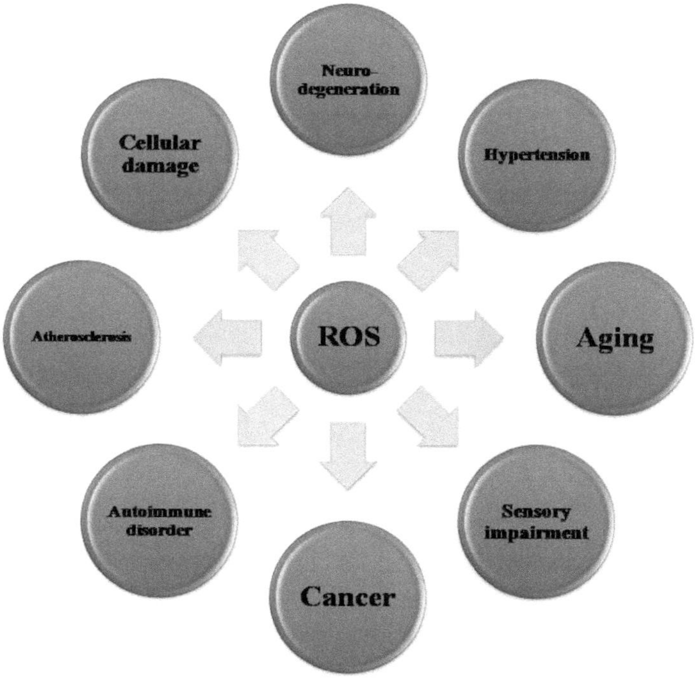

FIGURE 9.2 Involvement of ROS in pathological conditions.

fibrinolysis, and adiponectin (Al-Mohissen et al., 2010). However, only vitamin B3 niacin is found effective in dyslipidemia, but the non-flush niacin (inositol hexanicotinate-IHN) is not involved in the improvement of lipid profiles and hence, it is not recommended (Houston et al., 2009). Some side effects associated with niacin are hyperuricemia, gout, flushing, rash, pruritus, hyperpigmentation, gastritis, ulcers, bruising, tachycardia, and palpitations (Ruparelia et al., 2010; Al-Mohissen et al., 2010; Houston, 2012).

9.2.2 PHYTOSTEROLS

Phytosterols are plant-derived naturally occurring sterols or their derivatives that possess a wide range of biological activities. β-sitosterol is considered the most abundant phytosterol that helps in the treatment of prostatic hyperplasia (Patch et al., 2006; Othman & Moghadasian, 2011). It has been observed that phytosterols are significantly absorbed compared to plant stanols. In a study by Demonty (2009), it was reported that an average daily consumption of 2.15 g of phytosterols decreases LDL levels by 8.8%. The higher affinity of phytosterols towards micelles results in poor incorporation of dietary and biliary cholesterol. Additionally, interaction with enterocyte ATP-binding cassette transport proteins (ABCG8 and ABCG 5) also helps in lowering cholesterol levels by taking it back to the intestinal lumen (Patch et al., 2006; Houston et al., 2009). Phytosterols also have anti-inflammatory activity and are therefore able to decrease inflammatory cytokines like high sensitivity C-reactive protein (hs-CRP), interleukin-6 (IL-6), interleukin-1β, tumor necrosis factor (TNF), phospholipase A2, and fibrinogen. However, the anti-inflammatory potential varies among different phytosterols.

9.2.3 SOY

The mild improvements in serum lipids with soy have been reported in a number of studies. However, in such studies, few conflicts arise due to differences in the type and dose of soy (Harland et al., 2008). Soy reduces the micellar content and absorption of lipids via a combination of fiber, isoflavones, and phytoestrogens (Harland et al., 2008; Houston et al., 2009).

9.2.4 GREEN TEA

The bioactive components of green tea like catechins reported to have several health benefits including improvement of lipid profile via involvement in micellar solubilization of cholesterol in the gastrointestinal tract and decreased absorption (Houston et al., 2009). Epigallocatechin gallate

(EGCG) is a well-known compound that has gained attention due to its positive effects on health. It reduces the expression of fatty acid genes, inhibits HMGCoA reductase activity, increases mitochondrial energy expenditure, upregulates the LDL receptor, decreases the secretion of Apo B lipoprotein, and improves endothelial dysfunction (Singh et al., 2009; Brown et al., 2011).

9.2.5 OMEGA 3 FATTY ACID

Numerous observational, epidemiologic, and clinical trials have shown significant reductions in serum TGs, VLDL, and LDL levels with omega-3 fatty acids (Saremi & Arora, 2009). In a study done by Houston et al. (2009), it was reported that a rich diet of omega-3 fatty acids in CHD patients led to a lower mortality rate.

9.2.6 FLAX SEED

Flax seeds mainly contain fiber and lignans which increase endothelial nitric oxide synthase, improve endothelial dysfunction, decrease smooth muscle hypertrophy, prevent oxidative damage, and the development of atherosclerosis (Bioedon et al., 2008; Prasad, 2009).

9.2.7 MONOUNSATURATED FATS

In some studies, it has been reported that monounsaturated fats (MUFAs) like olive oil and nuts are capable of reducing low-density lipoprotein (LDL) triglycerides (TGs), oxidation reaction, and inflammatory response. On the other hand, they are also found to increase HDL levels and improve erectile dysfunction (Covas, 2007; Bester et al., 2010). MUFAs are considered one of the most potential agents to decrease oxidized LDL (oxLDL), which is associated with coronary artery disease (CAD).

9.2.8 SESAME

Sesame (*Sesamum indicum*) belongs to the family *Pedaliaceae*. It is one of the earliest domesticated oilseed plants known to have several beneficial effects. In India, it has been used in several religious practices since ancient times (Weiss, 1971). Sesame oil consists of numerous antioxidant compounds like sesamin, sesamolin, and tocopherols that act as nutraceuticals and prevent oxidative damage, hence regarded as the 'queen of oilseeds.' The major content of sesame oil is unsaturated fatty acids (83–90%), including glycerides of oleic acid (36–54%) and linoleic acid (38–49%). The saturated fatty acids include 0.1% myristic acid, 8–12% palmitic acid, 3.5–7% stearic acid, and 0.5–1% arachidonic acid. The unsaponifiable content like sesamin (0.1–0.6%) and sesamolin (0.25–0.3%) provide resistance to oil against rancidity (Pathak et al., 2019).

9.2.9 TOCOTRIENOLS

It is a family of unsaturated forms of vitamin E named alpha, beta, gamma, and delta. In a study done by Qureshi et al. (2001); McRae et al. (2005) reported the ability of gamma and delta tocotrienols to reduce the total cholesterol level by up to 17%, LDL by 24%, Apo B by 15%, and lipoprotein(a) by 17%, while the minimum changes reported in HDL or Apo A1. Furthermore, gamma and delta tocotrienols inhibit cholesterol synthesis by suppression of HMG-CoA reductase activity (Prasad, 2014; Houston et al., 2009).

9.2.10 PANTETHINE

Pantethine is a dimeric derivative of pantothenic acid held together by a disulfide bond. It is metabolized to cystamine-SH, which has transglutaminase (TG2) inhibition activity and is used in the treatment of dyslipidemia (Derosa et al., 2020). Pantethine prevents the peroxidation of lipids and deposition of lipids in the coronary arteries (McRae, 2005; Horvath & Vecsei, 2009). It can also inhibit cholesterol synthesis and enhance fatty acid metabolism by inhibiting hepatic acetyl-CoA carboxylase and increasing cytoplasmic CoA levels that stimulate the oxidation of acetate and thus increase Krebs cycle activity.

9.2.11 RESVERATROL

Resveratrol is a polyphenolic phytoalexin that was first isolated from the roots of Veratrum grandiflorum O. Loes (white hellebore) and identified in 1939 (Takaoka, 1940). It has also been found in various edible parts of plants such as grapes, berries, peanuts, pistachios, and plums. An abundant amount of resveratrol is found in the skin of fresh grapes at concentrations of 50–100 mg/g. During the last three decades, resveratrol has received considerable attention for its beneficial health effects on human health (Kopp, 1998). Resveratrol is reported to prevent several diseases like obesity, diabetes, cancer, metabolic disorders, hypertension, cardiovascular diseases, kidney disorders, and inflammatory diseases. Such activities are due to its ability to modulate different cell signaling molecules such as cytokines, caspases, metalloproteinases, Wnt ligand Notch, protein kinase, intercellular adhesion molecule, vascular cell adhesion molecule, and several others (Singh et al., 2019).

9.2.12 N-ACETYLCYSTEINE

N-acetylcysteine (NAC) was patented in 1960, while its medicinal use was reported in 1967. NAC is a sulfhydryl-containing compound that shows mucolytic properties. Naturally, cysteine is present in various products like fish, meat, grains, dairy, soybeans, and eggs. A small amount of NAC is also found naturally in some fruits and vegetables (Demirkol et al., 2004). It has been observed that NAC is involved in scavenging free radicals, improving glutathione activity, stabilizing protein structure, and has anti-inflammatory and mucolytic activity.

9.2.13 CURCUMIN

Curcumin is a polyphenolic low molecular weight compound. It is lipophilic in nature and therefore, insoluble in water as well as in ether. However, it is soluble in some organic solvents like ethanol and dimethylsulfoxide. Curcumin has long been used in the traditional system of medicine and is considered one of the most important medicinal herbs due to its wide range of biological activities such as antioxidant (Rheim et al., 2015), antimicrobial (Prasad et al., 2014), anti-inflammatory (Gómez-Estaca et al., 2017), and anti-mutagenic effect (Noorafshan & Ashkani-Esfahani, 2013). Particularly in the Indian traditional system of medicine, curcumin has been used in the treatment of various ailments like rheumatoid arthritis, conjunctivitis, skin diseases, wound infections, urinary tract infections (UTI), and liver diseases (Rathore et al., 2020).

9.2.14 POMEGRANATE JUICE

Pomegranate is considered an abundant source of dietary fiber that supplies various health-promoting nutrients such as vitamins (A, C, and folic acid) and minerals potassium. It is also a rich source of numerous phenolic compounds and alkaloids, triterpenes, and sterols which are well-known for their medicinal properties (Giménez-Bastida et al., 2021). Pomegranates are also rich in unsaturated fatty acids like omega-5 punicic acid which constitutes about 70% of pomegranate seed oil (Sreekumar et al., 2014; Zaouay et al., 2012). Numerous *in vitro* studies have reported the ability of pomegranate-related products (fruit, juice, and flower) to modulate the risk of cardiovascular disease.

9.2.15 CITRUS BERGAMOT

Bergamot and its products have been reported to have significant activity against several pathogens. Bergamot fruit possesses anti-fungal and bacteriostatic properties (Jin et al., 2016; Scuteri et al., 2018) while bergamot essential oil (BEO) is widely used in many cosmetic and perfumery industries (Verma et al., 2016). BEO has also been used in the pharmaceutical industry due to its antibacterial and antioxidant properties (Jiang et al., 2015; Watanabe et al., 2015). Moreover, in the recent scenario, BEO is being utilized for the preservation of food and is therefore considered a good alternative to chemical preservatives (Avila-Sosa et al., 2015).

9.2.16 VITAMIN C

Vitamin C (ascorbic acid) is one of the most vital micronutrients, which contributes to several important physiological processes inside the human body. Humans are not capable of producing vitamin C endogenously due to the mutation in the GULO gene and hence totally depend on dietary intake. It acts as a cofactor for numerous enzymatic reactions. Moreover, it can prevent oxidative damage to cells and work as an antioxidant (Van Gorkom et al., 2019). There are several possible mechanisms behind the action of vitamin C; however, one of the most important mechanisms is that vitamin C serves as a pro-oxidant and stimulates the generation of hydrogen peroxide, which leads to the formation of reactive oxygen species (ROS) that produce a cytotoxic effect on tumor cells (Chen et al., 2008).

9.3 TREATMENT MECHANISM OF DYSLIPIDEMIA INDUCE VASCULAR DISEASE

For treating dyslipidemia-induced vascular diseases different kinds of mechanisms are known some of which are summarized in Figure 9.3.

9.4 USE OF NUTRITIONAL SUPPLEMENTS TO TREAT DYSLIPIDEMIA INDUCED VASCULAR DISEASES

Dyslipidemia can induce different kinds of vascular disease, and to counter them apart from medication, humans are required to change their dietary habits so that it may curb these perilous diseases. There are different nutritional supplements that may counter dyslipidemia-induced vascular

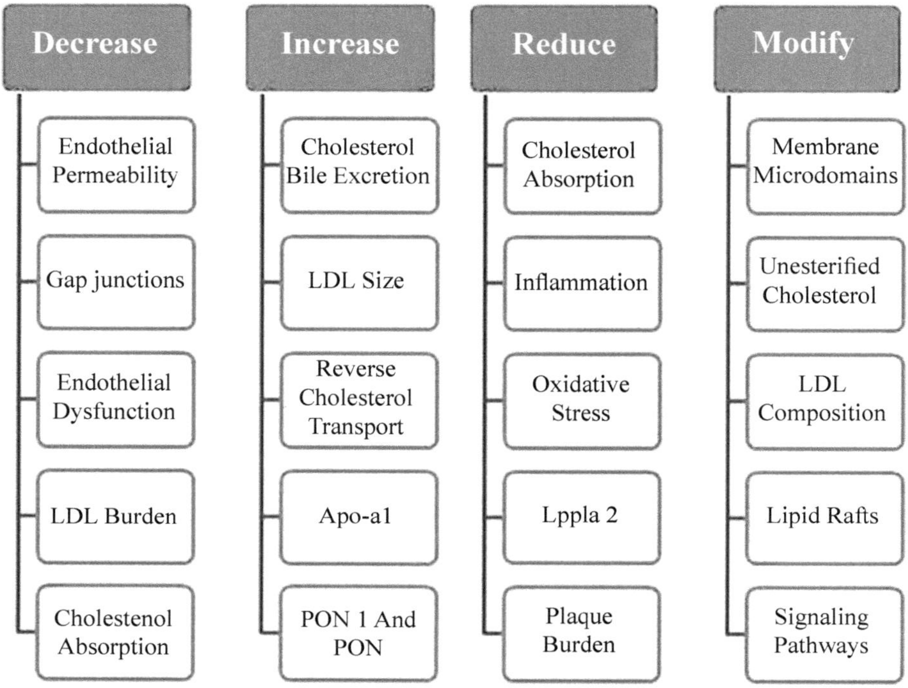

FIGURE 9.3 Different modes of action for decreasing dyslipidemia.

disease like Niacin, Green tea, Pantetheine, Garlic, Citrus fruits, etc., followed by some specific kinds of chemical inhibitors for the prevention like Carnosine, Histidine, Myricetin, Kaempferol, etc. The detailed mechanisms of action of different nutritional supplements are illustrated in Figures 9.4 and 9.5.

9.5 WAY FORWARD

The use of some lipid-lowering nutraceuticals (and their association) is supported by preclinical and clinical evidence of efficacy and safety. However, the use of nutraceuticals should never substitute the use of conventional drugs when their prescription is indicated by international guidelines.

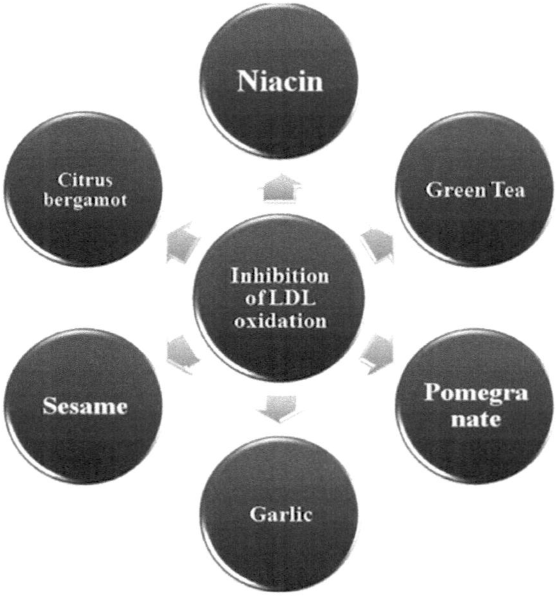

FIGURE 9.4 Food supplements are used to inhibit LDL oxidation.

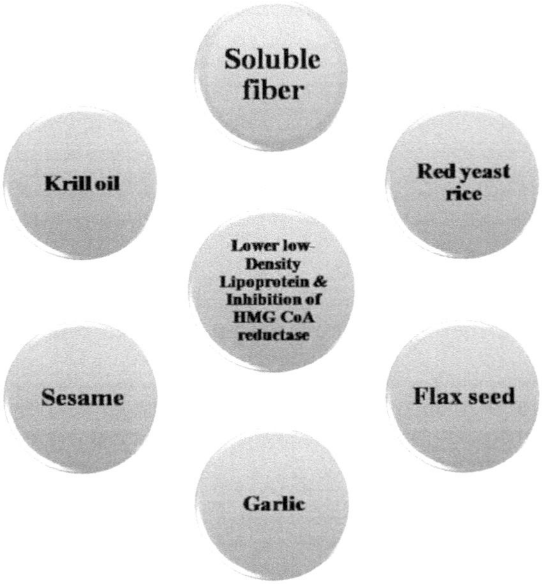

FIGURE 9.5 Food supplements inhibit HMG CoA reductase as well as lowering the density of lipoproteins.

KEYWORDS

- **cardiovascular disease**
- **classification**
- **coronary artery disease**
- **dyslipidemia**
- **lipid management**
- **low-density lipoprotein**
- **nutraceuticals**
- **triglycerides**
- **tumor necrosis factor**

REFERENCES

Adelaja, A. O., & Schilling, B. J. (1999). Nutraceutical: blurring the line between food and drugs in the twenty-first century. *Magazine of Food and Farm Resources, 14*, 35–40.

Al-Mohissen, M. A., Pun, S. C., & Frohlich, J. J. (2010). Niacin: from mechanisms of action to therapeutic uses. *Mini Reviews in Medicinal Chemistry, 10*, 204–217.

Bester, D., Esterhuyse, A. J., Truter, E. J., & van Rooven, J. (2010). Cardiovascular effects of edible oils: a comparison between four popular edible oils. *Nutrition Research Reviews, 23*, 334–348.

Bioedon, L. T., Balikai, S., Chittams, J., Cunnane, S. C., Berlin, J. A., Rader, D. J., Szapary, P. O., et al. (2008). Flaxseed and cardiovascular risk factors: results from a double-blind, randomized controlled clinical trial. *Journal of the American College of Nutrition, 27*, 65–74.

Brower, V. (1998). Nutraceuticals: poised for a healthy slice of the healthcare market? *Nature Biotechnology, 16*, 728–731.

Brown, A. L., Lane, J., Holyoak, C., Nicol, B., Mayes, A. E., & Dadd, T. (2011). Health effects of green tea catechins in overweight and obese men: a randomized controlled cross-over trial. *British Journal of Nutrition, 7*, 1–10.

Bull, E. (2000). What is nutraceutical? *Pharmaceutical Journal, 265*, 57–58.

Chen, Q., Espey, M. G., Sun, A. Y., Pooput, C., Kirk, K. L., Krishna, M. C., Khosh, D. B., et al. (2008). Pharmacologic doses of ascorbate act as a prooxidant and decrease growth of aggressive tumor xenografts in mice. *Proceedings of the National Academy of Sciences, 105*, 11105–11109.

Covas, M. I. (2007). Olive oil and the cardiovascular system. *Pharmacological Research, 55*, 175–186.

Das, L., Bhaumik, E., Raychaudhuri, U., & Chakraborty, R. (2012). Role of nutraceuticals in human health. *Journal of Food Science and Technology, 49*(2), 173–183.

Demirkol, O., Adams, C., & Ercal, N. (2004). Biologically important thiols in various vegetables and fruits. *Journal of Agricultural and Food Chemistry*, *52*(26), 8151–8154.
Demonty, I., Ras, R. T., van der Knaap, H. C., Duchateau, G. S., Meijer, L., Zock, P. L., Geleijnse, J. M., & Trautwein, E. A. (2009). Continuous dose-response relationship of the LDL cholesterol lowering effect of phytosterol intake. *Journal of Nutrition*, *139*, 271–284.
Derosa, G., Colletti, A., Maffioli, P., D'Angelo, A., Lupi, A., Zito, G. B., Mureddu, G. F., et al. (2020). Lipid-lowering nutraceuticals update on scientific evidence. *Journal of Cardiovascular Medicine*, *21*(11), 845–859.
Dureja, H., Kaushik, D., & Kumar, V. (2003). Developments in nutraceuticals. *Indian Journal of Pharmacology*, *35*, 363–372.
Giménez-Bastida, J. A., Ávila-Gálvez, M. Á., Espín, J. C., & González-Sarrías, A. (2021). Evidence for health properties of pomegranate juices and extracts beyond nutrition: A critical systematic review of human studies. *Trends in Food Science & Technology*, *114*, 410–423.
Gómez-Estaca, J., Balaguer, M. P., López-Carballo, G., Gavara, R., & Hernández-Muñoz, P. (2017). Improving antioxidant and antimicrobial properties of curcumin by means of encapsulation in gelatin through electrohydrodynamic atomization. *Food Hydrocolloids*, *70*, 313–320.
Harland, J. I., & Haffner, T. A. (2008). Systematic review, meta-analysis and regression of randomized controlled trials reporting an association between an intake of circa 25 g soya protein per day and blood cholesterol. *Atherosclerosis*, *200*, 13–27.
Horvath, Z., & Vecsei, L. (2009). Current medical aspects of pantethine. *Ideggyógyászati Szemle*, *8*, 220–229.
Houston, M. (2012). The role of nutraceutical supplements in the treatment of dyslipidemia. *Journal of Clinical Hypertension*, *14*(2), 121–132.
Houston, M. C., Fazio, S., Chilton, F. H., Wise, D. E., Jones, K. B., Barringer, T. A., & Bramlet, D. A. (2009). Non pharmacologic treatment of dyslipidemia. *Progress in Cardiovascular Diseases*, *52*, 61–94.
Jiang, T., Luo, Z., & Ying, T. (2015). Fumigation with essential oils improves sensory quality and enhances antioxidant ability of shiitake mushroom (*Lentinus edodes*). *Food Chemistry*, *172*, 692–698.
JIN, W. F. (2016). Research progress on bergamot essential oil and its related product development. *Chinese Traditional and Herbal Drugs*, *47*, 857–861.
Kalia, A. N. (2005). Textbook of Industrial Pharmacognosy. CBS Publisher and Distributor. pp.285. ISBN: 9788123912400.
Kannel, W. B., Castelli, W. P., Gordon, T., & McNamara, P. M. (1971). Serum cholesterol, lipoproteins, and the risk of coronary heart disease: the Framingham Study. *Annals of Internal Medicine*, *74*(1), 1–12.
Keservani, R. K., Kesharwani, R. K., Sharma, A. K., Vyas, N., & Chadoker, A. (2010b). Nutritional Supplements: An Overview. *International Journal of Current Pharmaceutical Review and Research*, *1*(1), 59–75.
Keservani, R. K., Kesharwani, R. K., Vyas, N., Jain, S., Raghuvanshi, R., & Sharma, A. K. (2010a). Nutraceutical and functional food as future food: a review. *Der Pharmacia Lettre*, *2*(1), 106–116.
Keservani, R. K., Sharma, A. K., & Kesharwani, R. K. (2017). An overview and therapeutic applications of nutraceutical and functional foods. In R. K. Keservani, A. K. Sharma, &

R. K. Kesharwani (Eds.), *Recent Advances in Drug Delivery Technology* (pp. 160–201). ISBN:9781522507543.

Keservani, R. K., Sharma, A. K., & Kesharwani, R. K. (Eds.). (2020). Nutraceuticals and Dietary Supplements: Applications in Health Improvement and Disease Management, Apple Academic Press, CRC Press. Pp. 1–344. ISBN: 9781771888738.

Kokate, C. K., Purohit, A. P., & Gohkale, S. B. (2002) Pharmacognosy. In: *Terpenoids*, 21st Edition, Nirali Prakashan, Pune, 377–378.

Kopp, P. (1998). Resveratrol, a phytoestrogen found in red wine. A possible explanation for the conundrum of the "French paradox"? *European Journal of Endocrinology*, *138*(6), 619–620.

Maddi, V. S., Aragade, P. D., Digge, V. G., & Nitaliker, M. N. (2007). Importance of nutraceuticals in health management. *Pharmacognosy Reviews*, *1*, 377–379.

Malik, A., Kumar, P., Kaushik, N., & Singh, A. (2008). The potentials of nutraceuticals. *Pharmainfo.net*, *6*, 151–183.

McRae, M. P. (2005). Treatment of hyperlipoproteinemia with pantethine: A review and analysis of efficacy and tolerability. *Nutrition Research*, *25*, 319–333.

Noorafshan, A., & Ashkani-Esfahani, S. (2013). A review of therapeutic effects of curcumin. *Current Pharmaceutical Design*, *19*(11), 2032–2046.

Othman, R. A., & Moghadasian, M. H. (2011). Beyond cholesterol-lowering effects of plant sterols: Clinical and experimental evidence of anti-inflammatory properties. *Nutrition Reviews*, *69*, 371–382.

Pandey, M., Verma, R. K., & Saraf, S. A. (2010). Nutraceuticals: New era of medicine and health. *Asian Journal of Pharmaceutical and Clinical Research*, *3*, 11–15.

Patch, C. S., Tapsell, L. C., Williams, P. G., & Gordon, M. (2006). Plant sterols as dietary adjuvants in the reduction of cardiovascular risk: Theory and evidence. *Vascular Health and Risk Management*, *2*, 157–162.

Pathak, N., Bhaduri, A., & Rai, A. K. (2019). Sesame: Bioactive compounds and health benefits. In *Bioactive Molecules in Food* (pp. 181–200).

Prasad, K. (2009). Flaxseed and cardiovascular health. *Journal of Cardiovascular Pharmacology*, *54*, 369–377.

Prasad, S., Tyagi, A. K., & Aggarwal, B. B. (2014). Recent developments in delivery, bioavailability, absorption and metabolism of curcumin: The golden pigment from golden spice. *Cancer Research and Treatment*, *46*(1), 2.

Qureshi, A. A., Sami, S. A., Salser, W. A., & Khan, F. A. (2001). Synergistic effect of tocotrienol-rich fraction (TRF 25) of rice bran and lovastatin on lipid parameters in hypercholesterolemic humans. *Journal of Nutritional Biochemistry*, *12*, 318–329.

R. Avila-Sosa, A. R. Navarro-Cruz, M. E. Sosa-Morales, A. López-Malo, & E. Palou. (2016). Chapter 27 – bergamot (*Citrus bergamia*) oils. *Essential Oils in Food Preservation Flavor & Safety*, pp. 247–252.

Rathore, S., Mukim, M., Sharma, P., Devi, S., Nagar, J. C., & Khalid, M. (2020). Curcumin: A review for health benefits. *International Journal of Research and Review*, *7*(1), 273–290.

Rheim, F. A., Ragab, A. A., Hamdy, H. E. D., & Hammam, F. M. (2015). Evaluation of DNA damage in-vivo by comet assay and chromosomal aberrations for pyrethroid insecticide and the antimutagenic: Role of curcumin. *Egyptian Journal of Hospital Medicine*, *59*, 172–181.

Ruparelia, N., Digby, J. E., & Choudhury, R. P. (2010). Effects of niacin on atherosclerosis and vascular function. *Current Opinion in Cardiology*, *26*(1), 66.

Saremi, A., & Arora, R. (2009). The utility of omega-3 fatty acids in cardiovascular disease. *American Journal of Therapeutics*, *16*, 421–436.

Scuteri, D., Crudo, M., Rombolà, L., Watanabe, C., Mizoguchi, H., Sakurada, S., Sakurada, T., Greco, R., Corasaniti, M. T., Morrone, L. A., & Bagetta, G. (2018). Antinociceptive effect of inhalation of the essential oil of bergamot in mice. *Fitoterapia*, *129*, 20–24.

Singh, A. P., Singh, R., Verma, S. S., Rai, V., Kaschula, C. H., Maiti, P., & Gupta, S. C. (2019). Health benefits of resveratrol: Evidence from clinical studies. *Medicinal Research Reviews*, *39*(5), 1851–1891.

Singh, D. K., Banerjee, S., & Porter, T. D. (2009). Green and black tea extracts inhibit HMG-CoA reductase and activate AMP kinase to decrease cholesterol synthesis in hepatoma cells. *Journal of Nutritional Biochemistry*, *20*, 816–822.

Sreekumar, S., Sithul, H., Muraleedharan, P., Azeez, J. M., & Sreeharshan, S. (2014). Pomegranate fruit as a rich source of biologically active compounds. *BioMed Research International*, *2014*, 1–12.

Takaoka, M. (1940). Of the phenolic substrate of hellebore (*Veratrum grandiflorum* Loes. fil.). *Journal of Faculty of Science, Hokkaido Imperial University*, *3*, 1–16.

Tian, N., Penman, A. D., Mawson, A. R., Manning Jr, R. D., & Flessner, M. F. (2010). Association between circulating specific leukocyte types and blood pressure: the atherosclerosis risk in communities (ARIC) study. *Journal of Hypertension*, *4*(6), 272–283.

Ungvari, Z., Kaley, G., De Cabo, R., Sonntag, W. E., & Csiszar, A. (2010). Mechanisms of vascular aging: new perspectives. *The Journals of Gerontology: Series A, Biological Sciences and Medical Sciences*, *65*, 1028–1041.

van Gorkom, G. N., Lookermans, E. L., Van Elssen, C. H., & Bos, G. M. (2019). The effect of vitamin C (ascorbic acid) in the treatment of patients with cancer: a systematic review. *Nutrients*, *11*(5), 977.

Verma, S. K., Goswami, P., Verma, R. S., Padalia, R. C., Chauhan, A., Singh, V. R., & Darokar, M. P. (2016). Chemical composition and antimicrobial activity of bergamot-mint (*Mentha citrata* Ehrh.) essential oils isolated from the herbage and aqueous distillate using different methods. *Industrial Crops and Products*, *91*, 152–160.

Watanabe, E., Kuchta, K., Kimura, M., Rauwald, H. W., Kamei, T., & Imanishi, J. (2015). Effects of bergamot (*Citrus bergamia* (Risso) Wright & Arn.) essential oil aromatherapy on mood states, parasympathetic nervous system activity, and salivary cortisol levels in 41 healthy females. *Journal of Complementary Medicine Research*, *22*(1), 43–49.

Weiss, E. A. (1971). Sesame, Castor and Safflower. Barnes and Noble, World Crop Series, Leonard Hill, New York. Pp. 311–525.

Wildman, R. E. C. (Ed.). (2001). *Handbook of Nutraceuticals and Functional Foods*. CRC Press, Boca Raton, pp. 1–568. ISBN: 9780429195570.

Zaouay, F., Mena, P., Garcia-Viguera, C., & Mars, M. (2012). Antioxidant activity and physico-chemical properties of Tunisian grown pomegranate (*Punica granatum* L.) cultivars. *Industrial Crops and Products*, *40*, 81–89.

CHAPTER 10

ROLE OF NUTRACEUTICALS IN HYPERTENSION

ABABIO GRACE K.

University of Ghana Medical School, Medical Biochemistry, Ghana, Africa

ABSTRACT

Nutraceuticals have proven beyond reasonable doubt their potency and efficacy. Their success depends on quality and safety maintenance. However, there remains a need for long-term safety data with the lowest risk-benefit ratio and the best cost-effectiveness for wider population coverage. As efforts are made to avoid toxicity, the ultimate choice involves a paradigm shift towards nutraceuticals to improve long-term compliance in the dietary management of hypertension.

10.1 INTRODUCTION

10.1.1 GENERAL OVERVIEW

Despite vast therapeutic approaches in hypertension, cardiovascular events remain one of the leading causes of death worldwide, and this is a public health concern. The urgent shift to nutraceuticals was in accordance with the fact that nutraceuticals provided benefits in the treatment of hypertension. Mediterranean diets and Dietary Approaches to Stop Hypertension (DASH) remain the widely utilized lifestyle approaches. Lots of evidence supports some nutraceuticals such as flavonoids, vitamins C and D, beetroot juice, some probiotics, garlic, and coffee to largely decrease cardiovascular events.

Antioxidants as Nutraceuticals. Nayan A. Gujarathi, Raj K. Keservani, Rajesh K. Kesharwani, Bhushan R. Rane, Yogeeta Sameer Goyal (Eds.)

However, other nutraceuticals such as flaxseed and green tea lack adequate findings. Quality and safety of nutraceuticals normally require consistent and reliable data in clinical trials. Attempts are made to avoid toxicity as nutraceuticals pass through regulatory control bodies.

10.1.2 NUTRACEUTICALS

A nutraceutical is a medicinal food that modulates immunity and enhances health (Abuajah et al., 2015). Nutraceuticals range from processed products of cereals, isolated nutrients, herbal products, dietary supplements, and genetically engineered foods. Nutraceuticals' therapeutic potential ranges from anti-sleep disorders to, the prevention of certain cancers, hypertension, osteoporosis, cholesterol control, diabetes, and depression. In the past few decades, there has been a surge in to production of nutraceuticals since it undoubtedly has a large market.

10.1.3 CLASSIFICATION OF NUTRACEUTICALS

Nutraceuticals are classified based on availability (Singh & Sinha, 2012) in the market and can be natural or synthetic.

Major classes include the following:

- Polyphenols
- Spices
- Dietary Fiber
- Antioxidants
- Probiotics
- Polyunsaturated fatty acids
- Prebiotics

10.1.4 THE VARIOUS CLASSES OF NUTRACEUTICALS AND THEIR EFFECTS ON HYPERTENSION

10.1.4.1 POLYPHENOLS

Polyphenols are phytochemicals (Stevenson & Hurst, 2007; Upadhyay & Dixit, 2015) comprising cereals, coffee, cocoa, fruits, wine, vegetables, legumes, whole grains, lignans, flavonoids (Ndiaye et al., 2008), stilbenes, and phenolic acids. Hydroxybenzoic derivatives (garlic, protocatechuic acid, p-hydroxybenzoic acid) and hydroxycinnamic acid derivatives (coumaric, caffeic acid, ferulic, chlorogenic acid, sinapic acid) are the two types of phenolic acids. Cherry, pear, berry fruits, kiwi, apple, chicory, and coffee contain phenolic acids. Anthocyanins, flavones, flavonols, isoflavones, and flavanones make up flavonoids. Anthocyanins are found in red wine, berries, red cabbage, strawberry, and black grape (Ndiaye et al., 2004). Grapes and wine decrease oxidative stress (Micallef et al., 2007; Pari & Suresh, 2008), inhibit platelet aggregation (Vitseva et al., 2005; Keevil et al., 2000; Dohadwala & Vita, 2009), and decrease LDL oxidation (Dohadwala & Vita, 2009). Even though the mechanism of grapes and wine is not well understood, it is thereby proposed in this write-up that grapefruit inhibits cytochrome P450 (Guo & Yamazoe, 2004; Edwards et al., 1996; Tassaneeyakul et al., 2000) interaction system, especially CYP3A4 (Veronese et al., 2003; Paine et al., 2005; Ho et al., 2001; Paine et al., 2004). CYP3A4 metabolizes statin drugs. Statins are lipid-lowering drugs. Statins inhibit HMG-CoA reductase (Istvan & Deisenhofer, 2001; Istvan, 2003; Istvan, 2002). Thus, it is logical to note that when CYP3A4 is inhibited by grapefruit, statins would not be metabolized or degraded by xenobiotics. Statins would then be free and could lower the higher lipid levels. Many studies have also indicated flavonoid properties ranging from anti-inflammatory, cardio-protective, and antioxidants (Nile et al., 2018). Notwithstanding the added input, there have been conflicting results with the association between flavonoid intake and total coronary heart disease.

10.1.4.2 SPICES

Spices have been indispensable since antiquity. Apart from seasoning and flavor, spices are used in indigenous medicines (Sharif et al., 2018), beverages, aromatherapy, cosmetics, perfumes, preservatives, natural colors, dental preparations, and pesticides. One unique and widely marketed spicy product in India is Chyawanprash (Sharma et al., 2019; Aryal, 2021) and it is composed of clove, cinnamon, *Curcuma spp.,* long pepper, and saffron. Chyawanprash boosts immunity, prevents cough, asthma, heart disease, fever, and impotency, increases digestion, and prevents coarse speech. Saffron (*Crocus sativus*) as a complexion skin promoter due to crocin and cicrocrocin found in saffron. Turmeric, clove, red pepper, ginger, black pepper, garlic, rosemary, coriander, and cinnamon have been indicated to act against neurodegenerative diseases (Kannappan et al., 2011; Bhagya & Raveendra, 2017). Turmeric regulates sebum in human skin. Allicin in garlic (Londhe et al., 2011) makes it cardio-protective (Banerjee & Maulik, 2002), an inhibitor of platelet aggregation (Rahman, 2007), a vasodilator, and aids in fibrinolysis.

10.1.4.3 DIETARY FIBER

Lignins and non-digestible carbohydrates in humans are termed dietary fibers (Mudgil & Barak, 2013; Champ et al., 2003). Total fiber equals dietary plus functional fiber. Functional fiber has beneficial effects in humans as shown in Table 10.1. Dietary Reference Intake (DRI) of fiber is 38 grams/day for men and 25 grams/day for women.

TABLE 10.1 Characteristics of Dietary Fiber

Physiological Characteristics	Effects	Benefits
Fermentation	Enables the growth of bacteria Ensures short-chain fatty acid production	Decrease glucose levels, insulin levels, and lipid levels after meals
Interaction	Interact with digestive enzymes	Defense against colorectal cancer and inflammation
Soluble dietary fiber	Delays or prevent nutrient uptake Inhibit reabsorption of bile acids Delays gastric emptying	Decrease glucose levels, insulin levels, and lipid levels after meals Prevent breast cancer
Insoluble dietary fiber	Increase stool transit time and stool weight	Decrease colorectal cancer and decrease the time taken for nutrient absorption

10.1.4.4 ANTIOXIDANTS

The known classes of antioxidants (Abourashed, 2013) include:

- Antioxidant enzymes, such as glutathione peroxidase, superoxide dismutase, and glutathione reductase, are involved in mopping up reactive oxidant species.

- Metal binding proteins, e.g., albumin, ferritin, ceruloplasmin, lactoferrin.
- Antioxidant phytonutrients from food.
- Physiological antioxidants:
- Endogenous: Bilirubin and thiols, e.g., lipoic acid, glutathione, N-acetyl cysteine.
- Dietary antioxidants, e.g., ascorbic acid (vitamin C), tocopherols and tocotrienols (vitamin E), carotenoids, and other low molecular weight compounds such as glutathione and lipoic acid.

Studies have indicated that decreased levels of vitamin E were associated with an increase in cardiovascular events, while lower levels of vitamin C were likewise associated with increased cardiovascular events and vice versa (Jha, 1995). In a 17-week confirmatory study on controlled diet depletion-repletion of vitamin C, an inverse correlation between vitamin C levels and blood pressure was noted (EFSA Panel on Dietetic Products, 2015). The recommended daily intake of vitamin C is 100 mcg/L. Vitamin C decreases angiotensin I receptor binding (Leclerc et al., 2008) without modifying its maximal binding capacity and affinity of angiotensin II receptor.

Lower levels of vitamin D have also been implicated in the inverse relationship with coronary heart disease (Anagnostis et al., 2010). Vitamin D, from sunlight as well, is involved in calcium-phosphate homeostasis (Taylor & Bushinsky, 2009). Low sunlight and low levels of vitamin D have been implicated in increased risk of myocardial infarction, heart failure, peripheral vascular disease, and stroke. Even though authors have duly indicated the relationship between vitamin D and heart diseases, there have not been any randomized clinical studies to confirm or affirm these facts. Much work is needed in this regard.

Among carotenoids (the same family to which vitamin A belongs), lycopene remains the major antioxidant compound. Lycopene is found in tomatoes, red peppers, watermelon, red fruits, and vegetables like papayas. Even though several studies have related lycopene to a decreased incidence of cardiovascular events (Arab & Steck, 2000; Rao, 2002; Mordente et al., 2011; Riccioni et al., 2008), the effect of its supplementation remains unconfirmed.

10.1.4.5 PROBIOTICS

Yeast and live bacteria are types of probiotics (Czerucka et al., 2007) that are good for our digestive system. Probiotics naturally occur in our bodies.

One may also find probiotics in foods and supplements. Lactobacillus is the most common probiotic (Pace et al., 2015) found in fermented foods and yogurt. Bifidobacterium is another probiotic (Pace et al., 2015) found in dairy products. Bifidobacterium is used to treat infectious diarrhea (caused by viruses, parasites, or bacteria), oral health, irritable bowel syndrome, allergies, eczema, common cold, inflammatory bowel disease, antibiotic-related diarrhea, and urinary and vaginal health.

10.1.4.6 POLYUNSATURATED FATTY ACIDS (PUFA)

ω-3 and ω-6 fatty acids are the known polyunsaturated fatty acids (Panda et al., 2022). ω-3 increases LDL and HDL cholesterol slightly as well as decreasing triglycerides only at high concentrations. ω-3 decreases free fatty acids delivery to the liver and decreases the activity of triglyceride-synthesizing enzymes. It is not so surprising to see conflicting results regarding the relationship between PUFA and cardiovascular events. Notwithstanding the added input, long-chain ω-3 PUFAs inhibit the synthesis of thromboxanes (a vasoconstrictor). ω-3 PUFA enhances the release of nitric oxide & acts as a vasodilator (Luo & Liu, 2020). Epigenetics in ω-3 PUFA genes of individuals could account for the difference in response.

10.1.4.7 PREBIOTICS

Even though prebiotics are fiber (Slavin, 2013), not all fibers are prebiotics. Prebiotics resist the acidic nature in the gastrointestinal tract, prevent hydrolysis by enzymes, and inhibit upper gastrointestinal tract absorption. A good prebiotic should be fermented by intestinal flora. Again, prebiotics should selectively stimulate the growth and activity of intestinal flora. Prebiotics decrease inflammation and symptoms associated with inflammatory bowel disease (Steed et al., 2008). Prebiotics prevent colon cancer (Wollowski et al., 2001); enable the uptake of magnesium, calcium, and iron; and decrease the risk of cardiovascular events. Prebiotics prevent obesity.

10.2 CONCLUSION

This write-up indicated the importance of nutraceuticals in the treatment of hypertension with a coherent improvement in diet and lifestyle.

ACKNOWLEDGMENT

The author is grateful to the University of Ghana Medical School for the online platform of varying resources.

KEYWORDS

- **antioxidants**
- **dietary fibers**
- **dietary reference intake**
- **hypertension**
- **nutraceuticals**
- **polyphenols**
- **polyunsaturated fatty acids**
- **prebiotics**
- **probiotics**

REFERENCES

Abourashed, E. A. (2013). Bioavailability of plant-derived antioxidants. *Antioxidants*, *2*(4), 309–325.

Abuajah, C. I., Ogbonna, A. C., & Osuji, C. M. (2015). Functional components and medicinal properties of food: A review. *Journal of Food Science and Technology*, *52*(5), 2522–2529.

Anagnostis, P., Athyros, V. G., Adamidou, F., Florentin, M., & Karagiannis, A. (2010). Vitamin D and cardiovascular disease: a novel agent for reducing cardiovascular risk? *Current Vascular Pharmacology*, *8*(5), 720–730.

Arab, L., & Steck, S. (2000). Lycopene and cardiovascular disease. *The American Journal of Clinical Nutrition*, *71*(6), 1691S–1695S.

Aryal, B., Paudyal, P., Ghimire, K., Sharma, S., & Khanal, D. P. (2021). Quality Assessment of Five Different Brands of Chyawanprash Marketed in Nepal. *Journal of Food Quality*, 2021.

Banerjee, S. K., & Maulik, S. K. (2002). Effect of garlic on cardiovascular disorders: a review. *Nutrition Journal*, *1*(1), 1–14.

Bhagya, H. P., & Raveendra, Y. C. (2017). Multi-beneficial uses of spices: A brief review.

Champ, M., Langkilde, A. M., Brouns, F., Kettlitz, B., & Collet, Y. L. B. (2003). Advances in dietary fibre characterisation. 1. Definition of dietary fibre, physiological relevance, health benefits and analytical aspects. *Nutrition Research Reviews*, *16*(1), 71–82.

Czerucka, D., Piche, T., & Rampal, P. (2007). Yeast as probiotics–*Saccharomyces boulardii*. *Alimentary Pharmacology and Therapeutics*, *26*(6), 767–778.
Dohadwala, M. M., & Vita, J. A. (2009). Grapes and cardiovascular disease. *The Journal of Nutrition*, *139*(9), 1788S–1793S.
Edwards, D. J., Bellevue, F. H., & Woster, P. M. (1996). Identification of 6,'7'-dihydroxybergamottin, a cytochrome P450 inhibitor, in grapefruit juice. *Drug Metabolism and Disposition*, *24*(12), 1287–1290.
EFSA Panel on Dietetic Products, Nutrition and Allergies (NDA). (2015). Scientific opinion on dietary reference values for magnesium. *EFSA Journal*, *13*(7), 4186.
Guo, L. Q., & Yamazoe, Y. (2004). Inhibition of cytochrome P450 by furanocoumarins in grapefruit juice and herbal medicines. *Acta Pharmacologica Sinica*, *25*(2), 129–136.
Ho, P. C., Saville, D. J., & Wanwimolruk, S. (2001). Inhibition of human CYP3A4 activity by grapefruit flavonoids, furanocoumarins and related compounds. *J Pharm Pharm Sci*, *4*(3), 217–27.
Istvan, E. (2003). Statin inhibition of HMG-CoA reductase: A 3-dimensional view. *Atherosclerosis Supplements*, *4*(1), 3–8.
Istvan, E. S. (2002). Structural mechanism for statin inhibition of 3-hydroxy-3-methylglutaryl coenzyme A reductase. *American Heart Journal*, *144*(6), S27–S32.
Istvan, E. S., & Deisenhofer, J. (2001). Structural mechanism for statin inhibition of HMG-CoA reductase. *Science*, *292*(5519), 1160–1164.
Jha, P., Flather, M., Lonn, E., Farkouh, M., & Yusuf, S. (1995). The antioxidant vitamins and cardiovascular disease: a critical review of epidemiologic and clinical trial data. *Annals of Internal Medicine*, *123*(11), 860–872.
Kannappan, R., Gupta, S. C., Kim, J. H., Reuter, S., & Aggarwal, B. B. (2011). Neuroprotection by spice-derived nutraceuticals: you are what you eat! *Molecular Neurobiology*, *44*(2), 142–159.
Keevil, J. G., Osman, H. E., Reed, J. D., & Folts, J. D. (2000). Grape juice, but not orange juice or grapefruit juice, inhibits human platelet aggregation. *The Journal of Nutrition*, *130*(1), 53–56.
Leclerc, P. C., Proulx, C. D., Arguin, G., Bélanger, S., Gobeil Jr, F., Escher, E., & Guillemette, G. (2008). Ascorbic acid decreases the binding affinity of the AT1 receptor for angiotensin II. *American Journal of Hypertension*, *21*(1), 67–71.
Londhe, V. P., Gavasane, A. T., Nipate, S. S., Bandawane, D. D., & Chaudhari, P. D. (2011). Role of garlic (*Allium sativum*) in various diseases: An overview. *Angiogenesis*, 12, 13.
Luo, Y., & Liu, J. Y. (2020). Pleiotropic functions of cytochrome P450 monooxygenase-derived eicosanoids in cancer. *Frontiers in Pharmacology*, *11*, 1–13.
Micallef, M., Lexis, L., & Lewandowski, P. (2007). Red wine consumption increases antioxidant status and decreases oxidative stress in the circulation of both young and old humans. *Nutrition Journal*, *6*(1), 1–8.
Mordente, A., Guantario, B., Meucci, E., Silvestrini, A., Lombardi, E., Martorana, G. E., & Bohm, V. (2011). Lycopene and cardiovascular diseases: an update. *Current Medicinal Chemistry*, *18*(8), 1146–1163.
Mudgil, D., & Barak, S. (2013). Composition, properties and health benefits of indigestible carbohydrate polymers as dietary fiber: A review. *International Journal of Biological Macromolecules*, 61, 1–6.
Ndiaye, M., Chataigneau, T., Chataigneau, M., & Schini-Kerth, V. B. (2004). Red wine polyphenols induce EDHF-mediated relaxations in porcine coronary arteries through the

redox-sensitive activation of the PI3-kinase/Akt pathway. *British Journal of Pharmacology, 142*(7), 1131–1136.
Nile, S. H., Keum, Y. S., Nile, A. S., Jalde, S. S., & Patel, R. V. (2018). Antioxidant, anti-inflammatory, and enzyme inhibitory activity of natural plant flavonoids and their synthesized derivatives. *Journal of Biochemical and Molecular Toxicology, 32*(1), e22002.
Pace, F., Pace, M., & Quartarone, G. (2015). Probiotics in digestive diseases: focus on *Lactobacillus GG*. *Minerva Gastroenterologica e Dietologica, 61*(4), 273–292.
Paine, M. F., Criss, A. B., & Watkins, P. B. (2004). Two major grapefruit juice components differ in intestinal CYP3A4 inhibition kinetic and binding properties. *Drug Metabolism and Disposition, 32*(10), 1146–1153.
Paine, M. F., Criss, A. B., & Watkins, P. B. (2005). Two major grapefruit juice components differ in time to onset of intestinal CYP3A4 inhibition. *Journal of Pharmacology and Experimental Therapeutics, 312*(3), 1151–1160.
Panda, C., Varadharaj, S., & Voruganti, V. S. (2022). PUFA, genotypes and risk for cardiovascular disease. *Prostaglandins, Leukotrienes and Essential Fatty Acids, 176*, 102377.
Pari, L., & Suresh, A. (2008). Effect of grape (*Vitis vinifera* L.) leaf extract on alcohol-induced oxidative stress in rats. *Food and Chemical Toxicology, 46*(5), 1627–1634.
Rahman, K. (2007). Effects of garlic on platelet biochemistry and physiology. *Molecular Nutrition & Food Research, 51*(11), 1335–1344.
Rao, A. V. (2002). Lycopene, tomatoes, and the prevention of coronary heart disease. *Experimental Biology and Medicine, 227*(10), 908–913.
Riccioni, G., Mancini, B., Di Ilio, E., Bucciarelli, T., & D Orazio, N. (2008). Protective effect of lycopene in cardiovascular disease. *European Review for Medical and Pharmacological Sciences, 12*(3), 183.
Sharif, M. K., Ejaz, R., & Pasha, I. (2018). Nutritional and therapeutic potential of spices. In *Therapeutic, Probiotic, and Unconventional Foods* (pp. 181–199). Academic Press.
Sharma, R., Martins, N., Kuca, K., Chaudhary, A., Kabra, A., Rao, M. M., & Prajapati, P. K. (2019). Chyawanprash: a traditional Indian bioactive health supplement. *Biomolecules, 9*(5), 161.
Singh, J., & Sinha, S. (2012). Classification, regulatory acts and applications of nutraceuticals for health. *International Journal of Pharma and Bio Sciences, 2*(1), 177–187.
Slavin, J. (2013). Fiber and prebiotics: mechanisms and health benefits. *Nutrients, 5*(4), 1417–1435.
Steed, H., Macfarlane, G. T., & Macfarlane, S. (2008). Prebiotics, symbiotic and inflammatory bowel disease. *Molecular Nutrition & Food Research, 52*(8), 898–905.
Stevenson, D. E., & Hurst, R. D. (2007). Polyphenolic phytochemicals–just antioxidants or much more? *Cellular and Molecular Life Sciences, 64*(22), 2900–2916.
Tassaneeyakul, W., Guo, L. Q., Fukuda, K., Ohta, T., & Yamazoe, Y. (2000). Inhibition selectivity of grapefruit juice components on human cytochromes P450. *Archives of Biochemistry and Biophysics, 378*(2), 356–363.
Taylor, J. G., & Bushinsky, D. A. (2009). Calcium and phosphorus homeostasis. *Blood Purification, 27*(4), 387–394.
Upadhyay, S., & Dixit, M. (2015). Role of polyphenols and other phytochemicals on molecular signaling. *Oxidative Medicine and Cellular Longevity*. Pp. 1–15.
Veronese, M. L., Gillen, L. P., Burke, J. P., Dorval, E. P., Hauck, W. W., Pequignot, E., & Greenberg, H. E. (2003). Exposure-dependent inhibition of intestinal and hepatic CYP3A4 in vivo by grapefruit juice. *The Journal of Clinical Pharmacology, 43*(8), 831–839.

Vitseva, O., Varghese, S., Chakrabarti, S., Folts, J. D., & Freedman, J. E. (2005). Grape seed and skin extracts inhibit platelet function and release of reactive oxygen intermediates. *Journal of Cardiovascular Pharmacology*, *46*(4), 445–451.

Wollowski, I., Rechkemmer, G., & Pool-Zobel, B. L. (2001). Protective role of probiotics and prebiotics in colon cancer. *The American Journal of Clinical Nutrition*, *73*(2), 451s–455s.

CHAPTER 11

DIETARY SUPPLEMENTATION AND CARDIAC HEALTH

BHUSHAN R. RANE,[1] NIDHI S. KATE,[1] AKASH J. AMKAR,[1] JAFFAR SHAIK,[2] AMIT KUMAR NAYAK,[3] and RAJ K. KESERVANI[4]

[1]*Shri D.D. Vispute College of Pharmacy and Research Center, Devad-Vichumbe, Panvel, Navi Mumbai, Maharashtra, India*

[2]*Research Scholar, Department of Biochemistry, Acharya Nagarjuna University, Guntur, Andhra Pradesh, India*

[3]*Department of Pharmacy, School of Medical and Allied Sciences, GD Goenka University, Gurgaon, Haryana, India*

[4]*Faculty of B. Pharmacy, CSM Group of Institutions, Prayagraj, Uttar Pradesh, India*

ABSTRACT

Cardiovascular disease (CVD) is a major cause of death in the world. Cardiac health problems or CVDs are greatly correlated with dietary or nutritional factors, which are important in daily life. Due to the inadequacy of dietary supplements, it impacts cardiac health. CVDs can be prevented by quitting smoking, consuming a specific diet, controlling blood pressure, increasing physical exercise, and maintaining a healthy weight. Furthermore, it has been reported that certain dietary supplements contain a variety of active components that have shown promise in the management and/or prevention of cardiac health problems or acquired CVDs. The significance of dietary supplements such as Fish oil, Ginseng, Garlic, Green tea, Co-enzyme Q, Omega-3 fatty acid, Vitamin C, and Vitamin E as cardioprotective agents is

Antioxidants as Nutraceuticals. Nayan A. Gujarathi, Raj K. Keservani, Rajesh K. Kesharwani, Bhushan R. Rane, Yogeeta Sameer Goyal (Eds.)

discussed, with claims that they can reduce CVD risk and that they should be included in daily diets.

11.1 INTRODUCTION

The major cause of death in the world is cardiovascular disease (CVD). Heart attacks, peripheral arterial disorder, rheumatic heart disease, deep vein thrombosis, strokes, congenital heart disorders, and pulmonary embolism are only a few of the conditions that are thought to be included in the group of conditions known as cardiovascular diseases (Abdel-Sattar et al., 2017).

According to the World Health Organization, CVD led to the deaths of 17.9 million individuals worldwide in 2019, accounting for 32% of all deaths. Heart attacks and strokes were responsible for 85% of these deaths. Around three-quarters of CVD mortality occurs in low and middle-income countries. CVDs were accountable for 38% of the 17 million fatalities caused by noncommunicable diseases (under the age of 70) in 2019. Behavioral risk factors such as cigarette use, smoking, obesity and poor diet, physical inactivity, and alcohol misuse can all be avoided. It is important to diagnose cardiovascular diseases as soon as possible to begin counseling and medication.

Poor food quality is closely linked to high morbidity and mortality from cardiovascular disease (Atkins et al., 2014). This scientific statement emphasizes the importance of dietary patterns over specific foods or nutrients, emphasizes the importance of nutrition early in life, presents features of heart-healthy dietary patterns, and highlights structural barriers to adherence to heart-healthy dietary patterns (Lichtenstein et al., 2021). Researchers have examined the close relationship between food and other lifestyle factors and certain diseases. In this regard, CVDs have received a lot of attention since vessel walls are constantly exposed to harmful food metabolites. This triggered research into the "protective" properties of plant-based foods and drinks with the aim of creating secure "nutritional remedies" for the management and prevention of CVDs (Abdel-Sattar et al., 2017).

Recent developments in our expertise of the pathways that lead to CVD provide a useful framework for supplement selections. CVD is characterized by poor circulation, which can be caused by a lack of cardiac output, a block obstructing the free flow of blood through the vascular system, or both. Increased heart strength to improve pumping action, dilatation of blood vessels, decreased peripheral resistance, and increased vascular tone are all therapeutic techniques for boosting cardiac output and venous return. Approaches to enhance blood flow through the vessels center around avoiding atherosclerotic plaque build-up and occlusion by reducing endothelial injury and inflammation, reducing dietary fat uptake, lowering the production and oxidation of low-density lipoprotein cholesterol (LDL-C), decreasing the possibility of thrombus formation, and minimizing the damage caused by oxidative damage (DeBusk & Ruth, 2000).

Dietary adjustments have been reported to lower the risk of premature CHD by 82% (Stampfer et al., 2000), whereas nutrition-related measures alone may lower the risk by 60% (Lichtenstein et al., 2006). Dietary supplements are non-food supplements that offer a concentrated variety of a presumed bioactive element (nutraceutical) from a food in a non-food matrix (often in solid dosage form) to improve health in dosages that are higher than those found in normal food. Polyphenols, phytoestrogens, organosulfur compounds, peptides, and vitamins are among the chemical entities covered by nutraceutical ingredients (Keservani et al., 2017, 2020). Bioactive ingredients, which are generally of plant origin, are of interest in combating dyslipidemia and, as a result, lowering the risk of cardiovascular disease (Vasanthi et al., 2010).

11.2 CARDIOVASCULAR DISEASE

Cardiovascular diseases (CVDs) are a collection of disorders that have an impact on the blood vessels and heart (Keservani et al., 2016a). It includes a condition where the blood vessels that supply the heart muscle are affected, known as coronary heart disease; cerebrovascular disease is a disorder of the blood vessels that supply the brain; and peripheral arterial disease is a disorder of the blood vessels that supply the limbs and legs. Streptococcal bacteria in rheumatic fever cause significant damage to the muscle and valves of the heart in rheumatic heart disease; congenital heart disease is a birth defect brought on by structural flaws in the heart from conception, which affect the heart's ability to develop and function normally; deep vein thrombosis and pulmonary embolism are terms for blood clots in the legs that can move and migrate to the heart and lungs (Abdel-Sattar et al., 2017). The various types of acquired CVDs that are likely to be positively influenced by dietary items are briefly detailed here (Abdel-Sattar et al., 2017).

11.2.1 ACQUIRED CARDIOVASCULAR DISEASES

11.2.1.1 CORONARY ARTERY DISEASE AND CORONARY HEART DISEASE

Coronary artery disease is a condition that causes blood flow to be obstructed in the blood arteries that supply the heart muscles. Due to the development of myocardial ischemia (reduction in blood flow to muscles of the heart), the symptoms are also referred to as "ischemic heart disease." Coronary thrombosis (blood clot formation), coronary spasm, and the hemodynamic (blood-flow) demands of the heart muscle are all elements that can turn coronary artery disease into coronary heart disease. Influences inside the heart muscle itself may raise the demand for blood flow over what is available, exposing the myocardium to changes in function, contractility, and the ability to maintain a regular rhythm (Senior et al., 2010).

Coronary heart disease encompasses all symptoms that arise as a result of advanced coronary artery disease due to myocardial ischemia, which is the major cause of death. It also covers a variety of disorders, the most important of which is atherosclerosis, which is defined as the formation of plaque on the artery walls. This may lead to blood vessels narrowing and reduced blood flow, which could lead to the formation of a blood clot. In this instance, the heart muscle supplied by that artery begins to die, resulting in a heart attack or stroke. Cigarette smoking, hypercholesterolemia, and hypertension are the three main risk factors for coronary heart disease (Senior et al., 2010).

The gut microbiota is associated with mediating basic metabolic processes, such as cholesterol metabolism, uric acid metabolism, oxidative stress, and inflammatory mediators, through its metabolites, which can contribute to the development of atherosclerosis and coronary heart disease (Liu et al., 2020). According to recent studies, blood TMAO concentrations are substantially linked to the risk of coronary heart disease (Wang et al., 2015). TMAO has also been proven in clinical investigations to increase the risk of cardiovascular disease (Otto & Rahimi, 2016). One of the independent potential risk factors for coronary heart disease may be the level of serum uric acid (Brown & Hazen, 2018).

11.2.1.2 ANGINA PECTORIS

Angina pectoris is a chest pain or spasm caused by the heart muscle's inability to receive enough oxygen due to occluded coronary arteries. The angina discomfort is generally accompanied by a feeling of suffocation. As a result of the imbalance in heart muscle demand and supply, myocardial ischemia develops (Senior et al., 2010).

11.2.1.3 HEART ATTACK (MYOCARDIAL INFARCTION)

Heart attack (myocardial infarction) is an acute disorder of necrosis that occurs in response to an imbalance between coronary blood supply and myocardial demand, resulting in what is called coronary thrombosis or coronary occlusion (Senior et al., 2010). Myocardial infarction is also seen as a complex condition that affects the heart's mechanical, electrical, structural, and biochemical aspects (Ruiz Petrich et al., 1996) (Bakheet et al., 2014). Acute myocardial infarction, cardiogenic shock, and death are all increased by TMAO, which increases the risk of cardiovascular disease (Otto & Rahimi, 2016). Chest aches or discomfort that can spread to the jaw, arm, shoulder, neck, or back are its defining symptoms (Azab & Elsayed, 2017). Acute myocardial infarction, along with non-ST-elevation myocardial infarction and unstable angina, is a disorder that falls under the term of coronary syndromes. About 90% of myocardial infarctions are brought on by an acute thrombus that blocks an atherosclerotic coronary artery (Domma & Gamal, 2015).

11.2.1.4 RHEUMATIC HEART DISEASE

Rheumatic heart disease is caused by Streptococcal bacteria causing rheumatic fever, which damages the heart muscle and valves. Rheumatic heart disease (RHD) is characterized by long-term damage to the heart's valves, which occurs as a major complication of recurrent episodes of acute rheumatic fever (ARF) (Katzenellenbogen et al., 2017). Acute rheumatic fever is driven by a complex interaction between group A streptococcus (GAS) and a vulnerable host. The joints and heart are usually affected. Carditis is a complication of cardiac involvement. Acute rheumatic carditis may resolve or develop into a chronic form of rheumatic heart disease (Arvind & Ramakrishnan, 2020).

11.2.1.5 CARDIAC ARRHYTHMIA

In cardiac arrhythmia, the heartbeat becomes irregular, either too slow (Bradycardia), too fast (tachycardia), or irregular (abnormal heart rhythm). In such circumstances, the heart might not be capable of pumping enough blood. Cardiac arrhythmias are more common as people get older, contributing to higher morbidity and mortality in the elderly. The prevalence of cardiac arrhythmias, particularly atrial fibrillation (AF) and ventricular tachyarrhythmia, is expected to rise as the population ages, putting a strain on healthcare resources (Mirza et al., 2012).

11.2.1.6 CEREBROVASCULAR DISEASE

Cerebrovascular disease affects the blood vessels that transport blood to the brain. It is also known as "ischemic stroke" (the most common variety), and it occurs when a blood vessel feeding the brain becomes clogged, causing brain cells to die (Paul & Candelario-Jalil, 2021). When blood vessels in the brain burst, it causes a "hemorrhagic stroke," which is almost always caused by hypertension (Abdel-Sattar et al., 2018).

11.2.1.7 PERIPHERAL ARTERIAL DISEASE

Peripheral arterial disease affects the blood vessels that deliver blood to the arms and legs (Abdel-Sattar et al., 2017). The narrowing and obstruction of antegrade flow of major systemic arteries other than those of the cerebral and coronary circulations is known as peripheral arterial disease (PAD) or peripheral vascular disease (PVD). In addition to atherosclerosis, other potential causes of PAD include degenerative disorders, dysplastic syndrome, vasculitis, thrombosis, and thromboembolism (Conte & Vale, 2018).

11.2.1.8 DEEP VEIN THROMBOSIS AND PULMONARY EMBOLISM

Venous thromboembolism can cause deep vein thrombosis and pulmonary embolism. Although deep vein thrombosis most commonly affects the legs, it can also affect the deep veins of the arms, the splanchnic veins, and the cerebral veins (Di Nisio et al., 2016). VTE is most common in places with low blood flow, such as venous valves and sinuses, where fibrin aggregates stimulate clotting factors locally, causing thrombus formation and propagation via the coagulation factors (Wenger et al., 2021).

11.3 OXIDATIVE STRESS-INDUCED CARDIOVASCULAR DISEASE

"A disturbance in the pro-oxidant/antioxidant balance that favors oxidation" is defined as oxidative stress (Sies et al., 1985). The brain and eye, as well as the respiratory, circulatory, and reproductive systems, are the organs and/or systems most vulnerable to oxidative injury. Oxidative damage puts a strain on the body's regular activities and can lead to the development of a variety of disorders (Vijayalakshmi & Chandrasekhar, 2008). The fundamental mechanism for several cardiovascular risk factors (diabetes and obesity) has been identified as oxidative stress (Seres et al., 2006) and has an impact on the development of several severe diseases, such as cardiovascular disease, some cancers, and neurodegenerative disorders (Ferrari & Torres, 2003).

Many free radicals found in living systems are unstable and extremely reactive, disrupting the balance of biological systems by destroying important constituent molecules, eventually leading to cell death. These radicals can be produced by NADP oxidase, xanthine oxidase, lipoxygenase, mitochondria, or the uncoupling of nitric oxide synthase in vascular cells, and they can harm the cell's lipids, membranes, proteins, and DNA (Parabathina et al., 2010). Free radicals can also react with serum low-density lipoproteins and eventually oxidize LDL, harming the arterial wall (Vijayalakshmi & Chandrasekhar, 2008). Oxygen-free radicals and their derivatives capable of causing oxidative damage, commonly referred to as active or reactive oxygen species, can be cytotoxic when in excess. NADPH oxidase, a critical enzyme in the formation of reactive oxygen species (ROS) that is expressed by a variety of cell types in both the artery wall and the blood, has been linked to hypercholesterolemia pathogenesis (Cave et al., 2006; Keaney et al., 2005; Stokes et al., 2007).

11.4 CANCER THERAPY-INDUCED CARDIOTOXICITY

Cardiotoxicity is caused by a combination of "on-target" and "off-target" consequences in cancer therapy. These effects are the result of redundancy in key signaling pathways that promote cancer cell growth while also protecting cardiomyocytes and endothelial cells, especially in stress reactions. Effective therapeutics for cancer therapy-induced cardiotoxicity must either take advantage of tissue-specific differences between malignant tissues and cardiomyocytes/cardiac endothelium or, more specifically, target cardiotoxic processes without interrupting antitumor pathways (Hahn et al., 2014).

Cardiotoxicity is divided into two types based on the presence of structural abnormalities and the degree of reversibility. Cardiotoxicity caused by type 1 is characterized by myocardial injury and is more likely to be irreversible, whereas cardiac dysfunction caused by type 2 cardiotoxicity has a larger chance of recovery if the offending agent is discontinued (Wickramasinghe et al., 2016).

Furthermore, anticancer drug combinations can result in both types of cardiotoxicity in the same patient. The 'multiple-hit' hypothesis implies that genetic and patient characteristics such as pre-existing cardiovascular risk factors (i.e., diabetes mellitus, hypertension, dyslipidemia) are substantial predictors of cardiovascular disease (CVD) development after chemotherapy. This is compounded by cancer treatment itself, which has both direct and indirect negative effects on cardiovascular reserve by altering dietary and lifestyle factors, as well as lowering adherence to potentially cardioprotective medications, increasing the overall cardiotoxicity risk in this patient group (Jones et al., 2007).

11.5 DIETARY SUPPLEMENTS

Healthy eating habits and food choices are regarded as key environmental variables in the prevention of noncommunicable chronic diseases over the life course; their adjustable characteristics offer a reduced socioeconomic global burden load in aging societies (Robinson et al., 2018).

In 1994, the United States Congress established the Dietary Supplement Health and Education Act (DSHEA), which provided a definition of the word "dietary supplement." As a result, a dietary supplement is defined as a product that is used orally and contains a "dietary ingredient" that is intended to supplement the diet. Vitamins, minerals, amino acids, herbs, or other botanical products, as well as enzymes, glandular, and organ tissues, and metabolites, are instances of dietary constituents (Stohs & Kitchens, 2019). It may also include a concentrate, an extract, a metabolite, a component, or a mix of the above-mentioned, but no human tissue or pathogenic germs should be present (Scarbrough et al., 2007).

Dietary supplements can be in the shape of capsules, tablets, powders, liquids, gel caps, soft gels, or bars, and can also be extracts or concentrates. Because they are a distinct category of "foods" and not medications, they must be labeled as dietary supplements. Dietary supplements are defined differently in the United States than they are in Europe, where the terminology refers to vitamins and minerals while herbal products are categorized as herbal medications or herbal remedies (Keservani et al., 2010a, b; Goldstein et al., 2007; Stohs & Preuss, 2017).

Dietary supplements are now widely used to assist in meeting nutritional requirements. Initially, this practice was recognized to avoid deficiencies in some essential micronutrients and their adverse health consequences, and its use was not questioned. This practice seems now to have gained the role of comforting consumers facing an ever-rising and nutritionally insufficient food supply. As a result, the use of dietary supplements has become a type of food behavior, and consumers, manufacturers, and regulatory officials need to assess and evaluate their safety, efficacy, and quality (Féart et al., 2020).

Dietary supplement regulation is complicated by the lack of global agreement on how the category of products called various dietary supplements, natural health products, complementary medicines, or food supplements is defined in different nations. A product, for example, that is categorized as a dietary supplement and governed as food in the United States may be categorized as a therapeutic good (complementary medicine or prescription medication), food supplement, or even a banned substance in another nation (Dwyer et al., 2018).

In reality, the FDA has more power over dietary supplements than it does over ordinary foods. Athletes, healthcare practitioners, and the general public all need to know how dietary supplements are regulated and what defines a dietary supplement (Stohs & Preuss, 2017; Stohs & Kitchens, 2019).

The projected benefits of a dietary supplement are less significant than those of a medicine, and the target group may differ (e.g., healthy or unhealthy) (Zeilstra et al., 2018).

It should have been noted that a portion of 1% of individuals ingesting dietary supplements witness adverse events, with most being classified as minor. Adulteration of supplements with medications and chemicals that are not recognized as supplements is the leading cause of adverse effects (Brown et al., 2017). Iron, magnesium (Nelson et al., 2010), sodium, zinc (Kreider et al., 2010), calcium, vitamin D (Larson-Meyer et al., 2013), vitamin C, vitamin E, and vitamin A (Machefer et al., 2007) are examples of nutritional deficiencies that have been specifically observed among athletes.

11.6 DIETARY SUPPLEMENTS IN CARDIOVASCULAR HEALTH

Some examples are hereby mentioned:

11.6.1 FISH OIL

Long-chain omega-3 (n–3) polyunsaturated fatty acids are obtained from fish oil. Eicosapentaenoic acid and docosahexaenoic acid are much more important. A fatty acid molecule has a chain that is 18 to 22 carbon atoms long, with the first double bond originating at the third carbon atom. Due to the existence of many double bonds, these are extremely curved structures. The positive effects of fish oil on coronary artery disease have been documented numerous times in the literature. The Japanese people and the Eskimos of Greenland had lower rates of death related to coronary heart disease, which has been attributed to their heavy consumption of fish (Tummala et al., 2019). Individuals are encouraged to consume a balanced diet with two meals of fatty fish each week, based on current data. Apart from ω-3 PUFAs, a food-based approach provides various other important nutrients. Fish oil supplements containing EPA and DHA have an excellent safety profile and may be a suitable option for those who can't eat fish, especially in patients with pre-existing heart failure, CVD, and hypertriglyceridemia (Goel et al., 2018). A total of 4,27,678 men and women between the ages of 40 and 69 who had no CVD or cancer were included in a cohort study. This study concluded that, in the general population, fish oil supplementation is linked to a 13% lower risk of all-cause death, a 16% reduced risk of CVD mortality, and a 7% lower risk of CVD events.

11.6.2 GINSENG

The Greek word "Panax" comes from the Latin word "panacea," which means "to treat all diseases," and ginseng has been shown to offer a wide range of medical advantages, including cardiovascular and aging-related disorders, among others. Preclinical and clinical investigations in recent years have indicated that ginseng has compelling positive benefits in a variety of neurological illnesses, including stroke, hypertension, cancer, and immune system hemostasis maintenance, including various protective pathways (Liu et al., 2019). The activities of ROS-regulating enzymes in the brain tissue of rats were considerably elevated after pre-treatment with *P. quinquefolium* and protopanaxadiol (PPD) saponins at doses of (25 and 50 mg/kg bw). These findings suggest that Panax extract may protect against stroke due to its antioxidant characteristics (Szczuka et al., 2019). Through inhibition of cardiac adrenergic responses, the administration of American Ginseng extract to rats prevented hypertrophy and heart failure caused by isoproterenol (Tang et al., 2016). Ginseng consumption reduced blood phospholipids, lysophosphatidylcholines and associated enzymes, high blood pressure variables, and cytokines while also increasing vasodilation. Furthermore, ginseng consumption reduced kidney oxidized glutathione levels. According to the findings, ginseng consumption can improve blood vessel health by modulating vasodilation, oxidative stress, and pro-inflammatory cytokines. Furthermore, the reduction in renal oxidized glutathione suggested that ginseng consumption is linked to a decrease in oxidative stress-induced renal impairment (Lee et al., 2020). The antiplatelet effects of red ginseng extract (RGE) and fermented red ginseng extract (FRG) were studied in research. Platelet aggregation, calcium mobilization, dense granule secretion, integrin-mediated fibrinogen binding, and fibrinogen adhesion were all markedly reduced by RGE and FRG. RGE-treated mice had much greater thrombosis survival than FRG-treated animals, with no effect on hemostasis, but a modest increase in bleeding duration in FRG-treated mice. Both extracts, particularly RGE, are excellent supplements for maintaining cardiovascular health and could be used to treat and prevent platelet-related cardiovascular diseases (Irfan et al., 2022).

11.6.3 GARLIC

Allium sativum, often known as garlic, has been utilized for a variety of purposes around the world since ancient times, particularly for its cardio-protective characteristics, which include blood pressure-lowering benefits. Supplementing garlic at a dosage of 600–900 mg/day has been shown to have strong benefits on blood pressure in hypertensive persons, but not in normotensive ones, according to more than 10 trials using Kwai garlic powder (Matsutomo et al., 2020). Based on a study, a 12-week treatment with a supplementary diet based on garlic homogenate only achieved a significant decrease in both systolic and diastolic blood pressure in patients with hypertension (Nakasone et al., 2013). AGE has been proven to substantially lower blood pressure in people with uncontrolled hypertension, suggesting it could be a useful adjunct therapy (Ried et al., 2016). AGE has also been proven to enhance peripheral circulation in hypertensive rats, raise NO levels in mice plasma levels, and cause endothelium-dependent vasorelaxation in isolated rat aortic rings (Takashima et al., 2017). It can also enhance cardiovascular parameters such as coronary artery calcium, microcirculation, epicardial and periaortic adipose tissue, carotid intima-media thickness, etc. Garlic can be used to prevent and treat CVD risk factors for these reasons (Imaizumi et al., 2022). Inhibiting cholesterol biosynthesis, suppressing low-density lipoprotein oxidation, controlling blood pressure, preventing platelet aggregation, lowering plasma fibrinogen levels, and increasing fibrinolytic activity are all known effects of garlic-based preparations that have clinically significant cardioprotective and anti-atherosclerotic effects (Sobenin et al., 2019).

11.6.4 GREEN TEA

Green tea (Kesharwani et al., 2016), made from the Camellia sinensis plant, is a popular beverage all over the world and has long been used as a medicine in Asian countries. The flavonoid-like (Keservani et al., 2016b) polyphenol contents in green tea, such as catechins, are largely responsible for its positive effects. The most prevalent green tea extracts that have been demonstrated to be helpful to human health are epigallocatechin gallate (EGCG), epicatechin gallate, epigallocatechin, and epicatechin (Xu et al., 2020). Tea phytochemicals help prevent heart disease by inhibiting LDL oxidation and acting as an antioxidant, anti-inflammatory, anti-thrombotic, and endothelial protective agent. Steaming newly picked leaves can inactivate heat-sensitive enzymes (polyphenol oxidase), preventing catechin oxidation and resulting in a stable product, green tea (Fang et al., 2019). Several meta-analysis studies have shown that green tea drinking and cardiovascular disease mortality have found a reduction in risk of 18% to 33%. Also, stroke incidence was comparable, with a reduced risk of 17% to 36% (Abe et al., 2021). In another meta-analysis (14 prospective studies with 5,13,804 individuals and a median follow-up of 11.5 years), it was discovered that drinking 3 cups of tea per day was related to a decreased risk of stroke (13%) and ischemic stroke (24%) (Casas et al., 2018). According to Harvard University research, persons who consume at least one cup of tea every day have a 44% lower risk of a heart attack. Green tea also boosts the antioxidant capacity of the blood, which helps to protect LDL cholesterol particles from oxidation, which is a risk factor for heart disease (Vishnoi et al., 2018).

11.6.5 COENZYME Q

Coenzyme Q (CoQ) is an antioxidant found in plasma membranes and lipoproteins. It plays an important role in the electron transport chain in mitochondria. A highly controlled process involving a mitochondrial multiprotein complex produces it endogenously in all cells. CoQ protects cell membranes and plasma lipoproteins against free radicals. It reduces the amount of lipid peroxidation in low-density lipoprotein (LDL) particles, which contributes to atherosclerosis (Hernández-Camacho et al., 2018). This endogenous antioxidant could be used to prevent and treat cardiovascular diseases, including hypertension, hyperlipidemia, heart failure, and coronary artery disease (Sarter et al., 2002). With 2400 mg of CoQ10 per day, CoQ is generally safe and well tolerated in treating people with early-stage Huntington's disease (Hernández-Camacho et al., 2018). Clinical evidence demonstrates that supplementing with CoQ10 at dosages of 200 mg/day or more for lengthy periods is safe, well-tolerated, and considerably increases CoQ10 concentration in plasma, as well as reducing oxidative stress and cardiovascular mortality. By improving mitochondrial respiration and raising myocardial tolerance to oxidative stress, CoQ10 supplementation improves heart failure symptomatology and clinical outcomes in patients undergoing coronary artery bypass graft surgery. Dietary CoQ10 has an anti-atherogenic action, which prevents LDL from accumulating in arteries, reduces vascular stiffness and hypertension, improves endothelial dysfunction, and boosts NO levels for vasodilation (Rabanal-Ruiz et al., 2021). Because of its safety profile and apparent efficacy, CoQ10 is used as an adjunctive therapy by many patients around the world. It is presently the third most popular dietary supplement in developing nations, owing to its anti-inflammatory qualities as well as its ability to alleviate endothelium and mitochondrial dysfunction in patients with ischemic heart disease when given at doses ranging from 60 mg to 300 mg per day (Sue-Ling et al., 2022). CoQ10 can currently be considered a safe adjunct to established therapy in cardiovascular disease due to the lack of clinically relevant side effects and anticipated therapeutic effectiveness (Pepe et al., 2007).

11.6.6 OMEGA-3 FATTY ACID

Omega-3 fatty acids have been studied in a variety of medical disorders including gastrointestinal, rheumatic, mental, metabolic, renal, dermatologic, and pulmonary problems. They are most commonly used for the prevention of cardiovascular disease. Eicosapentaenoic acid (EPA) and docosahexaenoic acid (DHA), both with 20 and 22 carbons, respectively, are the two most common long-chain omega-3 fatty acids. Seafood consumption is the main source of EPA and DHA (Mohebi-Nejad et al., 2014). There is a lot of evidence that EPA and DHA protect against cardiovascular disease, especially in people who already have heart disease or stroke. Omega-3 fatty acids have antithrombotic, anti-inflammatory, and antioxidative properties, and they benefit a variety of risk factors including blood pressure, blood vessel function, heart function, and blood lipids. Medications and omega-3 fatty acids do not interact negatively. Individuals with high blood triglyceride levels and patients with coronary heart disease should take omega-3 fatty acid supplements (Mori et al., 2017; Bäck et al., 2017). The antithrombotic function of EPA was first discovered — it inhibits the formation of thromboxane A2, which induces platelet aggregation and vasoconstriction by reducing platelet adhesion and reactivity, resulting in increased bleeding time. Blood flow irregularities can be influenced by omega-3 fatty acids; omega-3 fatty acids increase forearm blood flow in smokers and patients with chronic heart failure. Younger males tended to have more substantial impacts on fish oil than older men, but further research is needed in this area (Trebatická et al., 2017).

11.6.7 VITAMIN C

Vitamin C is a potent antioxidant and vital vitamin. Vitamin C intake has been found to have an inverse connection with major cardiovascular events and CVD risk variables in observational studies (Al-Khudairy et al., 2017). Vitamin C, being a powerful antioxidant and radical scavenger, protects cell constituents from oxidative stress caused by reactive oxygen species (ROS) and free radicals, which is one of the many biological tasks for which it is responsible (Morelli et al., 2020). Although it is generally recognized that vitamin C suppresses LDL-protein oxidation, hence lowering atherosclerosis, the cardiovascular consequences of this and other vitamin C effects are yet unknown. This topic has been studied in both randomized controlled trials and observational cohort studies, with varied results (Moser et al., 2016). Vitamin C is engaged in a number of processes involved in the pathogenesis of cardiovascular diseases, according to both preclinical and clinical studies available in the literature. However, significant limitations must be taken into account when evaluating the results of studies looking at how Vitamin C affects human health; for example, dietary assessment methods such as questionnaires or food diaries are imprecise and inaccurate, and they do not account for other factors that can affect Vitamin C levels and homeostasis (Morelli et al., 2020).

11.6.8 VITAMIN E

Vitamin E (a fat-soluble vitamin) plays an important role in the prevention and treatment of various disorders. α-tocopherol, the biologically most active form of vitamin E, has been the subject of several *in vitro/ in vivo* and clinical studies. Vitamin E exists in two forms: tocopherols and tocotrienols, each with four analogs: α, β, γ, and δ. The atheroprotective benefits of vitamin E have also been investigated in animal models. Supplementation of vitamin E in the diets of mice (with palm, olive, or sunflower oil) was found to be linked to smaller atherosclerotic lesions in the aorta. Research on vitamin E also focuses on inflammation. In cell culture and animal studies, α-tocopherol has been shown to possess anti-inflammatory properties (Sozen et al., 2019). Overall, extensive research has explored vitamin E's potential to reduce cardiovascular events. Promising associations have been found between higher vitamin E intake and plasma levels, and a reduced risk of cardiovascular events, as well as associations between vitamin E intake/plasma levels and cardiovascular disease risk factors such as hypertension, hyperlipidemia, and venous thrombosis, based on data from observational studies (Ziegler et al., 2020).

11.7 CONCLUSION

Multiple scientific studies now back up the classic Hippocratic saying, "Let thy food be thy medicine and thy medicine be thy food." Because of rising interest in personal health, the aging population, and promising tailored care solutions, the market for nutritional supplements has grown and will continue to rise. Several herbs and nutritional supplements, such as garlic, CoQ10, and vitamins, have shown promise in the treatment of cardiovascular risk factors and should be investigated further in large randomized primary and secondary prevention trials.

11.8 FUTURE PERSPECTIVES

Because of the expanding importance of these dietary supplements, researchers may be able to conduct ad hoc studies to better understand their role and the relative importance of each one in determining cardiovascular risk and CVD. Furthermore, more clinical studies can be done to set common grounds for the dosage of dietary supplements for various cardiovascular diseases.

KEYWORDS

- **acute rheumatic fever**
- **antioxidant**
- **atherosclerosis**
- **cardiovascular disease**
- **dietary supplements**
- **group A streptococcus**
- **lipoprotein cholesterol**
- **polyunsaturated fatty acids**
- **reactive oxygen species**
- **rheumatic heart disease**

REFERENCES

Abdel-Sattar, E., El Zalabani, S. M., & Sabry, M. M. (2017). Role of Dietary Supplements in Cardiovascular Diseases. In *Cardioprotective Natural Products* (pp. 193–246).

Abe, S. K., & Inoue, M. (2021). Green Tea and Cancer and Cardiometabolic Diseases: A Review of the Current Epidemiological Evidence. *European Journal of Clinical Nutrition, 75*(6), 865–876. https://doi.org/10.1038/s41430-020-00710-7.

Abe, S. K., Research Group for the Development and Evaluation of Cancer Prevention Strategies in Japan, Saito, E., Sawada, N., Tsugane, S., Ito, H., & Inoue, M. (2019). Green Tea Consumption and Mortality in Japanese Men and Women: A Pooled Analysis of Eight Population-Based Cohort Studies in Japan. *European Journal of Epidemiology, 34*(10), 917–926. https://doi.org/10.1007/s10654-019-00545-y

Al-Khudairy, L., Flowers, N., Wheelhouse, R., Ghannam, O., Hartley, L., Stranges, S., & Rees, K. (2017). Vitamin C Supplementation for the Primary Prevention of Cardiovascular Disease. *Cochrane Database of Systematic Reviews, 3*(3), CD011114. https://doi.org/10.1002/14651858.CD011114.pub2.

Arvind, B., & Ramakrishnan, S. (2020). Rheumatic fever and rheumatic heart disease in children. *The Indian Journal of Pediatrics, 87*(4), 305–311.

Atkins, J. L., Whincup, P. H., Morris, R. W., Lennon, L. T., Papacosta, O., & Wannamethee, S. G. (2014). High Diet Quality Is Associated with a Lower Risk of Cardiovascular Disease and All-Cause Mortality in Older Men. *The Journal of Nutrition, 144*(5), 673–680.

Azab, A. E., & Elsayed, A. S. (2017). Acute myocardial infarction risk factors and correlation of its markers with serum lipids. *Journal of Applied Biotechnology & Bioengineering, 3*(4), 00075.

Bäck, M. (2017). Omega-3 Fatty Acids in Atherosclerosis and Coronary Artery Disease. *Future Science OA, 3*(4), FSO236. https://doi.org/10.4155/fsoa-2017-0067.

Bakheet, M. S., Soltan, S., Gadalla, A., Haredy, H. H., & Shakoor, M. A. (2014). Antioxidants (vitamin E and gallic acid) as valuable protective factors against myocardial infarction. *Basic Research Journal of Medicine and Clinical Sciences*, 11, 109–122.

Balk, E. M., Adam, G. P., Langberg, V., Halladay, C., Chung, M., Lin, L., & Trikalinos, T. A. (2016). Omega-3 Fatty Acids and Cardiovascular Disease: An Updated Systematic Review. *Agency for Healthcare Research and Quality*, Vol 1, pp. 1–25.

Bowen, K. J., Harris, W. S., & Kris-Etherton, P. M. (2016). Omega-3 Fatty Acids and Cardiovascular Disease: Are There Benefits? *Current Treatment Options in Cardiovascular Medicine*, *18*(11), 69. https://doi.org/10.1007/s11936-016-0487-1.

Brown, A. C. (2017). An overview of herb and dietary supplement efficacy, safety and governmental regulations in the United States with suggested improvements. Part 1 of 5 parts. *Food and Chemical Toxicology*, *107*, 449–471.

Brown, J. M., & Hazen, S. L. (2018). Microbial Modulation of Cardiovascular Disease. *Nature Reviews Microbiology*, *16*(3), 171–181.

Casas, R., Castro-Barquero, S., Estruch, R., & Sacanella, E. (2018). Nutrition and Cardiovascular Health. *International Journal of Molecular Sciences*, *19*(12), 3988. https://doi.org/10.3390/ijms19123988.

Cave, A. C., Brewer, A. C., Narayanapanicker, A., Ray, R., Grieve, D. J., Walker, S., & Shah, A. M. (2006). NADPH Oxidases in Cardiovascular Health and Disease. *Antioxidants & Redox Signaling*, *8*(5–6), 691–728.

Chan, W.-J. J., McLachlan, A. J., Luca, E. J., & Harnett, J. E. (2020). Garlic (*Allium Sativum* L.) in the Management of Hypertension and Dyslipidemia – A Systematic Review. *Journal of Herbal Medicine*, *19*(100292), 100292. https://doi.org/10.1016/j.hermed.2019.100292.

Conte, S. M., & Vale, P. R. (2018). Peripheral arterial disease. *Heart, Lung and Circulation*, *27*(4), 427–432.

DeBusk, R. M. (2000). Dietary supplements and cardiovascular disease. *Current Atherosclerosis Reports*, *2*(6), 508–514.

Di Nisio, M., Van Es, N., & Büller, H. R. (2016). Deep vein thrombosis and pulmonary embolism. *The Lancet*, *388*(10063), 3060–3073.

Domma, A. M., & Gamal, M. A. (2015). Association between acute myocardial infarction, lipid profile and smoking habit. *Journal of Dental and Medical Sciences*, *14*(6), 47–51.

Dwyer, J. T., Coates, P. M., & Smith, M. J. (2018). Dietary supplements: Regulatory challenges and research resources. *Nutrients*, *10*(1), 41.

Fang, J., Sureda, A., Silva, A. S., Khan, F., Xu, S., & Nabavi, S. M. (2019). Trends of Tea in Cardiovascular Health and Disease: A Critical Review. *Trends in Food Science & Technology*, 88, 385–396. https://doi.org/10.1016/j.tifs.2019.04.001.

Féart, C. (2020). Dietary Supplements: Which Place between Food and Drugs? *Nutrients*, *12*(1), 204.

Fernandez, M. L., Blomquist, S. A., Hallmark, B., & Chilton, F. H. (2021). Omega-3 Supplementation and Heart Disease: A Population-Based Diet by Gene Analysis of Clinical Trial Outcomes. *Nutrients*, *13*(7), 2154. https://doi.org/10.3390/nu13072154.

Ferrari, C. K. B., & Torres, E. A. F. S. (2003). Biochemical Pharmacology of Functional Foods and Prevention of Chronic Diseases of Aging. *Biomedicine & Pharmacotherapy*, *57*(5–6), 251–260.

Goel, A., Pothineni, N. V., Singhal, M., Paydak, H., Saldeen, T., & Mehta, J. L. (2018). Fish, Fish Oils and Cardioprotection: Promise or Fish Tale? *International Journal of Molecular Sciences*, *19*(12), 3703. https://doi.org/10.3390/ijms19123703.

Goldstein, H., Elias, M., Ron-Avraham, G., Biniaurishvili, B. Z., Madjar, M., Kamargash, I., & Golik, A. (2007). Consumption of herbal remedies and dietary supplements amongst patients hospitalized in medical wards. *British Journal of Clinical Pharmacology, 64*, 373–380.

Gutierrez-Mariscal, F. M., de la Cruz-Ares, S., Torres-Peña, J. D., Alcalá-Diaz, J. F., Yubero-Serrano, E. M., & López-Miranda, J. (2021). Coenzyme Q10 and Cardiovascular Diseases. *Antioxidants, 10*(6), 906. https://doi.org/10.3390/antiox10060906.

Hahn, V. S., Lenihan, D. J., & Ky, B. (2014). Cancer therapy–induced cardiotoxicity: basic mechanisms and potential cardioprotective therapies. *Journal of the American Heart Association, 3*(2), e000665.

Hanaki, Y., Sugiyama, S., Ozawa, T., & Ohno, M. (1993). Coenzyme Q10 and Coronary Artery Disease. *Clinical Investigator, 71*(8 Suppl), S112–S115. https://doi.org/10.1007/bf00226850.

Hernández-Camacho, J. D., Bernier, M., López-Lluch, G., & Navas, P. (2018). Coenzyme Q10 Supplementation in Aging and Disease. *Frontiers in Physiology, 9*, 44. https://doi.org/10.3389/fphys.2018.00044.

Imaizumi, V. M., Laurindo, L. F., Manzan, B., Guiguer, E. L., Oshiiwa, M., Otoboni, A. M. M. B., & Barbalho, S. M. (2022). Garlic: A Systematic Review of the Effects on Cardiovascular Diseases. *Critical Reviews in Food Science and Nutrition, 63*(24), 1–23. https://doi.org/10.1080/10408398.2022.2043821.

Irfan, M., Lee, Y. Y., Lee, K. -J., Kim, S. D., & Rhee, M. H. (2022). Comparative antiplatelet and antithrombotic effects of red ginseng and fermented red ginseng extracts. *Journal of Ginseng Research, 46*(3), 387–395. https://doi.org/10.1016/j.jgr.2021.05.010.

Isola, G., Polizzi, A., Muraglie, S., Leonardi, R., & Lo Giudice, A. (2019). Assessment of Vitamin C and Antioxidant Profiles in Saliva and Serum in Patients with Periodontitis and Ischemic Heart Disease. *Nutrients, 11*(12), 2956. https://doi.org/10.3390/nu11122956.

Jones, L. W., Haykowsky, M. J., Swartz, J. J., Douglas, P. S., & Mackey, J. R. (2007). Early breast cancer therapy and cardiovascular injury. *Journal of the American College of Cardiology, 50*(15), 1435–1441.

Katzenellenbogen, J. M., Ralph, A. P., & Wyber, R., & Carapetis, J. R. (2017). Rheumatic heart disease: infectious disease origin, chronic care approach. *BMC Health Services Research, 17*(1), 1–6.

Keaney, J. F. (2005). Oxidative Stress and the Vascular Wall. *Circulation, 112*(17), 2585–2588.

Keservani, R. K., Kesharwani, R. K., Sharma, A. K., Vyas, N., & Chadoker, A. (2010). Nutritional Supplements: An Overview. *International Journal of Current Pharmaceutical Review and Research, 1*(1), 59–75.

Keservani, R. K., Kesharwani, R. K., Vyas, N., Jain, S., Raghuvanshi, R., & Sharma, A. K. (2010). Nutraceutical and functional food as future food: a review. *Der Pharmacia Lettre, 2*(1), 106–116.

Keservani, R. K., Sharma, A. K., & Kesharwani, R. K. (2016). Medicinal effect of nutraceutical fruits for the cognition and brain health. *Scientifica*, 2016, Article ID 3109254, 10 pages. doi:10.1155/2016/3109254.

Keservani, R. K., Sharma, A. K., & Kesharwani, R. K. (2016). Nutraceutical and Functional Foods for Cardiovascular Health. In A. K. Sharma & R. K. Kesharwani (Eds.), *Food Process Engineering* (pp. 257–278). Apple Academic Press, CRC Press. ISBN: 9781771884020.

Keservani, R. K., Sharma, A. K., & Kesharwani, R. K. (2017). An overview and therapeutic applications of nutraceutical and functional foods. In *Recent Advances in Drug Delivery Technology* (pp. 160–201). ISBN: 9781522507543.
Keservani, R. K., Sharma, A. K., & Kesharwani, R. K. (Eds.). (2020). *Nutraceuticals and Dietary Supplements: Applications in Health Improvement and Disease Management*, 1–344. CRC Press. ISBN: 9781771888738.
Kesharwani, R. K., Singh, P., & Keservani, R. K. (2016). Green Coffee Bean Extract and Chlorogenic Acids: Chemistry and Novel Antioxidant Benefits. In D. Bagchi, H. Moriyama, & A. Swaroop (Eds.), *Green Coffee Bean Extract in Human Health* (Chapter 1, pp. 1–17). Boca Raton, Taylor and Francis, USA. ISBN: 9781498716376.
Kreider, R. B., Wilborn, C. D., Taylor, Campbell, B., Almada, A. L., Collins, R., Cooke, M., & Greenwood, M. (2010). ISSN exercise & sport nutrition review: research & recommendations. *Journal of the International Society of Sports Nutrition*, *7*, 1–35.
Kumar, A., Kaur, H., Devi, P., & Mohan, V. (2009). Role of Coenzyme Q10 (CoQ10) in Cardiac Disease, Hypertension and Meniere-like Syndrome. *Pharmacology & Therapeutics*, *124*(3), 259–268. https://doi.org/10.1016/j.pharmthera.2009.07.003.
Larson-Meyer, E. (2013). Vitamin D supplementation in athletes. *Nestle Nutrition Institute Workshop Series*, *75*, 109–121.
Lau, S., Georgousopoulou, E., Kellett, J., Thomas, J., McKune, A., Mellor, D., & Naumovski, N. (2016). The effect of dietary supplementation of green tea catechins on cardiovascular disease risk markers in humans: A systematic review of clinical trials. *Beverages*, *2*(2), 16. https://doi.org/10.3390/beverages2020016.
Lee, H. -J., Kim, B. -M., Lee, S. H., Sohn, J. -T., Choi, J. W., Cho, C. -W., & Kim, H. -J. (2020). Ginseng-induced changes to blood vessel dilation and the metabolome of rats. *Nutrients*, *12*(8), 2238. https://doi.org/10.3390/nu12082238.
Li, Z. -H., Zhong, W. -F., Liu, S., Kraus, V. B., Zhang, Y. -J., Gao, X., & Mao, C. (2020). Associations of habitual fish oil supplementation with cardiovascular outcomes and all-cause mortality: Evidence from a large population-based cohort study. *BMJ*, *368*, m456. https://doi.org/10.1136/bmj.m456.
Lichtenstein, A. H., Appel, L. J., Brands, M., Carnethon, M., Daniels, S., Franch, H. A., & Wylie-Rosett, J. (2006). Diet and Lifestyle Recommendations Revision 2006. *Circulation*, *114*(1), 82–96.
Lichtenstein, A. H., Appel, L. J., Vadiveloo, M., Hu, F. B., Kris-Etherton, P. M., Rebholz, C. M., & Wylie-Rosett, J. (2021). 2021 Dietary guidance to improve cardiovascular health: a scientific statement from the American heart association. *Circulation*, *144*(23), 472–487.
Liu, H., Zhuang, J., Tang, P., Li, J., Xiong, X., & Deng, H. (2020). The role of the gut microbiota in coronary heart disease. *Current Atherosclerosis Reports*, *22*(12), 1–7.
Liu, L., Anderson, G. A., Fernandez, T. G., & Doré, S. (2019). Efficacy, and mechanism of panax ginseng in experimental stroke. *Frontiers in Neuroscience*, *13*, 294. https://doi.org/10.3389/fnins.2019.00294.
Lorenzo, J. M., & Munekata, P. E. S. (2016). Phenolic Compounds of Green Tea: Health Benefits and Technological Application in Food. *Asian Pacific Journal of Tropical Biomedicine*, *6*(8), 709–719. https://doi.org/10.1016/j.apjtb.2016.06.010.
Lundy, B. (2011). Nutrition for synchronized swimming: a review. *International Journal of Sport Nutrition and Exercise Metabolism*, *21*, 436–445.

Machefer, G., Groussard, C., Zouhal, H., Vincent, S., Youssef, H., Faure, H., & Gratas-Delamache, A. (2007). Nutritional and plasmatic antioxidant vitamins status of ultra-endurance athletes. *Journal of the American College of Nutrition, 26*, 311–316.

Martelli, A., Testai, L., Colletti, A., & Cicero, A. F. G. (2020). Coenzyme Q10: Clinical Applications in Cardiovascular Diseases. *Antioxidants (Basel), 9*(4), 341. https://doi.org/10.3390/antiox9040341.

Matsutomo, T. (2020). Potential benefits of garlic and other dietary supplements for the management of hypertension. *Experimental and Therapeutic Medicine, 19*(2), 1479–1484. https://doi.org/10.3892/etm.2019.8375.

Mirza, M., Strunets, A., Shen, W. K., & Jahangir, A. (2012). Mechanisms of arrhythmias and conduction disorders in older adults. *Clinics in Geriatric Medicine, 28*(4), 555–573.

Mohebi-Nejad, A., & Bikdeli, B. (2014). Omega-3 supplements and cardiovascular diseases. *Tanaffos, 13*(1), 6–14.

Morelli, M. B., Gambardella, J., Castellanos, V., Trimarco, V., & Santulli, G. (2020). Vitamin C and cardiovascular disease: An update. *Antioxidants (Basel), 9*(12), 1227. https://doi.org/10.3390/antiox9121227.

Mori, T. A. (2017). Marine OMEGA-3 fatty acids in the prevention of cardiovascular disease. *Fitoterapia, 123*, 51–58. https://doi.org/10.1016/j.fitote.2017.09.015.

Moser, M. A., & Chun, O. K. (2016). Vitamin C and heart health: A review based on findings from epidemiologic studies. *International Journal of Molecular Sciences, 17*(8), 1328. https://doi.org/10.3390/ijms17081328.

Nakasone, Y., Nakamura, Y., Yamamoto, T., & Yamaguchi, H. (2013). Effect of a traditional Japanese garlic preparation on blood pressure in prehypertensive and mildly hypertensive adults. *Experimental and Therapeutic Medicine, 5*(2), 399–405. https://doi.org/10.3892/etm.2012.819.

Nelson, F. H. (2010). Magnesium, inflammation, and obesity in chronic disease. *Nutrition Reviews, 68*, 333–340.

Nielsen, F. H., & Lukaski, H. L. (2006). Update on the relationship between magnesium and exercise. *Magnesium Research, 19*, 1801–1809.

Otto, C. M., & Rahimi, K. (2016). Heartbeat: The gut microbiota and heart failure. *Heart, 102*(11), 811–812.

Parabathina, R. K., Raja, G. V., Rao, M. N., Rao, G. S., & Rao, K. S. (2010). Cardioprotective effects of vitamin E, morin, rutin and quercetin against doxorubicin induced oxidative stress of rabbits: A biochemical study. *Journal of Chemical and Pharmaceutical Research, 2*(3), 754–765.

Paul, S., & Candelario-Jalil, E. (2021). Emerging neuroprotective strategies for the treatment of ischemic stroke: An overview of clinical and preclinical studies. *Experimental Neurology, 335*, 113518.

Pepe, S., Marasco, S. F., Haas, S. J., Sheeran, F. L., Krum, H., & Rosenfeldt, F. L. (2007). Coenzyme Q10 in cardiovascular disease. *Mitochondrion, 7*(Suppl), S154–S167. https://doi.org/10.1016/j.mito.2007.02.005.

Rabanal-Ruiz, Y., Llanos-González, E., & Alcain, F. J. (2021). The use of coenzyme Q10 in cardiovascular diseases. *Antioxidants (Basel), 10*(5), 755. https://doi.org/10.3390/antiox10050755.

Ried, K., Travica, N., & Sali, A. (2016). The effect of aged garlic extracts on blood pressure and other cardiovascular risk factors in uncontrolled hypertensives: The AGE at Heart Trial. *Integrated Blood Pressure Control, 9*, 9–21. https://doi.org/10.2147/IBPC.S93335.

Robinson, S. M. (2018). Improving nutrition to support healthy ageing: What are the opportunities for intervention? *Proceedings of the Nutrition Society*, *77*(3), 257–264.

Ruiz Petrich, E., Schanne, O. F., & Ponce Zumino, A. (1996). Electrophysiological responses to ischemia and reperfusion. In *Myocardial ischemia: Mechanisms, reperfusion, protection* (pp. 115–133).

Sarter, B. (2002). Coenzyme Q10 and cardiovascular disease: A review. *Journal of Cardiovascular Nursing*, *16*(4), 9–20. https://doi.org/10.1097/00005082-200207000-00003.

Scarbrough, B. (2004). Dietary supplements: a review of United States regulation with emphasis on the Dietary Supplement Health and Education Act of 1994 and subsequent activity. *1,* 1–3.

Senior, K. R. (2010). Blood: Physiology and Circulation. The Rosen Publishing Group. Pp. 1–240. ISBN: 9781615301218.

Seres, L. B. (2006). Oxidative stress in cardiovascular diseases and in experimental models (PhD thesis). *2006*. 5, *2006*.

Sies, H. (1985). Hydroperoxides and thiol oxidants in the study of oxidative stress in intact cells and organs. In *Oxidative Stress* (pp. 73–90).

Sobenin, I. A., Myasoedova, V. A., Iltchuk, M. I., Zhang, D.-W., & Orekhov, A. N. (2019). Therapeutic effects of garlic in cardiovascular atherosclerotic disease. *Chinese Journal of Natural Medicines*, *17*(10), 721–728. https://doi.org/10.1016/S1875-5364(19)30088-3.

Sozen, E., Demirel, T., & Ozer, N. K. (2019). Vitamin E: Regulatory role in the cardiovascular system. *IUBMB Life*, *71*(4), 507–515. https://doi.org/10.1002/iub.2020.

Sperling, L. S., & Nelson, J. R. (2016). History and future of omega-3 fatty acids in cardiovascular disease. *Current Medical Research and Opinion*, *32*(2), 301–311. https://doi.org/10.1185/03007995.2015.1120190.

Stachowicz, M., & Lebiedzinska, A. (2016). The role of vitamin D in health preservation and exertional capacity of athletes. *Postępy Higieny i Medycyny Doświadczalnej*, *70*, 637–643.

Stampfer, M. J., Hu, F. B., Manson, J. E., Rimm, E. B., & Willett, W. C. (2000). Primary prevention of coronary heart disease in women through diet and lifestyle. *New England Journal of Medicine*, *343*, 16–17.

Stohs, S. J., & Kitchens, E. K. (2019). Nutritional supplementation in health and sports performance. *Nutrition and Enhanced Sports Performance*, 3–9.

Stohs, S. J., & Preuss, H. G. (2017). What health care professionals should know about the regulation and safety of dietary supplements. *Journal of the American College of Nutrition*, *36*, 306–309.

Stokes, K. Y., Russell, J. M., Jennings, M. H., Alexander, J. S., & Granger, D. N. (2007). Platelet-associated NAD(P)H oxidase contributes to the thrombogenic phenotype induced by hypercholesterolemia. *Free Radical Biology and Medicine*, *43*(1), 22–30.

Sue-Ling, C. B., Abel, W. M., & Sue-Ling, K. (2022). Coenzyme Q10 as adjunctive therapy for cardiovascular disease and hypertension: A systematic review. *The Journal of Nutrition*, *152*(7), 1666–1674, https://doi.org/10.1093/jn/nxac079.

Sunkara, A., & Raizner, A. (2019). Supplemental vitamins and minerals for cardiovascular disease prevention and treatment. *Methodist DeBakey Cardiovascular Journal*, *15*(3), 179–184. https://doi.org/10.14797/mdcj-15-3-179.

Szczuka, D., Nowak, A., Zakłos-Szyda, M., Kochan, E., Szymańska, G., Motyl, I., & Blasiak, J. (2019). American ginseng (*Panax quinquefolium* L.) as a source of bioactive phytochemicals with pro-health properties. *Nutrients*, *11*(5), 1041. https://doi.org/10.3390/nu11051041.

Takashima, M., Kanamori, Y., Kodera, Y., Morihara, N., & Tamura, K. (2017). Aged garlic extract exerts endothelium-dependent vasorelaxant effect on rat aorta by increasing nitric oxide production. *Phytomedicine*, *24*, 56–61. https://doi.org/10.1016/j.phymed.2016.11.016.

Tang, J., Zheng, J.-S., Fang, L., Jin, Y., Cai, W., & Li, D. (2015). Tea consumption and mortality of all cancers, CVD and all causes: A meta-analysis of eighteen prospective cohort studies. *British Journal of Nutrition*, *114*(5), 673–683. https://doi.org/10.1017/s0007114515002329.

Tang, X., Gan, X. T., Rajapurohitam, V., Huang, C. X., Xue, J., Lui, E. M. K., & Karmazyn, M. (2016). North American ginseng (*Panax quinquefolius*) suppresses β-adrenergic-dependent signaling, hypertrophy, and cardiac dysfunction. *Canadian Journal of Physiology and Pharmacology*, *94*, 1325–1335. https://doi.org/10.1139/cjpp-2016-0337.

Trebatická, J., Dukát, A., Ďuračková, Z., & Muchová, J. (2017). Cardiovascular diseases, depression disorders and potential effects of omega-3 fatty acids. *Physiological Research*, *66*(3), 363–382. https://doi.org/10.33549/physiolres.933430.

Tummala, R., Ghosh, R. K., Jain, V., Devanabanda, A. R., Bandyopadhyay, D., Deedwania, P., & Aronow, W. S. (2019). Fish oil and cardiometabolic diseases: Recent updates and controversies. *The American Journal of Medicine*, *132*(10), 1153–1159.

Vasanthi, H. R., Kartal-Özer, N., Azzi, A., & Das, D. K. (2010). Dietary supplements, cholesterol and cardiovascular disease. In *Modern Dietary Fat Intakes in Disease Promotion* (pp. 227–247).

Vijayalakshmi, B., & Chandrasekhar, M. (2008). Oxidative stress and their resultant products as the target molecules in clinical diagnosis of age-related disease. *Current Trends in Biotechnology and Pharmacy*, *2*(2), 239–250.

Vishnoi, H., Bodla, R. B., & Kant, R. (2018). Green tea (*Camellia sinensis*) and its antioxidant property: A review. *International Journal of Pharmaceutical Sciences Research*, *9*(5), 1723–1736. https://doi.org/10.13040/IJPSR.0975-8232.9(5).1723-36.

Volpe, S. (2015). Magnesium and the athlete. *Current Sports Medicine Reports*, *14*, 279–283.

Wang, Z., Roberts, A. B., Buffa, J. A., Levison, B. S., Zhu, W., Org, E., Gu, X., Huang, Y., Zamanian-Daryoush, M., Culley, M. K., DiDonato, A. J., Fu, X., Hazen, J. E., Krajcik, D., DiDonato, J. A., Lusis, A. J., & Hazen, S. L. (2015). Non-lethal inhibition of gut microbial trimethylamine production for the treatment of atherosclerosis. *Cell*, *163*(7), 1585–1595.

Watanabe, Y., & Tatsuno, I. (2017). Omega-3 polyunsaturated fatty acids for cardiovascular diseases: Present, past and future. *Expert Review of Clinical Pharmacology*, *10*(8), 865–873. https://doi.org/10.1080/17512433.2017.1333902.

Wenger, N., Sebastian, T., Engelberger, R. P., Kucher, N., & Spirk, D. (2021). Pulmonary embolism and deep vein thrombosis: Similar but different. *Thrombosis Research*, *206*, 88–98.

Wickramasinghe, C. D., Nguyen, K. L., Watson, K. E., Vorobiof, G., & Yang, E. H. (2016). Concepts in cardio-oncology: Definitions, mechanisms, diagnosis and treatment strategies of cancer therapy-induced cardiotoxicity. *Future Oncology*, *12*(6), 855–870.

Xu, R., Yang, K., Ding, J., & Chen, G. (2020). Effect of green tea supplementation on blood pressure: A systematic review and meta-analysis of randomized controlled trials. *Medicine*, *99*(6), e19047. https://doi.org/10.1097/md.0000000000019047.

Zeilstra, D., Younes, J. A., Brummer, R. J., & Kleerebezem, M. (2018). Perspective: Fundamental limitations of the randomized controlled trial method in nutritional research: The example of probiotics. *Advances in Nutrition*, *9*, 561–571.

Zhang, C., Qin, Y.-Y., Wei, X., Yu, F.-F., Zhou, Y.-H., & He, J. (2015). Tea consumption and risk of cardiovascular outcomes and total mortality: A systematic review and meta-analysis of prospective observational studies. *European Journal of Epidemiology, 30*(2), 103–113. https://doi.org/10.1007/s10654-014-9960-x.

Ziegler, M., Wallert, M., Lorkowski, S., & Peter, K. (2020). Cardiovascular and metabolic protection by vitamin E: A matter of treatment strategy? *Antioxidants (Basel), 9*(10), 935. https://doi.org/10.3390/antiox9100935.

CHAPTER 12

CARDIOPROTECTIVE EFFECTS OF BEE PRODUCTS: AN EVIDENCE-BASED REVIEW

MYRENE ROSELYN D'SOUZA

Department of Biochemistry, Mount Carmel College Autonomous, Karnataka, India

ABSTRACT

Since the beginning of human history, the honeybee has held a place of critical significance in human society. There is currently a wide variety of bee products on the market that can be utilized in conventional and alternative treatments, collectively referred to as apitherapy. Honeybee products and the apitherapeutic benefits they offer will be the topic of discussion in this chapter. Honey, bee pollen, propolis, bee bread, royal jelly, and bee venom are all valuable natural products that contain a variety of active biological properties. Some of these properties include antioxidant, anti-inflammatory, antimicrobial, antiviral, and antitumor properties. These biological activities are largely fluctuating and depend on a wide variety of factors, including geographical location, floral sources, environmental conditions, the performance of the beekeeper, and the species of bees involved. This chapter discusses the composition of a variety of natural bee products, as well as the active biological effects in ameliorating symptoms of cardiovascular disease.

12.1 INTRODUCTION

As per the World Health Organization's record of the top 10 reasons for death in 2019, seven out of them were non-communicable ailments such

Antioxidants as Nutraceuticals. Nayan A. Gujarathi, Raj K. Keservani, Rajesh K. Kesharwani, Bhushan R. Rane, Yogeeta Sameer Goyal (Eds.)

as diabetes mellitus, ischemic heart disease, stroke, Alzheimer's disease, cancers, and kidney disease (WHO, 2020). It has been demonstrated that metabolic syndrome, also known as MetS, significantly raises the risk of a variety of chronic diseases (Borshchev et al., 2019). When compared to a patient who does not have MetS, the financial burden that a patient with MetS places on the healthcare system is typically several times greater (Scholze et al., 2010). MetS and the chronic diseases with which it is associated also significantly raise the risk of morbidity and mortality in patients with viral infections like COVID-19 (Dietz et al., 2020; McGurnaghan et al., 2020). As a direct result of this, metabolic syndrome has developed into a significant problem for the general public's health all over the world.

MetS is a syndrome including a cluster of risk factors related to lifestyle and diet such as increased triglycerides, abdominal obesity, increased blood pressure, reduced HDL, and increased fasting glucose (Iqbal et al., 2020). These days, there is widespread interest in products made from natural ingredients all over the world. Dietary supplements containing these substances are utilized to prevent and treat several diseases, as well as lifestyle-related conditions such as atherosclerosis (Forbes-Hernández et al., 2017; Dsouza et al., 2018). Nutraceutical supplementations with pro- and prebiotics, micronutrients, plant extracts, polyphenols, and other natural products are effective in ameliorating the severity of MetS symptoms (Sirtori et al., 2017). At this point, the majority of human health protection is focused on medical prophylaxis, a field of expertise aiming at preventing disease development and also at controlling the risk of their development (Forbes-Hernández et al., 2017; Moghadasian et al., 2017).

12.2 PARAMETERS OF CARDIOVASCULAR HEALTH

The condition known as atherosclerosis is characterized by a persistent inflammation of the aorta and the arteries of medium size. The dysfunction of the endothelial cells is the primary event that kickstarts the formation of vascular wall lesions. Increased oxidative stress can have the effect of impairing endothelial function, which can be seen as abnormal vasodilation, intensification of the inflammatory process, increased macromolecule permeability, increased pro-thrombotic activity, and smooth muscle proliferation (Viola & Soehnlein, 2015; Megson et al., 2016). The decreased formation of nitrogen oxide is related to a disruption in the vascular wall vasodilation function. Endothelial nitric oxide synthase is the enzyme responsible for the production of nitric oxide (eNOS). Since it plays an essential anti-inflammatory role and also causes the endothelium to dilate, this molecule can be considered an endothelial anti-atherosclerotic molecule (Falk, 2006). The body produces an excessive amount of substances that inhibit endothelial nitric oxide synthase (eNOS) and reduce the bioavailability of NO as a result of oxidative stress. Asymmetric dimethylarginine (Pacurari et al., 2014), ox-LDL (Desai et al., 2012), angiotensin-converting enzyme, and angiotensin II (Steyers & Miller, 2014) are some examples of these factors.

Ischemic heart disease, in particular, is associated with oxidative stress, which can lead to an excessive synthesis or accumulation of free radicals or their oxidative products, called reactive oxygen species (ROS) (Tsutsui et al., 2011). As a free radical antioxidant defense system, endogenous enzymes such as superoxide dismutase (SOD), glutathione reductase (GRx), glutathione-S-transferase (GST), glutathione peroxidase (GPx), and catalase are produced to combat ROS (Maksimenko et al., 2012; Hana et al., 2019; Shediwah et al., 2019). Proteins, lipids, and DNA can all suffer oxidative damage when there is an excess of ROS. After the disruption of the permeability of the lipid membrane and the modification in the activity of the cardiac enzyme caused by the oxidants, the damage is ultimately manifested as myocardial infarction. The measurement of ROS as well as endogenous antioxidant enzymes is therefore an excellent analyst of cardiovascular disease risk (Marrocco et al., 2017).

An imbalance in lipid metabolism can result in an increase in total cholesterol (TC), triglyceride levels (TG), and low-density lipoprotein (LDL). A disproportionate amount of ROS can react with the elevated LDL, which can eventually lead to the formation of atherosclerotic plaque (Linton et al., 2000; Shediwah et al., 2019). In the long run, the plaque occludes the blood supply to the myocardium, which will result in a hypoxic state that has the potential to cause necrosis of the myocardial tissue, which in turn disrupts the regular rhythm of the heartbeat if the myocardium is affected. Therefore, electrocardiogram parameters like arrhythmia are employed as markers of CVD.

A low molecular weight protein known as cardiac troponin I (cTnI) is a component of the myofibrillary contractile apparatus that is found in cardiac muscle fiber. Following damage to the cardiac muscle, the uptake of these proteins into blood circulation can be demonstrated by the presence of cTnI in the serum, a highly specific marker for the identification of heart attacks (Ásthildur et al., 2018). The cTnI level increases between 4 and 6 hours after the injury and persists for 5–10 days after that. Some of the enzymes present in the myocardium include aspartate aminotransferase (AST), creatine kinase MB (CK-MB), and alanine aminotransferase (ALT) (Patibandla et al., 2020). These enzymes, when operating under normal physiological conditions, contribute to the production of ATP and the intracellular metabolism of cells. A myocardial infarction is a condition that can be clinically diagnosed when certain parts of the heart's circulation are deprived of oxygen. This results in the death of myocardial cells, which can then be diagnosed. Therefore, the death of cells in the myocardium causes these biochemical markers to be released, which is also a predictor of myocardial infarction (Mythili & Malathi, 2015).

12.3 NATURAL PRODUCTS FROM THE HONEYBEE AND ITS ROLE IN AMELIORATING CVD

The earliest documentation of human consumption of honey or other bee-derived products dates back to approximately 13,000 BCE. Recently, there has been a rapid increase in the use of bee products in both conventional and alternative forms of medicine. Apitherapy makes use of natural bee products like honey, bee pollen, propolis, and royal jelly which come from the bees themselves. Due to the effectiveness of bee products, there are currently a lot of studies looking into the specific health benefits and pharmacological properties of bee products. It is distinguished by its potent antioxidant effect as well as a wide range of biological activities, including bacteriostatic and bactericidal activities, detoxicative, hepatoprotective, and regenerative activities. In addition to this, it works to rev up the immune system and activates the metabolisms of both cells and the body as a whole (Kieliszek et al., 2018). This has led to an increase in the development of nutraceuticals and functional food from these products. When compared to traditional foods that have been remediated and are nutritional, foods that are considered to be functional are those that have the potential to improve a person's physiological or psychological health. These effects contribute favorably to excellent health maintenance, overall well-being, and a reduction in the risk of developing chronic illness.

12.3.1 HONEY

Honey's antilipidemic effect was discovered in a hypertriglyceridemia mouse model that was fructose-induced (Busserolles et al., 2002). This sparked the initial interest in the utilization of honey as a cardioprotective agent. Honey was found to have both antioxidative and protective effects against lipid peroxidation, according to the study. The imbalance that results from the generation of ROS and the inhibition of that production by endogenous antioxidant enzymes has been linked to the cardiovascular system. Regarding the inhibition of reactive oxygen species (ROS), one study that used neutrophils and macrophages that had been activated with bovine thrombin reported that honey completely inhibited ROS production (Ahmad et al., 2009).

High-fructose diets are linked to cardiovascular disease. Busserolles et al. (2002) investigated honey's influence on fructose-induced hypertriglyceridemia. Mice fed with fructose were found to possess increased TG levels, while those fed with honey demonstrated lowered TG despite its fructose content. Honey-fed mice had less lipid peroxidation than fructose-fed animals (Busserolles et al., 2002). Honey-fed mice exhibited greater levels of serum TG, HDL, and VLDL than control mice. In contrast, honey-fed mice had decreased total cholesterol (Alagwu et al., 2011). Pre-feeding honey prior to a high-fat diet increased HDL and HMG-CoA: mevalonate and decreased LDL and cholesterol (Erejuwa et al., 2018). In fructose-induced hypertriglyceridemia, mice had elevated nitric oxide and decreased α-tocopherol. Honey-fed mice had reduced NO and more α-tocopherol despite its fructose content (Busserolles et al., 2002). Honey therapy restored ascorbic acid, GSH, and SOD levels perturbed by epinephrine.

Honey's ability to reduce bovine thrombin-induced phagocytic oxidation may help halt cardiovascular disease progression. Honey suppressed ROS generation in thrombin-induced neutrophils and macrophages (Ahmad et al., 2009). Honey reverses the increase in venous blood pressure upon epinephrine induction, indicating honey modulates vasomotor function. The *ex vivo* cardiac arrhythmia model constructed in an isolated rat heart demonstrated an effect after reperfusion with honey following ischemia (Najafi et al., 2011). A reduction in VT, VEBs, VT, and total VF incidence was reported. Pre-treatment with honey was found to normalize parameters of the heart such as tachyarrhythmia, extrasystole, bradyarrhythmia, P-wave, and ST segment abnormalities (Najafi et al., 2011).

A substantial reduction in infarct size, dependent on honey concentration, was reported in *ex vivo* models of ischemia and reperfusion (Eteraf-Oskouei et al., 2013). Honey reduces inflammation and preserves cardiac muscle fiber shape, indicating a preventive effect against myocardial infarction (Khalil et al., 2015). Chrysin, a bioactive honey component, and myocardial damage restoration restore ISO-induced rats' impaired hemodynamic and ventricular functioning. It also reduces oxidative stress resulting from ISO induction,

PPAR-γ suppression, and artery ligation. Chrysin leads to the reversal of PPAR-γ inhibition and reduces NF-κBp65, RAGE, TNF-α, and IKK-β levels. Chrysin lowered cardiac injury indicators. Chrysin reduces apoptotic markers, protecting the heart. Histology confirms chrysin's myocardium-preservation action (Wu et al., 2018).

12.3.2 PROPOLIS

The Greek word "propolis" means "the beehive." Propolis also fills holes and crevices in the beehive, smooths the beehive's inner surface, maintains the temperature at 35°C, protects it from the elements and predators, and creates a sterile interior environment. Heat makes propolis malleable and sticky. It has been used in ethnomedicine since 300 BC for its several associated health benefits (Sung et al., 2017). Propolis comprises polyphenols, flavonoids, resins, fatty acids, essential oils, pollen, and wax in addition to important vitamins and minerals (Anjum et al., 2019). It has many therapeutic effects, including antioxidant, immunomodulatory, anti-inflammatory, antimicrobial, and antiproliferative functions (Silva-Carvalho et al., 2015).

Oral administration of Libyan propolis prevented a rise in blood cholesterol, TG, LDL, and VLDL levels in lead-acetate-intoxicated mice (Tolba et al., 2013). Croatian propolis reverses cholesterol transport, expresses ATP-binding cassette transporters A1 and G1 (Yu et al., 2011), and directly stimulates HDL production in high-fat diet-fed mice. In mice, artepillin C promotes the transformation of adipocytes from white to brown, suggesting its role in improving energy expenditure and in the prevention and treatment of metabolic diseases like diabetes and obesity (Nishikawa et al., 2016).

Propolis modulates lipids and interferes with plaque macrophages' vascular LDL handling. When it takes place early in the evolution of plaque, macrophage apoptosis is related to decreased cellularity and reduced lesion growth. Propolis made in ethanolic extracts may protect macrophages from oxLDL-mediated apoptosis. Propolis inhibits the matrix responsible for tissue remodeling, repair, and atherosclerotic plaque destabilization (Saavedra et al., 2016). It was also reported to inhibit atherosclerosis progression by reducing dysfunction of vascular endothelium via the inhibition of the human umbilical vein phospholipase C (HUVECs) implicated in atherosclerosis by ROS scavenging and NF-B suppressor actions (Xuan et al., 2014). Ethanolic extracts of propolis were found to inhibit ADP-induced platelet aggregation in young individuals with thrombophilia, with increased efficacy ascribed to low luteolin and/or pinocembrin-7-methyleter concentration (Bojić et al., 2018). Aqueous propolis extracts when mixed with human platelet-rich plasma were found to inhibit aggregation of platelets stimulated by ADP, collagen, and the thrombin receptor activator peptide. Comparable results were reported for several flavonoids from propolis like pinostrobin, chrysin, and galangin, by decreasing PAI-1, an inflammatory fibrinolysis inhibitor (Zhang et al., 2017).

Propolis' antihypertensive benefits in animal models have been attributed to its alteration of antioxidant and anti-inflammatory properties, in addition to modulation of the vascular tone (Silveira et al., 2019). This can be attributed to its ability to promote the activity of NO synthase (NOS) and block N(gamma)-nitro-L-arginine methyl ester (L-NAME)-induced hypertension and tyrosine hydroxylase-mediated catecholamine production (Gogebakan et al., 2012). Antihypertensive effects related to endothelium-dependent vasorelaxation are due to muscarinic receptor agonistic action or downstream pathway potentiation. Several investigations have shown vasoactive chemicals in propolis such as kaempferide, dihydrokaempferide, isosakuranetin, and dihydrochromen. Chrysin increases glutathione-S-transferase and glutathione reductase in L-NAME-induced hypertension in Wistar rats (Malarvili & Veerappan, 2014).

Inflammation and malignancy cause chronic and inappropriate angiogenesis leading to plaque development and hence atherosclerosis. Instability leads to intraplaque bleeding and plaque rupture. Propolis extracts limit the viability of endothelial cells by triggering apoptotic processes or reducing cell migration and proliferation (Dianat et al., 2018). Antiangiogenic activity can be attributed to artepillin C, kaempferol, galangin, and quercetin (Ahn et al., 2009).

Pre-treatment of human umbilical vein endothelial cells (HUVECs) with ethanolic extracts of Chinese propolis reduced NOX activation, malondialdehyde, and ROS production while enhancing antioxidant enzyme activity (Fang et al., 2014). In addition, oxLDL absorption by HUVECs was also inhibited by the attenuation of oxLDL-induced activation of LOX-1 (Sawamura et al., 1997). Increasing LDH release, activating caspase-3, and oxLDL-induced cell death dose-dependently maintained cell viability, indicating protection against oxLDL-mediated endothelial dysfunction. Protection was also afforded by Chinese poplar propolis opposed to oxLDL-mediated endothelial dysfunction by stimulating the PI3K/Akt/mTOR signaling pathway, reducing LOX-1/p38 MAPK level, and preserving the levels of MMPs to limit apoptotic processes and autophagy (Chang et al., 2018).

12.3.3 BEE POLLEN

Polyphenols present in bee pollen inhibit enzymes that catalyze ROS generation, chelate metal ions implicated in the formation of free radicals, scavenge free radicals to counteract peroxidation of lipids, and work synergistically with tocopherols and vitamin C.

Complementing a high-fat diet with ethanolic extract of bee pollen reduces liver ballooning. This hepatoprotective effect was linked to a 31% and 35% decrease in TC and LDL cholesterol (Rzepecka-Stojko et al., 2017). Such supplementation for a period of 16 weeks reduces ox-LDL in mice by 33% and 47%, respectively (Rzepecka-Stojko et al., 2017). These effects can be explained by enhanced adipokine regulation and insulin sensitivity, reduction in de novo lipogenesis, and an improvement in fatty acid oxidation (Steinberg & Witztum, 2010). Polyphenols can modulate lipid levels through various mechanisms, according to research. Flavonoids cause a reduction in hypercholesterolemic conditions by inhibiting hepatic apolipoprotein B synthesis (Loke et al., 2010). They inhibit prostaglandin E2 release and reduce pro-inflammatory cytokine gene expression in macrophages. Furthermore, inhibition of VLDL absorption, blocking of SR-A receptor, and impeding the metabolism of acylated LDL by macrophages take place (Widmer et al., 2013). It was found to reduce HNF4 expression, which affects apolipoprotein B secretion and glucose and lipid metabolism. Polyphenols in bee pollen also reduce VLDL acyl-CoA: cholesterol acyltransferase (ACAT) activity (Böger, 2003).

High concentrations of asymmetric dimethylarginine (ADMA) cause endothelial dysfunction in various diseases. Endogenous dimethylarginine inhibits NOS. ADMA limits the bioavailability of NO, an anti-atherosclerotic endogenous substance. Stress, inflammation, and hypercholesterolemia reduce DDAH activity (Xu et al., 2006). ADMA increases endothelial dysfunction, oxidative stress, and monocyte adhesion by reducing NO synthesis. Elevation in ADMA levels has been reported in people with kidney disease, atherosclerosis, hypercholesterolemia, diabetes, hyperhomocysteinemia, and hypertension (Hou et al., 2012). This indicator changes early in atherosclerosis development in animals. During the entire observation period, C57BL6 mice on a high-fat diet had the highest ADMA level. Supplementing a high-fat diet with bee pollen lowers ADMA levels. EEP reduces endothelial dysfunction by increasing NO bioavailability, which prevents atherosclerosis (Rzepecka-Stojko et al., 2017).

Angiotensin II affects atherosclerosis and oxidative stress. It causes endothelial dysfunction, particularly in response to NO, and inhibits endothelial vasodilator function by stimulating ROS production, which forms ox-LDL. Supplementing a high-fat diet lowers angiotensin-converting enzyme by 17%. Based on the study results, polyphenol fraction from bee pollen may protect against cardiovascular disease by improving endothelial function by modulating the renin-angiotensin-aldosterone system (Rzepecka-Stojko et al., 2017).

12.3.4 ROYAL JELLY

Royal jelly (RJ) is classified as a functional food. It is used as a supplement and in cosmetics. It is a thick and milky substance secreted by young worker bees, *Apis mellifera* Linn (Ramadan & Al-Ghamdi, 2012). It is rich in the bioactive 10-hydroxy-2-decenoic acid (Nagai & Inoue, 2004). RJ protein contains several glycoproteins with N-terminal oligosaccharide bonds known as Major royal jelly proteins (MRJP 1–9) (Drapeau et al., 2006) – characterized using 2D SDS-PAGE: 46% MRJP1, 11% MRJP2, 13% MRJP3, and 30% of the other six MRJPs (Kashima et al., 2014). Research shows that RJ MRJPs contribute to various physiological functions (Schönleben et al., 2007). Previous work has linked the hypocholesterolemic effect of dietary proteins to bile acid binding and metabolism (Kashima et al., 2014). RJ improves the metabolism of lipoproteins in humans by an unknown underlying mechanism (Guo et al., 2007). This study aimed to show that protein-enriched RJ has the ability to regulate blood lipids by increasing the levels of DHEA-S in healthy mild hypercholesterolemic model organisms (Guo et al., 2007). SDS-PAGE analysis demonstrated hypocholesterolemic proteins MRJP1 and MRJP2 with molecular weights of 49 and 55 kDa, respectively as the major constituents (Kashima et al., 2014).

Three-month RJ or placebo interventions did not affect body weight, waist circumference, or body fat. Thus, RJ consumption did not cause physiological changes or discomfort. Healthy participants had normal postures. Guo et al. (2007) found that 6 g of RJ did not affect body weight, body fat composition, or waist circumference. Liver and kidney function markers were unaffected by the RJ or placebo. When rats were given a low dose of 100 mg/kg body weight of RJ, they exhibited similar serum glutamic oxaloacetic transaminase (GOT) and serum glutamic pyruvic transaminase (GPT) activities when compared to the control group (El-Nekeety et al.,

2007). Three months of continuous RJ intake did not cause hepatic or renal damage, proving it a safe drug without adverse effects.

Estradiol (E2), dehydroepiandrosterone sulfate (DHEA-S), and testosterone (T) exert anti-aging, hypocholesterolemic, anti-atherogenic, immunomodulatory, hypotensive, and cognitive effects, according to studies (Corona et al., 2011). CVD patients had lower E2, T, and DHEA-S levels than non-CVD patients (Shufelt et al., 2011). These parameters are measured to determine the link between RJ and CVD. Supplementation with RJ improved DHEA-S levels, but there were no significant changes during follow-up. In some models, MRJP and 10-hydroxy-2-decenoic acid possess estrogenic activity (Moutsatsou et al., 2010). The estrogenic activity of RJ increases DHEA-S levels. In experimental and placebo groups, E2 and T levels were unchanged. DHEA-S influences the activities of glucose 6-phosphate dehydrogenase and glycerol 3-phosphate dehydrogenase and stops NADPH synthesis. It also inhibits the synthesis of phospholipids, fatty acids, and cholesterol (Porsova-Dutoit et al., 2000). Elevated levels of DHEA-S may alter lipid metabolism by lowering TC and LDL-C (Tchernof et al., 1997).

A few trials show that high LDL-C and low HDL-C may increase CVD risk (Chiu et al., 2015). TC, LDL-C, and HDL-C must be evaluated. Dietary protein affects blood cholesterol (Madani et al., 2003). Due to MRJP1 and 2, RJ reduces TC and LDL-C. MRJP1 possesses a high bile acid binding capacity that hinders cholesterol absorption, and micelle formation, and represses lowering cholesterol and LDL-C levels (Nagaoka et al., 2010). In a rat model, MRJP1 significantly upregulates the levels of cholesterol 7-hydroxylase (CYP7A1) in hepatic cells (Kashima et al., 2014). RJ does not affect TG or HDL-C levels. Few clinical trials show RJ reduces TC, VLDL, and LDL-C (Morita et al., 2012).

12.4 CONCLUSION

It would appear that honey and other products made from bees may offer some degree of protection to the heart. Regrettably, despite the fact that this potential has been observed *in vitro*, in animal models, and human models, very few *in vivo* studies have been performed on human models. In addition, there is not yet any concrete clinical evidence to support the efficacy or safety of apitherapy treatments, nor are there any recommendations concerning the effective or safe doses of bee products for the prevention and treatment of CVDs. In addition, the studies that were examined used a variety of different kinds of bee products, some of which had an unknown chemical makeup. In spite of this, the findings of this chapter shed new light on the cardioprotective mechanisms of compounds that are present in bee products. Despite the fact that these mechanisms are complicated and, for the most part, are still a mystery, there is some evidence to suggest that phenolic compounds, in particular, may play an important role in these mechanisms. For instance, the phenolic components of propolis may lessen the production of ROS and NO, as well as lessen the activity of cyclooxygenase, phospholipase A2, and C. Propolis has been used for a variety of medicinal purposes. In addition, the phenolic compounds found in propolis have the potential to lower the expression of TLR4 and NF-κB. Nevertheless, additional research is required to shed light on the workings of their mechanisms of action. Even so, it is essential to make the point that even though none of the test subjects who were given bee products exhibited any negative side effects, it is possible for bee products to provoke allergic responses in some people. These kinds of reactions are able to take place in the cardiovascular system and have the potential to result in ischemia of the myocardium.

KEYWORDS

- **aminotransferase**
- **atherosclerosis**
- **glutathione reductase**
- **glutathione-s-transferase**
- **low-density lipoprotein**
- **metabolic syndrome**
- **reactive oxygen species**
- **royal jelly**
- **superoxide dismutase**

REFERENCES

Ahmad, A., Khan, R. A., & Mesaik, M. A. (2009). Anti-inflammatory effect of natural honey on bovine thrombin-induced oxidative burst in phagocytes. *Phytotherapy Research, 23*(6), 801–808. https://doi.org/10.1002/ptr.2725.

Ahn, M. R., Kunimasa, K., Kumazawa, S., Nakayama, T., Kaji, K., Uto, Y., Hori, H., Nagasawa, H., & Ohta, T. (2009). Correlation between antiangiogenic activity and antioxidant activity of various components from propolis. *Molecular Nutrition & Food Research, 53*(5), 643–651. https://doi.org/10.1002/mnfr.200800204.

Alagwu, E. A., Okwara, J. E., Nneli, R. O., & Osim, E. E. (2011). Effect of honey intake on serum cholesterol, triglycerides and lipoprotein levels in albino rats and potential benefits on risks of coronary heart disease. *Nigerian Journal of Physiological Sciences, 26*(2), 161–165. https://doi.org/10.4314/njps.v26i2.5.

Anjum, S. I., Ullah, A., Khan, K. A., Attaullah, M., Khan, H., Ali, H., Bashir, M. A., Tahir, M., Ansari, M. J., Ghramh, H. A., Adgaba, N., & Dash, C. K. (2019). Composition and functional properties of propolis (bee glue): A review. *Saudi Journal of Biological Sciences, 26*(7), 1695–1703. https://doi.org/10.1016/j.sjbs.2018.02.011.

Árnadóttir, Á., Vestergaard, K. R., Sölétormos, G., Steffensen, R., Goetze, J. P., & Iversen, K. (2018). Prediction of coronary heart disease or heart failure using high-sensitivity cardiac troponin T: A pilot study. *European Journal of Clinical Investigation, 48*(10), e13009. https://doi.org/10.1111/eci.13009.

Böger, R. H. (2003). The emerging role of asymmetric dimethylarginine as a novel cardiovascular risk factor. *Cardiovascular Research, 59*(4), 824–833. https://doi.org/10.1016/S0008-6363(03)00515-1.

Bojić, M., Antolić, A., Tomičić, M., Debeljak, Ž., & Maleš, Ž. (2018). Propolis ethanolic extracts reduce adenosine diphosphate induced platelet aggregation determined on whole blood. *Nutrition Journal, 17*(1), 52. https://doi.org/10.1186/s12937-018-0360-2.

Borshchev, Y. Y., Uspensky, Y. P., & Galagudza, M. M. (2019). Pathogenetic pathways of cognitive dysfunction and dementia in metabolic syndrome. *Life Sciences, 237*, 116932. https://doi.org/10.1016/j.lfs.2019.116932.

Busserolles, J., Gueux, E., Rock, E., Mazur, A., & Rayssiguier, Y. (2002). Substituting honey for refined carbohydrates protects rats from hypertriglyceridemic and prooxidative effects of fructose. *The Journal of Nutrition, 132*(11), 3379–3382. https://doi.org/10.1093/jn/132.11.3379.

Chang, H., Yuan, W., Wu, H., Yin, X., & Xuan, H. (2018). Bioactive components and mechanisms of Chinese poplar propolis alleviates oxidized low-density lipoprotein-induced endothelial cells injury. *BMC Complementary and Alternative Medicine, 18*(1), 142. https://doi.org/10.1186/s12906-018-2213-2.

Chiu, H. F., Chen, B. K., Lu, Y. Y., Han, Y. C., Shen, Y. C., Venkatakrishnan, K., Golovinskaia, O., & Wang, C. K. (2017). Hypocholesterolemic efficacy of royal jelly in healthy mild hypercholesterolemic adults. *Pharmaceutical Biology, 55*(1), 497–502. https://doi.org/10.1080/13880209.2016.1262442.

Corona, G., Rastrelli, G., Vignozzi, L., Mannucci, E., & Maggi, M. (2011). Testosterone, cardiovascular disease and the metabolic syndrome. *Best Practice & Research Clinical Endocrinology & Metabolism, 25*(2), 337–353. https://doi.org/10.1016/j.beem.2010.09.004.

Desai, A., Darland, G., Bland, J. S., Tripp, M. L., & Konda, V. R. (2012). META060 attenuates TNF-α-activated inflammation, endothelial-monocyte interactions, and matrix metalloproteinase-9 expression, and inhibits NF-κB and AP-1 in THP-1 monocytes. *Atherosclerosis, 223*(1), 130–136. https://doi.org/10.1016/j.atherosclerosis.2012.05.015.

Dianat, M., Saadatfard, S., Badavi, M., Pour, A. A., & Sadeghi, N. (2018). Corrigendum: The effect of caffeic acid phenethyl ester on development of left ventricular dysfunction in cirrhotic rats. *International Cardiovascular Research Journal, 12*(4), 179–184. https://doi.org/10.5812/icrj.159.

Dietz, W., & Santos-Burgoa, C. (2020). Obesity and its implications for COVID-19 mortality. *Obesity (Silver Spring, Md.), 28*(6), 1005. https://doi.org/10.1002/oby.22818.

Drapeau, M. D., Albert, S., Kucharski, R., Prusko, C., & Maleszka, R. (2006). Evolution of the Yellow/Major Royal Jelly Protein family and the emergence of social behavior in honey bees. *Genome Research, 16*(11), 1385–1394. https://doi.org/10.1101/gr.5012006.

Dsouza, M. R., Rufina, K., & Hana, D. (2018). Extraction of diosgenin from fenugreek and evaluation of its pharmacological role in alleviating metabolic syndrome in vitro. *Research Journal of Biotechnology, 13*(12), 10–17.

El-Nekeety, A. A., El-Kholy, W., Abbas, N. F., Ebaid, A., Amra, H. A., & Abdel-Wahhab, M. A. (2007). Efficacy of royal jelly against the oxidative stress of fumonisin in rats. *Toxicon, 50*(2), 256–269. https://doi.org/10.1016/j.toxicon.2007.03.017.

Erejuwa, O. O., Akpan, J. L., Uwaezuoke, N., Nwobodo, N. N., Ezeokpo, B. C., Erhiano, E., Araromi, E. J., Ude, U. N., AbdulWahab, M., & Sulaiman, S. A. (2018). Effects of honey on postprandial hyperlipidemia and oxidative stress in Wistar rats: Role of HMG-CoA reductase inhibition and antioxidant effect. *Nigerian Journal of Physiological Sciences, 33*(2), 129–138. https://doi.org/10.4314/njps.v33i2.3.

Eteraf-Oskouei, T., Shaseb, E., Ghaffary, S., & Najafi, M. (2003). Prolonged preconditioning with natural honey against myocardial infarction injuries. *Pakistan Journal of Pharmaceutical Sciences, 26*(4), 681–686.

Falk, E. (2006). Pathogenesis of atherosclerosis. *Journal of the American College of Cardiology, 47*(8 Suppl), C7–C12. https://doi.org/10.1016/j.jacc.2005.09.068.

Fang, Y., Li, J., Ding, M., Xu, X., Zhang, J., Jiao, P., Han, P., Wang, J., & Yao, S. (2014). Ethanol extract of propolis protects endothelial cells from oxidized low-density lipoprotein-induced injury by inhibiting lectin-like oxidized low-density lipoprotein receptor-1-mediated oxidative stress. *Experimental Biology and Medicine, 239*(12), 1678–1687. https://doi.org/10.1177/1535370214539348.

Forbes-Hernández, T. Y., Giampieri, F., Gasparrini, M., Afrin, S., Mazzoni, L., Cordero, M. D., Mezzetti, B., Quiles, J. L., & Battino, M. (2017). Lipid accumulation in HepG2 cells is attenuated by strawberry extract through AMPK activation. *Nutrients, 9*(6), 621. https://doi.org/10.3390/nu9060621.

Gogebakan, A., Talas, Z. S., Ozdemir, I., & Sahna, E. (2012). Role of propolis on tyrosine hydroxylase activity and blood pressure in nitric oxide synthase-inhibited hypertensive rats. *Clinical and Experimental Hypertension, 34*(6), 424–428. https://doi.org/10.3109/10641963.2012.673899.

Guo, H., Saiga, A., Sato, M., Miyazawa, I., Shibata, M., Takahata, Y., & Morimatsu, F. (2007). Royal jelly supplementation improves lipoprotein metabolism in humans. *Journal of Nutritional Science and Vitaminology, 53*(4), 345–348. https://doi.org/10.3177/jnsv.53.345.

Hana, C. D., Rufina, K., & Dsouza, M. R. (2019). Diosgenin from Dioscorea Alata: Extraction and potential effects on enzymes related to metabolic syndrome. *International Journal of Pharmacy and Biological Sciences, 9*, 177–185.

Hou, S. Z., Xu, S. J., Jiang, D. X., Chen, S. X., Wang, L. L., Huang, S., & Lai, X. P. (2012). Effect of the flavonoid fraction of Lithocarpus polystachyus Rehd. on spontaneously hypertensive and normotensive rats. *Journal of Ethnopharmacology, 143*(2), 441–447. https://doi.org/10.1016/j.jep.2012.06.032.

Iqbal, S. P., Ramadas, A., Fatt, Q. K., Shin, H. L., Onn, W. Y., & Kadir, K. A. (2020). Relationship of sociodemographic and lifestyle factors and diet habits with metabolic syndrome (MetS) among three ethnic groups of the Malaysian population. *PLoS ONE, 15*(3), e0224054. https://doi.org/10.1371/journal.pone.0224054.

Kashima, Y., Kanematsu, S., Asai, S., Kusada, M., Watanabe, S., Kawashima, T., Nakamura, T., Shimada, M., Goto, T., & Nagaoka, S. (2014). Identification of a novel hypocholesterolemic protein, major royal jelly protein 1, derived from royal jelly. *PLoS ONE, 9*(8), e105073. https://doi.org/10.1371/journal.pone.0105073.

Khalil, M. I., Tanvir, E. M., Afroz, R., Sulaiman, S. A., & Gan, S. H. (2015). Cardioprotective effects of Tualang honey: Amelioration of cholesterol and cardiac enzymes levels. *BioMed Research International*, 286051. https://doi.org/10.1155/2015/286051.

Kieliszek, M., Piwowarek, K., Kot, A. M., Błażejak, S., Chlebowska-Śmigiel, A., & Wolska, I. (2018). Pollen and bee bread as new health-oriented products: A review. *Trends in Food Science & Technology, 71*, 170–180. https://doi.org/10.1016/j.tifs.2017.10.021.

Linton, M., Yancey, P., Davies, S., Jerome, W., & Vickers, K. C. (2000). The role of lipids and lipoproteins in atherosclerosis. In *MDText.com, Inc., 1,* 1–200.

Loke, W. M., Proudfoot, J. M., Hodgson, J. M., McKinley, A. J., Hime, N., Magat, M., Stocker, R., & Croft, K. D. (2010). Specific dietary polyphenols attenuate atherosclerosis in apolipoprotein E-knockout mice by alleviating inflammation and endothelial dysfunction. *Arteriosclerosis, Thrombosis, and Vascular Biology, 30*(4), 749–757. https://doi.org/10.1161/ATVBAHA.109.197244.

Madani, S., Prost, J., Narce, M., & Belleville, J. (2003). VLDL metabolism in rats is affected by the concentration and source of dietary protein. *The Journal of Nutrition, 133*(12), 4102–4106. https://doi.org/10.1093/jn/133.12.4102.

Maksimenko, A. V., & Vavaev, A. V. (2012). Antioxidant enzymes as potential targets in cardioprotection and treatment of cardiovascular diseases. Enzyme antioxidants: the next stage of pharmacological counterwork to the oxidative stress. *Heart International, 7*(1), e3. https://doi.org/10.4081/hi.2012.e3.

Malarvili, T., & Veerappan, R. (2014). Effects of chrysin on free radicals and enzymatic antioxidants in Nω-nitro-l-arginine methyl ester: Induced hypertensive rats. *International Journal of Nutrition, Pharmacology, Neurological Diseases, 4*, 112. https://doi.org/10.4103/2231-0738.127724.

Marrocco, I., Altieri, F., & Peluso, I. (2017). Measurement and clinical significance of biomarkers of oxidative stress in humans. *Oxidative Medicine and Cellular Longevity, 2017*, 6501046. https://doi.org/10.1155/2017/6501046.

McGurnaghan, S. J., Weir, A., Bishop, J., Kennedy, S., Blackbourn, L., McAllister, D. A., Hutchinson, S., Caparrotta, T. M., Mellor, J., Jeyam, A., O'Reilly, J. E., Wild, S. H., Hatam, S., Höhn, A., Colombo, M., Robertson, C., Lone, N., Murray, J., Butterly, E., Petrie, J., & Scottish Diabetes Research Network Epidemiology Group. (2021). Risks of and risk factors for COVID-19 disease in people with diabetes: A cohort study of the total population of Scotland. *The Lancet Diabetes & Endocrinology, 9*(2), 82–93. https://doi.org/10.1016/S2213-8587(20)30405-8.

Megson, I. L., Whitfield, P. D., & Zabetakis, I. (2016). Lipids and cardiovascular disease: Where does dietary intervention sit alongside statin therapy? *Food & Function, 7*(6), 2603–2614. https://doi.org/10.1039/C5FO01515A.

Moghadasian, M. H., Zhao, R., Ghazawwi, N., Le, K., Apea-Bah, F. B., Beta, T., & Shen, G. X. (2017). Inhibitory effects of North American wild rice on monocyte adhesion and inflammatory modulators in low-density lipoprotein receptor-knockout mice. *Journal of Agricultural and Food Chemistry, 65*(41), 9054–9060. https://doi.org/10.1021/acs.jafc.7b02556.

Morita, H., Ikeda, T., Kajita, K., Fujioka, K., Mori, I., Okada, H., Uno, Y., & Ishizuka, T. (2012). Effect of royal jelly ingestion for six months on healthy volunteers. *Nutrition Journal, 11*, 77. https://doi.org/10.1186/1475-2891-11-77.

Moutsatsou, P., Papoutsi, Z., Kassi, E., Heldring, N., Zhao, C., Tsiapara, A., Melliou, E., Chrousos, G. P., Chinou, I., Karshikoff, A., Nilsson, L., & Dahlman-Wright, K. (2010). Fatty acids derived from royal jelly are modulators of estrogen receptor functions. *PLoS ONE, 5*(12), e15594. https://doi.org/10.1371/journal.pone.0015594.

Mythili, S., & Malathi, N. (2015). Diagnostic markers of acute myocardial infarction. *Biomedical Reports, 3*(6), 743–748. https://doi.org/10.3892/br.2015.510.

Nagai, T., & Inoue, R. (2004). Preparation and the functional properties of water extract and alkaline extract of royal jelly. *Food Chemistry, 84*(2), 181–186. https://doi.org/10.1016/S0308-8146(03)00202-6.

Nagaoka, S., Nakamura, A., Shibata, H., & Kanamaru, Y. (2010). Soystatin (VAWWMY), a novel bile acid-binding peptide, decreased micellar solubility and inhibited cholesterol absorption in rats. *Bioscience, Biotechnology, and Biochemistry, 74*(8), 1738–1741. https://doi.org/10.1271/bbb.100252.

Najafi, M., Shaseb, E., Ghaffary, S., Fakhrju, A., & Eteraf-Oskouei, T. (2011). Effects of chronic oral administration of natural honey on ischemia/reperfusion-induced arrhythmias in isolated rat heart. *Iranian Journal of Basic Medical Sciences, 14*(1), 75–81.

Nishikawa, S., Aoyama, H., Kamiya, M., Higuchi, J., Kato, A., Soga, M., Kawai, T., Yoshimura, K., Kumazawa, S., & Tsuda, T. (2016). Artepillin C, a typical Brazilian propolis-derived component, induces brown-like adipocyte formation in C3H10T1/2 cells, primary inguinal white adipose tissue-derived adipocytes, and mice. *PLoS ONE, 11*(9), e0162512. https://doi.org/10.1371/journal.pone.0162512.

Pacurari, M., Kafoury, R., Tchounwou, P. B., & Ndebele, K. (2014). The renin-angiotensin-aldosterone system in vascular inflammation and remodeling. *International Journal of Inflammation, 2014*, 689360. https://doi.org/10.1155/2014/689360.

Patibandla, S., & Alsayouri, K. (2020). Cardiac enzymes. In *StatPearls*, 1–2. StatPearls Publishing.

Porsová-Dutoit, I., Sulcová, J., & Stárka, L. (2000). Do DHEA/DHEAS play a protective role in coronary heart disease? *Physiological Research, 49*(Suppl 1), S43–S56.

Ramadan, M. F., & Al-Ghamdi, A. (2012). Bioactive compounds and health-promoting properties of royal jelly: A review. *Journal of Functional Foods, 4*(1), 39–52. https://doi.org/10.1016/j.jff.2011.12.007.

Rzepecka-Stojko, A., Stojko, J., Jasik, K., & Buszman, E. (2017). Anti-atherogenic activity of polyphenol-rich extract from bee pollen. *Nutrients, 9*(12), 1369. https://doi.org/10.3390/nu9121369.

Saavedra, N., Cuevas, A., Cavalcante, M. F., Dörr, F. A., Saavedra, K., Zambrano, T., Abdalla, D. S., & Salazar, L. A. (2016). Polyphenols from Chilean propolis and pinocembrin reduce MMP-9 gene expression and activity in activated macrophages. *BioMed Research International, 2016*, 6505383. https://doi.org/10.1155/2016/6505383.

Sawamura, T., Kume, N., Aoyama, T., Moriwaki, H., Hoshikawa, H., Aiba, Y., Tanaka, T., Miwa, S., Katsura, Y., Kita, T., & Masaki, T. (1997). An endothelial receptor for oxidized low-density lipoprotein. *Nature, 386*(6620), 73–77. https://doi.org/10.1038/386073a0.

Scholze, J., Alegria, E., Ferri, C., Langham, S., Stevens, W., Jeffries, D., & Uhl-Hochgraeber, K. (2010). Epidemiological and economic burden of metabolic syndrome and its consequences in patients with hypertension in Germany, Spain and Italy; a prevalence-based model. *BMC Public Health, 10*, 529. https://doi.org/10.1186/1471-2458-10-529.

Schönleben, S., Sickmann, A., Mueller, M. J., & Reinders, J. (2007). Proteome analysis of Apis mellifera royal jelly. *Analytical and Bioanalytical Chemistry, 389*(4), 1087–1093. https://doi.org/10.1007/s00216-007-1478-5.

Shediwah, F., Naji, K. M., Gumaih, H. S., Alhadi, F. A., Al-Hammami, A. L., & D'Souza, M. R. (2019). Antioxidant and antihyperlipidemic activity of Costus speciosus against atherogenic diet-induced hyperlipidemia in rabbits. *Journal of Integrative Medicine, 17*(3), 181–187. https://doi.org/10.1016/j.joim.2019.04.002.

Shufelt, C., Bretsky, P., Almeida, C. M., Johnson, B. D., Shaw, L. J., Azziz, R., Braunstein, G. D., Pepine, C. J., Bittner, V., Vido, D. A., Stanczyk, F. Z., & Bairey Merz, C. N. (2010). DHEA-S levels and cardiovascular disease mortality in postmenopausal women: Results from the National Institutes of Health–National Heart, Lung, and Blood Institute (NHLBI)-sponsored Women's Ischemia Syndrome Evaluation (WISE). *The Journal of Clinical Endocrinology & Metabolism, 95*(11), 4985–4992. https://doi.org/10.1210/jc.2010-0453.

Silva-Carvalho, R., Baltazar, F., & Almeida-Aguiar, C. (2015). Propolis: A complex natural product with a plethora of biological activities that can be explored for drug development. *Evidence-Based Complementary and Alternative Medicine: eCAM, 2015*, 206439. https://doi.org/10.1155/2015/206439.

Silveira, M., Teles, F., Berretta, A. A., Sanches, T. R., Rodrigues, C. E., Seguro, A. C., & Andrade, L. (2019). Effects of Brazilian green propolis on proteinuria and renal function in patients with chronic kidney disease: A randomized, double-blind, placebo-controlled trial. *BMC Nephrology, 20*(1), 140. https://doi.org/10.1186/s12882-019-1344-5.

Sirtori, C. R., Pavanello, C., Calabresi, L., & Ruscica, M. (2017). Nutraceutical approaches to metabolic syndrome. *Annals of Medicine, 49*(8), 678–697. https://doi.org/10.1080/07853890.2017.1343892.

Steinberg, D., & Witztum, J. L. (2010). Oxidized low-density lipoprotein and atherosclerosis. *Arteriosclerosis, Thrombosis, and Vascular Biology, 30*(12), 2311–2316. https://doi.org/10.1161/ATVBAHA.108.179697.

Steyers, C. M., 3rd, & Miller, F. J., Jr. (2014). Endothelial dysfunction in chronic inflammatory diseases. *International Journal of Molecular Sciences, 15*(7), 11324–11349. https://doi.org/10.3390/ijms150711324.

Sung, S. H., Choi, G. H., Lee, N. W., & Shin, B. C. (2017). External use of propolis for oral, skin, and genital diseases: A systematic review and meta-analysis. *Evidence-Based Complementary and Alternative Medicine: eCAM, 2017*, 8025752. https://doi.org/10.1155/2017/8025752.

Tchernof, A., Labrie, F., Bélanger, A., Prud'homme, D., Bouchard, C., Tremblay, A., Nadeau, A., & Després, J. P. (1997). Relationships between endogenous steroid hormones, sex hormone-binding globulin, and lipoprotein levels in men: Contribution of visceral obesity, insulin levels, and other metabolic variables. *Atherosclerosis, 133*(2), 235–244. https://doi.org/10.1016/S0021-9150(97)00020-9.

Tolba, M. F., Azab, S. S., Khalifa, A. E., Abdel-Rahman, S. Z., & Abdel-Naim, A. B. (2013). Caffeic acid phenethyl ester, a promising component of propolis with a plethora of biological activities: A review on its anti-inflammatory, neuroprotective, hepatoprotective, and cardioprotective effects. *IUBMB Life, 65*(8), 699–709. https://doi.org/10.1002/iub.1181.

Tsutsui, H., Kinugawa, S., & Matsushima, S. (2011). Oxidative stress and heart failure. *American Journal of Physiology – Heart and Circulatory Physiology, 301*(6), H2181–H2190. https://doi.org/10.1152/ajpheart.00554.2011.

Viola, J., & Soehnlein, O. (2020). Atherosclerosis – A matter of unresolved inflammation. *Seminars in Immunology, 27*(3), 184–193. https://doi.org/10.1016/j.smim.2015.03.013.

Widmer, R. J., Freund, M. A., Flammer, A. J., Sexton, J., Lennon, R., Romani, A., Mulinacci, N., Vinceri, F. F., Lerman, L. O., & Lerman, A. (2013). Beneficial effects of polyphenol-rich olive oil in patients with early atherosclerosis. *European Journal of Nutrition, 52*(3), 1223–1231. https://doi.org/10.1007/s00394-012-0430-7.

World Health Organization. (2020). Global health estimates. pp. 1–2. Available online: https://www.who.int/news-room/fact-sheets/detail/the-top-10-causes-of-death.

Wu, J., Xun, N., Yang, Y., Zeng, L., Li, Z., Yang, W., Liang, Y., Tang, H., & Ma, Z. (2018). Chrysin attenuates myocardial ischemia–reperfusion injury by inhibiting myocardial inflammation. *RSC Advances, 8*(25), 13739–13746. https://doi.org/10.1039/C8RA00417D.

Xu, Y. Y., Yang, C., & Li, S. N. (2006). Effects of genistein on angiotensin-converting enzyme in rats. *Life Sciences, 79*(9), 828–837. https://doi.org/10.1016/j.lfs.2006.03.030.

Xuan, H., Li, Z., Wang, J., Wang, K., Fu, C., Yuan, J., & Hu, F. (2014). Propolis reduces phosphatidylcholine-specific phospholipase C activity and increases annexin A7 level in oxidized-LDL-stimulated human umbilical vein endothelial cells. *Evidence-Based Complementary and Alternative Medicine: eCAM, 2014*, 465383. https://doi.org/10.1155/2014/465383.

Yu, Y., Si, Y., Song, G., Luo, T., Wang, J., & Qin, S. (2011). Ethanolic extract of propolis promotes reverse cholesterol transport and the expression of ATP-binding cassette transporter A1 and G1 in mice. *Lipids, 46*(9), 805–811. https://doi.org/10.1007/s11745-011-3575-7.

Zhang, Y. X., Yang, T. T., Xia, L., Zhang, W. F., Wang, J. F., & Wu, Y. P. (2017). Inhibitory effect of propolis on platelet aggregation in vitro. *Journal of Healthcare Engineering, 2017*, 3050895. https://doi.org/10.1155/2017/3050895.

Zhou, Y., Zheng, R., Tan, L., Xu, R., Wang, Z., & Fu, J. (2020). Protective effect of caffeic acid phenethyl ester against atherosclerosis and cardiac injury in apolipoprotein E-deficient mice. *Cardiovascular Toxicology, 20*(4), 366–375. https://doi.org/10.1007/s12012-019-09539-3.

Zhu, W., Li, Y. H., Chen, M. L., & Hu, Y. Z. (2011). Metabolism and pharmacokinetics of caffeic acid phenethyl ester in rats. *Journal of Pharmaceutical and Biomedical Analysis, 55*(2), 329–334. https://doi.org/10.1016/j.jpba.2011.01.022.

Zordoky, B. N. M., Robertson, I. M., & Dyck, J. R. B. (2015). Preclinical and clinical evidence for the role of resveratrol in the treatment of cardiovascular diseases. *Biochimica et Biophysica Acta (BBA) – Molecular Basis of Disease, 1852*(6), 1155–1177. https://doi.org/10.1016/j.bbadis.2014.10.016.

Zulet, M. A., Marti, A., & Martínez, J. A. (2009). Pro-inflammatory cytokines and adipose tissue. In C. Fantuzzi & T. Mazzone (Eds.), *Adipose Tissue and Inflammation* (pp. 183–204). Humana Press. https://doi.org/10.1007/978-1-60327-874-6_11.

Zwaka, T. P., Hombach, V., & Torzewski, J. (2001). C-reactive protein-mediated low density lipoprotein uptake by macrophages: implications for atherosclerosis. *Circulation, 103*(9), 1194–1197. https://doi.org/10.1161/01.CIR.103.9.1194.

PART III

CARDIOTONIC ACTIVITY OF POLYPHENOLS

CHAPTER 13

EFFECTS OF POLYPHENOLS ON HYPERTENSION

ABABIO GRACE K.

University of Ghana Medical School, Medical Biochemistry

ABSTRACT

This piece reviewed the biochemistry of polyphenols and its implications in hypertension. A working model or conceptual framework is duly suggested. Discussions were focused on advances and/or challenges for future research. It was well noted that the biological effects of polyphenols go beyond the modulation of oxidative stress. Their potency and efficacy as well depended on the amount of polyphenols consumed and bioavailability.

13.1 INTRODUCTION

13.1.1 POLYPHENOLS

Polyphenols are phytochemicals (Stevenson & Hurst, 2007), originating from plants like coffee, fruits, cereals, and vegetables (Sakakibara, 2003). Polyphenol subtypes (Figure 13.1) or classes include lignans, phenolic acids, stilbenes, flavonoids, and phenolic alcohols.

Most polyphenols are glycosides. Isoflavones, chalcones, and neoflavonoids are types of flavonoids (Tsao, 2010; Harborne, 1989; Alzand & Mohamed, 2012; Keservani & Sharma, 2014; Keservani et al., 2016a, b) seen in legumes. Chalcones are found in hops, apples, and beer as well. Taxifolin, another type of flavonoid, is found in citrus fruits. Seeds of blueberries, apples, and grapes have flavonoids; not forgetting cacao beans and tea leaves. Anthocyanidins form the main component of the colored pigments (purple,

Antioxidants as Nutraceuticals. Nayan A. Gujarathi, Raj K. Keservani, Rajesh K. Kesharwani, Bhushan R. Rane, Yogeeta Sameer Goyal (Eds.)

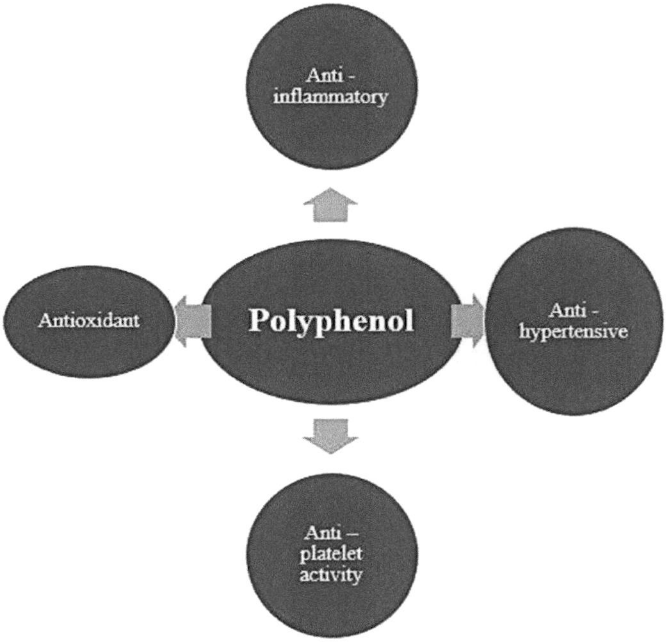

FIGURE 13.1 Structure of the subtypes of polyphenols.

Source: Adapted from Behl et al., 2020

red, blue) of flower petals, vegetables, fruits, and more so black rice. Lignans are found in seeds (e.g., sesame, flax, poppy, pumpkin, sunflower), whole grains (rye, barley, oats), bran (wheat, rye, oat), beans, vegetables, fruit (particularly berries), and beverages like tea, wine, and coffee. Stilbenes, on the other hand, are found in berries.

13.1.2 EXTRACTION TECHNIQUES USED FOR POLYPHENOLS

Nowadays, liquid-liquid partitioning and solid-liquid extraction of polyphenols are frequently utilized in laboratories. Even though the spectrophotometer had been a great tool in ages past, reversed-phase HPLC coupled with a diode array detector and/or mass spectrometric detector (LC-MS) is the preferred analytical quantification technique. Occasionally, polyphenols, e.g., isoflavones, are converted to methyl esters and analyzed by gas chromatography (GC).

13.1.3 KNOWN PROPERTIES OF POLYPHENOLS

Even though there has been massive corroborative *in vitro* antioxidant studies, mounting evidence depicts that polyphenols' role goes beyond the antioxidant functions *in vivo* (Hajilyani et al., 2009; Granato et al., 2016; Reis et al., 2021). This makes the phytochemical receive numerous attentions lately as its role is also being implicated in degenerative diseases, neurodegenerative diseases, and cardiovascular diseases.

Fatty streaks initiate most cardiovascular lesions, and anthocyanins as well as lignans reduce the formation of fatty streaks. Anthocyanins have vasodilation effects as well as anti-aggregative (Pataki et al., 2002; Reed, 2002). Anthocyanin dyes inhibit cyclooxygenase and inhibit vascular cell adhesion molecule (VCAM) as well as degranulation of mast cells.

Stilbenes are used in manufacturing dyes and optical brighteners and could act as phosphor luminescence as well as a scintillator.

Flavonoids act as visual attractors, antioxidants, feeding repellants, antimicrobials, light screening, and photoreceptors in plants (Harborne, 1989; Marias et al., 2006; Pietta, 2000). Several studies have shown the biological and pharmaceutical prowess of flavonoids, including cardio-protection, antioxidant, anticancer, cytotoxic, antibacterial, antiviral, antimalarial, hepatoprotective, antileishmanial, neuroprotective, anti-amebial, anti-trypanosomal properties (Harborne, 1989; Marias et al., 2006; Pietta, 2000; Harborne & Williams, 2000). Not until the mid-20th century were flavonoids known as plant metabolic waste. This notion was refuted by the myriad flavonoid functions (Harborne, 1989; Marias et al., 2006; Pietta, 2000).

13.2 CLINICAL INVESTIGATION

Despite advances made in the pathophysiology and pharmacotherapy of hypertension, interventional strategies are still problematic and this is of public health concern. Some studies have involved dietary changes in the treatment regimen, of which dietary polyphenols are no exception. There has also been an inverse relationship between cardiovascular events and polyphenol consumption (Kim & Je, 2017; Mendonça et al., 2019). However, the mechanism of the cardio-protective effects of polyphenols has not fully been established. In the PREDMED study, there were decreased rates of cardiovascular events after polyphenol consumption. HAPEE and EPIC were observational studies that had a unique relationship between polyphenol-rich diets and arterial blood pressure. Ras et al. (2013), conducted a double-blind study while Mongol et al. (2013), conducted a randomized clinical trial (Table 13.1). Even though Ras et al., 2013,

TABLE 13.1 Some Studies on Polyphenols

Study acronym (or1st author	Study name	Number of participants	Intervention	Primary endpoint observed	other parameters	References
PREDIMED	Prevention with Mediterranean diet	7447	2 different polyphenol-rich diets	Decerased rate of major cardiovascular events	Decerased systolic and diastolic blood pressure	Estruch et al ,2013: Medina-Remón et al.,2016 Grosso et al.,2016
HAPIEE	Health,Alcohol and Psychosocial factors In Eastern Europe cohort study	8821 (Polish)	Observational study	Amelioration of metabolic syndrome parameters (Body mass index waist circumference, blood pressure, triglycerides) in polyphenol-rich diets		
EPIC	European Prospective investigation into Cancer and Nutrition	20,343 (Greek cohort)	Observational study with evaluation of a Mediterranean Diet Score	Inverse correlation between olive oil intake and arterial blood pressure		Psaltopoulou et al 2004
Ras et al.	Effect of polyphenol-rich grape seed extract on ambulatory blood pressure in subject with pre-and stage I hypertension	35	Administration of polyphenol-rich grape seed extract in a double-bliud,Placebo controlled, randomized parallel-group trial	No lowering of blood pressure in untreated subject with pre-and stage I hypertension		Ras et al.,2013
Mogollon et al.	Blood pressure and endothelial fuction in healthy pregnant women after acute and daily consumption of flavanol-rich chocolate ;a Pilot, randomized controlled trial 23	23	Randomized controlled trial of acute and chronic consumption of flavanol-rich chocolate	No association with significant changes in systolic or diastolic blood pressure		Mogollon et al.,2013

seemed to follow the general trend, Mongol et al. (2013), did show significant changes in blood pressure but they could not establish any decisive association.

13.3 HYPERTENSION AND POLYPHENOLS

Hypertension is a non-communicable (Grabauskas, 1988) and a multifactorial disease with high morbidity and mortality. Despite vast therapeutic options, the prevalence of hypertension is still on the rise, and this is a public health concern.

Hypertension causes end-organ damage (Ferrara et al., 1997; Verbrugge et al., 2020; Papadopoulos et al., 2010) and results in an increase in cardiac output, an increase in systemic vascular resistance, or both. In the youth, the cardiac output is increased, while in the aged, increased stiffness of the vasculature and systemic vascular resistance are the main predictors of left ventricular hypertrophy and left ventricular diastolic dysfunction. Cytosolic calcium in vascular smooth muscle causes vasoconstriction, and there is therefore a need for vascular remodeling.

The British National Formulary recommends the following approach:

Blood pressure greater than 220/120 mm Hg: immediate therapy;

Blood pressure approximately 200–219/110–119 mm Hg: confirm over 1–2 weeks, then treat; and

Blood pressure around 160–199/100–109 mm Hg confirm over 3–4 weeks, then treat.

Even though many advances have been made in the resetting of baroreflexes (Lohmeier et al., 2005) and nature, regulatory mechanisms of hypertension remain elusive. Lately, the effects of polyphenols on hypertension have gained attention. Polyphenols can bind albumin and lipids (Jakobek, 2015; Poloni et al., 2019; Viljanen et al., 2004). There is a significant correlation between lipid profile and hypertension (Jakobek, 2015; Poloni et al., 2019; Viljanen et al., 2004). Even though lipid profiles are not the sole determinant of lipoprotein accumulation in arteries, they initiate lesions. Thus, polyphenols binding to lipids is a great breakthrough.

13.3.1 MECHANISM OF ACTION OF POLYPHENOLS IN HYPERTENSION

Walking through the schematic diagrams displayed below (Figures 13.2–13.4), it is thus clear that polyphenol is involved in curbing oxidative stress, cardiovascular events, diabetes, and reperfusion injury.

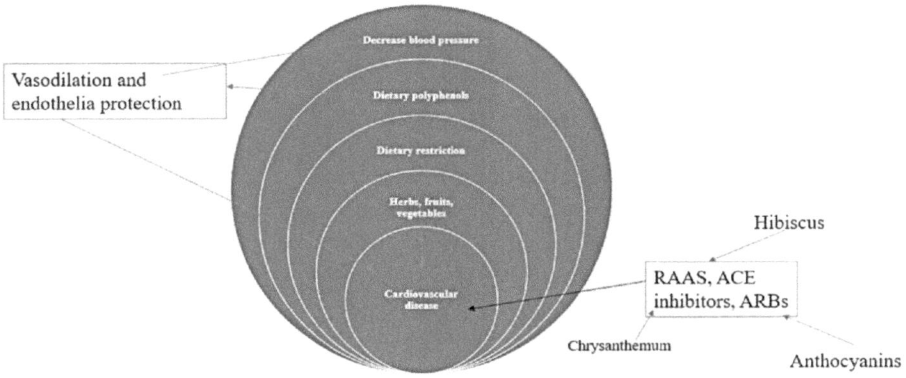

FIGURE 13.2 Polyphenol interaction with the endothelial cells.

Source: Adapted from Hugel et al., 2016

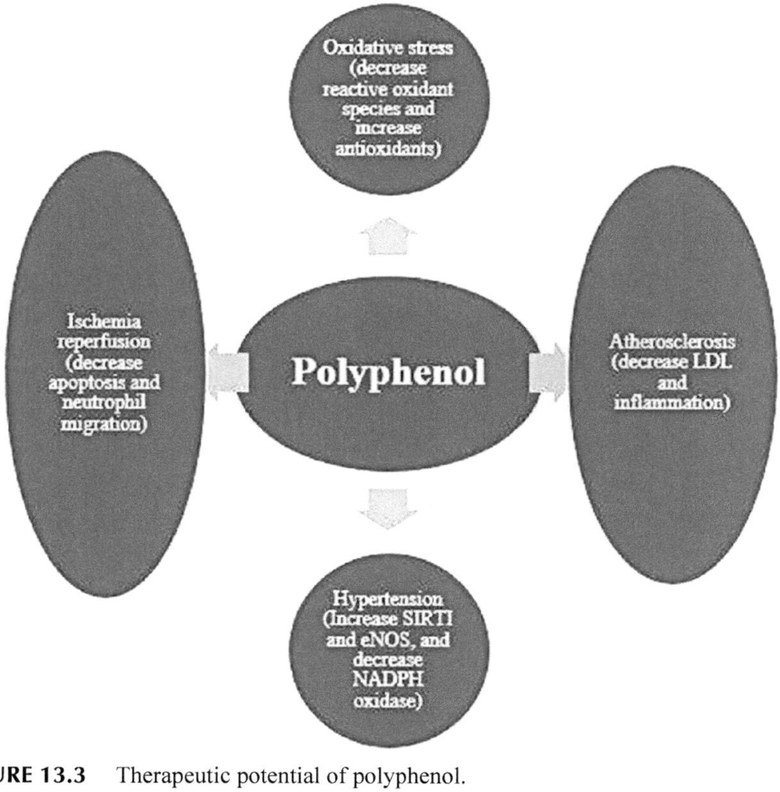

FIGURE 13.3 Therapeutic potential of polyphenol.

Source: Adapted from Khurana et al., 2013

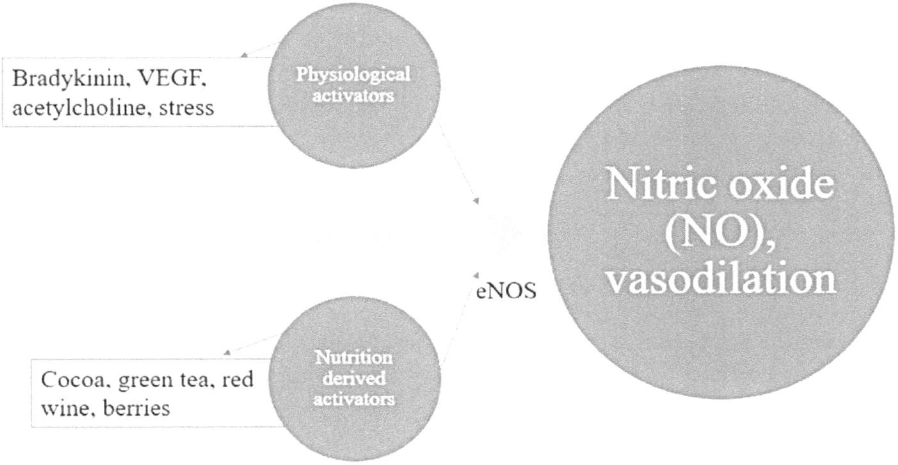

FIGURE 13.4 Cardio-protective nature of polyphenols.
Source: Adapted from Andriantsitohaina et al., 2012

Polyphenols, especially oligomeric procyanidins, suppress vasoconstrictor endothelin-1 synthesis (Caton et al., 2010), stimulate endothelium-dependent vasodilation, stimulate laminar shear stress response in endothelial cells, and inhibit the activity of metalloproteinases (MMPs) including angiotensin-converting enzyme (ACE), lowering blood pressure (Hügel et al., 2016).

It is well suggested that polyphenols stimulate endothelial nitric oxide synthase (eNOS) expression (Leikert et al., 2002; Wallerath et al., 2002; Räthel et al., 2007) by a number of signaling pathways and inhibit reactive oxygen species-producing enzymes (NADPH and/or xanthine oxidases), thereby increasing glutathione (GSSG).

It is therefore important to note that polyphenols upregulate NADPH dehydrogenase quinone 1 (NQO1) (Kim et al., 2012), superoxide dismutase, heme oxygenase-1, and glutathione peroxidase.

In this conceptual framework, it is proposed that, after decreasing reactive oxidant species through NADPH oxidase reduction, polyphenol then stimulates SIRT1 (an NAD-dependent deacetylase sirtuin-1) which deacetylates nitric oxide synthase, thereby making nitric oxide bioavailable. Deacetylation of nitric oxide synthase protects cells from apoptosis by inhibiting p53. The deacetylation process also inhibits NF-kB and FoxO1, thereby preventing inflammation and angiogenesis, respectively. SIRT1 can be a possible drug target for therapeutic purposes since it has also been noted to be involved in mitochondrial biosynthesis, glucose synthesis, insulin secretion, and fat production. The latter is implicated in hypertension.

A paradigm shift in the treatment of cardiovascular events is targeting reactive oxygen species produced as a consequence of increased angiotensin II, and this is the mainstay of angiotensin-converting enzyme inhibitors and angiotensin receptor blockers.

13.4 PLEIOTROPIC EFFECTS OF POLYPHENOLS

From the conceptual framework, it is noteworthy that data supporting the beneficial effects of polyphenols is duly applauded. The gene-coding polyphenols in plants seem to exert multiple phenotypic effects (Boudet, 2007) and this makes them pleiotropic. Beneficial actions include the inhibition of platelet aggregation, blood pressure reduction, ameliorating endothelial dysfunction (Leikert et al., 2002; Wallerath et al., 2002; Räthel et al., 2007), inhibition of the oxidation of low-density lipoprotein, and alleviating inflammatory responses. Recent data supports cardio-protective actions mediated by polyphenols (Zern & Fernandez, 2005) (Figure 13.5). However, these studies were inconclusive on outcomes due to variations in the dose and the lack of appropriate controls.

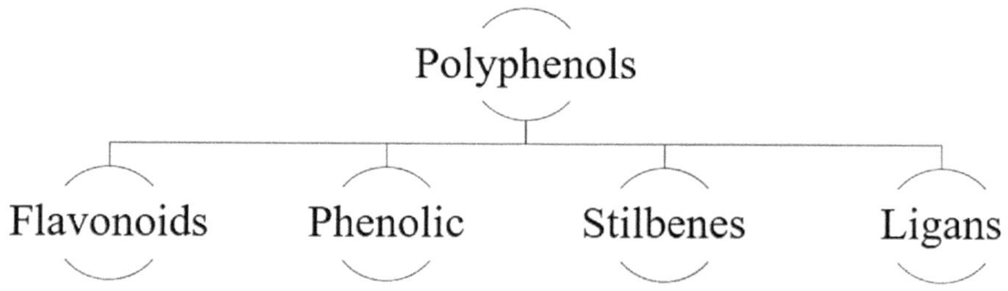

Losada Echenerria *et al.*, 2017 Modified significantly

FIGURE 13.5 Pleiotropic effects of polyphenols.

13.5 CONCLUSION

In the past few decades, increased awareness has steered polyphenol consumption to a greater percentage. Polyphenols gained prominence because of the vast plant-based and the negative correlation with hypertension. In this write-up, it was pointed out that polyphenols, through the SIRT1 pathway, make nitric oxide bioavailable for vasodilation, and this is cardio-protective.

ACKNOWLEDGMENT

The author is grateful to the University of Ghana Medical School for the online platform of varying resources.

KEYWORDS

- **angiotensin-converting enzyme**
- **cardio-protective**
- **gas chromatography**
- **hypertension**
- **metalloproteinase**
- **polyphenols**
- **reactive oxidant species**

REFERENCES

Alzand, K. I., & Mohamed, M. A. (2012). Flavonoids: Chemistry, biochemistry and antioxidant activity. *Journal of Pharmaceutical Research, 5*(40134012), 37.

Andriantsitohaina, R., Auger, C., Chataigneau, T., Étienne-Selloum, N., Li, H., Martínez, M. C., Schini-Kerth, V. B., & Laher, I. (2012). Molecular mechanisms of the cardiovascular protective effects of polyphenols. *British Journal of Nutrition, 108*(9), 1532–1549. https://doi.org/10.1017/S0007114512003406.

Behl, T., Bungau, S., Kumar, K., Zengin, G., Khan, F., Kumar, A., Kaur, R., Venkatachalam, T., Tit, D. M., Vesa, C. M., Barsan, G., & Mosteanu, D. E. (2020). Pleotropic effects of polyphenols in cardiovascular system. *Biomedicine and Pharmacotherapy, 130*, 110714. https://doi.org/10.1016/j.biopha.2020.110714.

Boudet, A. M. (2007). Evolution and current status of research in phenolic compounds. *Phytochemistry, 68*(22–24), 2722–2735. https://doi.org/10.1016/j.phytochem.2007.06.012.

Caton, P. W., Pothecary, M. R., Lees, D. M., Khan, N. Q., Wood, E. G., Shoji, T., Kanda, T., Rull, G., & Corder, R. (2010). Regulation of vascular endothelial function by procyanidin-rich foods and beverages. *Journal of Agricultural and Food Chemistry, 58*(7), 4008–4013. https://doi.org/10.1021/jf9036716.

Estruch, R., Ros, E., & Martinez-Gonzalez, M. A. (2013). Mediterranean diet for primary prevention of cardiovascular disease. *New England Journal of Medicine, 369*, 676–677. https://doi.org/10.1056/NEJMc1306659.

Ferrara, L. A., Guida, L., Pasanisi, F., Celentano, A., Palmieri, V., Iannuzzi, R., Gaeta, I., Leccia, G., & Crivaro, M. (1997). Isolated office hypertension and end-organ damage. *Journal of Hypertension, 15*(9), 979–985. https://doi.org/10.1097/00004872-199715090-00005.

Grabauskas, V. J. (1988). Glucose intolerance as a contributor to noncommunicable disease morbidity and mortality: WHO Integrated Program for Community Health in Noncommunicable Diseases. *Diabetes Care, 11*(3), 253–257. https://doi.org/10.2337/diacare.11.3.253.

Granato, D., de Magalhães Carrapeiro, M., Fogliano, V., & van Ruth, S. M. (2016). Effects of geographical origin, varietal and farming system on the chemical composition and functional properties of purple grape juices: A review. *Trends in Food Science & Technology, 52*, 31–48. https://doi.org/10.1016/j.tifs.2016.03.017.

Grosso, G., Stepaniak, U., Micek, A., Stefler, D., Bobak, M., & Pająk, A. (2017). Dietary polyphenols are inversely associated with metabolic syndrome in Polish adults of the HAPIEE study. *European Journal of Nutrition, 56*(4), 1409–1420. https://doi.org/10.1007/s00394-016-1170-6.

Hajialyani, M., Hosein Farzaei, M., Echeverría, J., Nabavi, S. M., Uriarte, E., & Sobarzo-Sánchez, E. (2009). Hesperidin as a neuroprotective agent: A review of animal and clinical evidence. *Molecules, 24*(3), 648. https://doi.org/10.3390/molecules24030648.

Harborne, J. B. (1989). Flavonoids. In *Natural Products of Woody Plants* (pp. 533–570). Springer, Berlin, Heidelberg. https://doi.org/10.1007/978-3-642-74075-6_10.

Harborne, J. B. (1989). General procedures and measurement of total phenolics. In *Methods in Plant Biochemistry, Vol. 1, Plant Phenolics, 1*, 1–28. Harborne, J. B., Ed., Academic Press, London, chap. 1.

Harborne, J. B., & Williams, C. A. (2000). Advances in flavonoid research since 1992. *Phytochemistry, 55*(6), 481–504. https://doi.org/10.1016/S0031-9422(00)00235-1.

Hügel, H. M., Jackson, N., May, B., Zhang, A. L., & Xue, C. C. (2016). Polyphenol protection and treatment of hypertension. *Phytomedicine, 23*(2), 220–231. https://doi.org/10.1016/j.phymed.2015.12.012.

Jakobek, L. (2015). Interactions of polyphenols with carbohydrates, lipids and proteins. *Food Chemistry, 175*, 556–567.

Keservani, R. K., & Sharma, A. K. (2014). Flavonoids: emerging trends and potential health benefits. *Journal of Chinese Pharmaceutical Sciences, 23*(12), 815.

Keservani, R. K., Sharma, A. K., & Kesharwani, R. K. (2016a). Nutraceutical and Functional Foods for Cardiovascular Health. In *Food Process Engineering* (pp. 291–312). Apple Academic Press, CRC Press, (pp. 257–278). ISBN: 9781771884020.

Keservani, R. K., Sharma, A. K., & Kesharwani, R. K. (2016b). Medicinal effect of nutraceutical fruits for the cognition and brain health. *Scientifica*, Article ID 3109254, 10 pages. doi:10.1155/2016/3109254.

Khurana, S., Piche, M., Hollingsworth, A., Venkataraman, K., & Tai, T. C. (2013). Oxidative stress and cardiovascular health: therapeutic potential of polyphenols. *Canadian Journal of Physiology and Pharmacology, 91*(3), 198–212.

Kim, J., Lee, S., Shim, J., Kim, H. W., Kim, J., Jang, Y. J., Park, J., Choi, S. H., Yoon, J. H., & Lee, H. J. (2012). Caffeinated coffee, decaffeinated coffee, and the phenolic phytochemical chlorogenic acid up-regulate NQO1 expression and prevent H2O2-induced apoptosis in primary cortical neurons. *Neurochemistry International, 60*(5), 466–474.

Kim, Y., & Je, Y. (2017). Flavonoid intake and mortality from cardiovascular disease and all causes: A meta-analysis of prospective cohort studies. *Clinical Nutrition ESPEN, 20*, 68–77.

Leikert, J. F., Räthel, T. R., Wohlfart, P., Cheynier, V., Vollmar, A. M., & Dirsch, V. M. (2002). Red wine polyphenols enhance endothelial nitric oxide synthase expression and subsequent nitric oxide release from endothelial cells. *Circulation, 106*(13), 1614–1617.

Lohmeier, T. E., & Iliescu, R. (2015). The baroreflex as a long-term controller of arterial pressure. *Physiology, 30*(2), 148–158.

Lohmeier, T. E., Hildebrandt, D. A., Warren, S., May, P. J., & Cunningham, J. T. (2005). Recent insights into the interactions between the baroreflex and the kidneys in hypertension. *American Journal of Physiology-Regulatory, Integrative and Comparative Physiology, 288*(4), R828–R836.

Marais, J. P. J., Deavours, B., Dixon, R. A., & Ferreira, D. (2006). The stereochemistry of flavonoids, in *The Science of Flavonoids*, 1–46. Grotewold, E., Ed., Springer Science, New York, Chapter 1.

Medina-Remón, A., Casas, R., Tresserra-Rimbau, A., Ros, E., Martínez-González, M. A., Fitó, M., Corella, D., Salas-Salvadó, J., Lamuela-Raventos, R. M., & Estruch, R. (2017). PREDIMED Study Investigators. Polyphenol intake from a Mediterranean diet decreases inflammatory biomarkers related to atherosclerosis: a substudy of the PREDIMED trial. *British Journal of Clinical Pharmacology, 83*(1), 114–128.

Mendonça, R. D., Carvalho, N. C., Martin-Moreno, J. M., Pimenta, A. M., Lopes, A. C. S., Gea, A., Martinez-Gonzalez, M. A., & Bes-Rastrollo, M. (2019). Total polyphenol intake, polyphenol subtypes and incidence of cardiovascular disease: The SUN cohort study. *Nutrition, Metabolism and Cardiovascular Diseases, 29*(1), 69–78.

Mogollon, J. A., Bujold, E., Lemieux, S., Bourdages, M., Blanchet, C., Bazinet, L., Couillard, C., Noël, M., & Dodin, S. (2013). Blood pressure and endothelial function in healthy, pregnant women after acute and daily consumption of flavanol-rich chocolate: a pilot, randomized controlled trial. *Nutrition Journal, 12*(1), 1–13.

Papadopoulos, D. P., Mourouzis, I., Thomopoulos, C., Makris, T., & Papademetriou, V. (2010). Hypertension crisis. *Blood Pressure, 19*(6), 328–336.

Pataki, T., Bak, I., Kovacs, P., Bagchi, D., Das, D. K., & Tosaki, A. (2002). Grape seed proanthocyanidins improved cardiac recovery during reperfusion after ischemia in isolated rat hearts. *American Journal of Clinical Nutrition, 5*, 894–899.

Pieatta, G. P. (2000). Flavonoids as antioxidant. *Journal of Natural Products, 63*, 1035.

Poloni, D. M., Dangles, O., & Vinson, J. A. (2019). Binding of plant polyphenols to serum albumin and LDL: Healthy implications for heart disease. *Journal of Agricultural and Food Chemistry, 67*(33), 9139–9147.

Psaltopoulou, T., Naska, A., Orfanos, P., Trichopoulos, D., Mountokalakis, T., & Trichopoulou, A. (2004). Olive oil, the Mediterranean diet, and arterial blood pressure: the Greek European Prospective Investigation into Cancer and Nutrition (EPIC) study. *American Journal of Clinical Nutrition, 80*, 1012–1018.

Ras, R. T., Zock, P. L., Zebregs, Y. E., Johnston, N. R., Webb, D. J., & Draijer, R. (2013). Effect of polyphenol-rich grape seed extract on ambulatory blood pressure in subjects with pre- and stage I hypertension. *British Journal of Nutrition, 110*, 2234–2241.

Räthel, T. R., Samtleben, R., Vollmar, A. M., & Dirsch, V. M. (2007). Activation of endothelial nitric oxide synthase by red wine polyphenols: Impact of grape cultivars, growing area, and the vinification process. *Journal of Hypertension, 25*(3), 541–549.
Reed, J. (2002). Cranberry flavonoids, atherosclerosis and cardiovascular health. *Critical Reviews in Food Science and Nutrition, 42*, Suppl. 3, 301–316.
Reis, A., Perez-Gregorio, R., Mateus, N., & de Freitas, V. (2021). Interactions of dietary polyphenols with epithelial lipids: Advances from membrane and cell models in the study of polyphenol absorption, transport, and delivery to the epithelium. *Critical Reviews in Food Science and Nutrition, 61*(18), 3007–3030.
Sakakibara, H., Honda, Y., Nakagawa, S., Ashida, H., & Kanazawa, K. (2003). Simultaneous determination of all polyphenols in vegetables, fruits, and teas. *Journal of Agricultural and Food Chemistry, 51*(3), 571–581.
Stevenson, D. E., & Hurst, R. D. (2007). Polyphenolic phytochemicals–just antioxidants or much more? *Cellular and Molecular Life Sciences, 64*(22), 2900–2916.
Tresserra-Rimbau, A., Guasch-Ferré, M., Salas-Salvadó, J., Toledo, E., Corella, D., Castañer, O., Guo, X., Gómez-Gracia, E., Lapetra, J., Arós, F., & Fiol, M. (2015). Intake of total polyphenols and some classes of polyphenols is inversely associated with diabetes in elderly people at high cardiovascular disease risk. *The Journal of Nutrition, 146*, 767–777.
Tsao, R. (2010). Chemistry and biochemistry of dietary polyphenols. *Nutrients, 2*(12), 1231–1246.
Verbrugge, F. H., Guazzi, M., Testani, J. M., & Borlaug, B. A. (2020). Altered hemodynamics and end-organ damage in heart failure: impact on the lung and kidney. *Circulation, 142*(10), 998–1012.
Viljanen, K., Kivikari, R., & Heinonen, M. (2004). Protein–lipid interactions during liposome oxidation with added anthocyanin and other phenolic compounds. *Journal of Agricultural and Food Chemistry, 52*(5), 1104–1111.
Wallerath, T., Deckert, G., Ternes, T., Anderson, H., Li, H., Witte, K., & Förstermann, U. (2002). Resveratrol, a polyphenolic phytoalexin present in red wine, enhances expression and activity of endothelial nitric oxide synthase. *Circulation, 106*(13), 1652–1658.
Zern, T. L., & Fernandez, M. L. (2005). Cardio – protective effects of dietary polyphenols. *The Journal of Nutrition, 135*(10), 2291–2294.

CHAPTER 14

CARDIOPROTECTIVE POTENTIAL OF DIETARY PHYTOCHEMICALS PRESENT IN THE MEDICINAL FOODS OF KERALA, SOUTH INDIA: A REVIEW

S. R. SUJA,[1] SHOBHA BHASKAR,[1] B. S. BIJUKUMAR,[2] and R. PRAKASHKUMAR[1]

[1]*Ethnomedicine and Ethnopharmacology Division, Jawaharlal Nehru Tropical Botanic Garden and Research Institute (JNTBGRI), Thiruvananthapuram, Kerala, India*

[2]*Post-Graduate Department of Zoology and Research Center, Mahatma Gandhi College, Thiruvananthapuram, Kerala, India*

ABSTRACT

There is an escalation in the occurrence of cardiovascular diseases (CVDs) owing to the sharp rise in developing countries which are experiencing rapid health transition. Nowadays, cardiovascular diseases (CVDs) are one of the main reasons for death, ranking first globally. The increase in incidences of cardiovascular disease is a manifestation of a chronic poor diet. International health organizations have proposed the promotion of traditional diets to tackle the growing global non-communicable diseases (NCDs) and obesity rates. Traditional foods are rich in nutrients, and consuming even small amounts of them can contribute significantly to dietary quality. A variety of fruits, grains, vegetables, and spices with medicinal properties are the major ingredients of Kerala's traditional cuisine, contributing to many health advantages. Ayurveda, an alternative system of medical practice

Antioxidants as Nutraceuticals. Nayan A. Gujarathi, Raj K. Keservani, Rajesh K. Kesharwani, Bhushan R. Rane, Yogeeta Sameer Goyal (Eds.)

popular in Kerala, offers significant knowledge on nutrition and health, as well as having distinctive concepts. The people of Kerala consider the month of 'Karkkidaka' (Saka year/Malayalam year), i.e., the middle of July to the middle of August, as a treatment month or the rejuvenating month. They used to follow a vegetarian food habit during this month and used a medicinal gruel known as 'Karkkidaka kanji' and a side dish prepared by 10 medicinal plants ('Dasapushpam') known as 'Marunnuthoran' which has much importance in the regulation of cardiac health. The constituents of the gruel include 'Njavara' rice (*Oryza sativa* L.), Mung bean (*Vigna radiata* (L) *Wilczek*), broken wheat (*Triticum aestivum* L.), fenugreek seeds (*Trigonella foenum-graceum* L.), cumin seeds (*Cuminum cyminum* L.), dried ginger powder (*Zingiber officinale* Roscoe), Garlic (*Allium sativum* L.), onion (*Allium cepa* L.), pepper (*Piper nigrum* L.) and coconut milk (*Cocos nucifera* L.). The side dish includes the leaves of 10 locally available medicinal plants. They are 'Cherula' (*Aerva lanata* (L.) Juss), 'Mukkutti' (*Biophytum sensitivum* (L.) DC), 'Uzhinja' (*Cardiospermum halicacabum* L.), 'Nilappana' (*Curculigo orchioides* Gaertn.), 'Karuka' (*Cynodon dactylon* (L.) Pers), 'Kayyonni' (*Eclipta prostate* (L.) L), 'Muyalcheviyan' (*Emilia sonchifolia* (L.) DC. ex-DC), 'Vishnukranthi' (*Evolvulus alsinoides* (L.) L.), 'Thiruthali' (*Ipomoea obscura* (L.) Ker Gawl.), 'Poovamkurunnila' (*Vernonia cinerea* Less.). Another traditional food of Kerala is Kerala Sadhya, a nutrition-dense vegetarian meal that has a great balance of antioxidants, anti-inflammatory, cardioprotective, immunomodulatory foods, vitamins, minerals, and all essential nutrients that make it a powerhouse of nutrients. For a better understanding of the future of medicine and healthcare, diseases, etc., understanding the linkage between traditional medicines and visualization of the future of medicine is very essential as it gives us 'new directions and possible solutions. This review highlighted the dietary phytochemicals with the cardioprotective potential present in the ingredients of some traditional foods of Kerala, their effects, and their mechanism of action.

14.1 INTRODUCTION

According to the World Health Organization (WHO), since 2000, cardiovascular disease has been the world's biggest killer and is responsible for 16% of the total deaths accounted for in 2019. Stroke and chronic obstructive pulmonary disease are the 2nd and 3rd leading causes of death, responsible for approximately 11% and 6% of total deaths, respectively. India has a rich history of using various herbs, spices, and herbal components for treating various diseases, and knowledge of plant-derived antioxidants and spices could reduce the cost of healthcare. In Kerala, the southern state of India, it is reported that 31.0% of total deaths are due to ailments in the circulatory system (Registrar General of India, 2019).

Cardiovascular Disease (CVD) includes a large number of pathologies, such as coronary heart disease, cerebrovascular diseases, peripheral arteriopathies, and rheumatic and congenital heart disease. Atherosclerosis, a multifactorial disease, is the common pathological process in most of them (Stevens et al., 2019). Physical inactivity, obesity, sedentary lifestyle, and metabolic dysfunction are risk factors for CVD. Pathological mechanisms associated with CVD include increased oxidative stress, inflammation, dyslipidemia, and insulin resistance. The imbalance between free radicals and natural antioxidants in the body leads to oxidative stress, which causes thrombogenesis, vascular inflammation, and endothelial dysfunction. This, in turn, leads to myocardial damage, ischemic episodes, and thrombosis, ultimately culminating in CVD (Yamagata & Yamori, 2020). Many currently used modern drugs do not have valid proven clinical utility when compared to traditional medicine. Herbal drugs are known to exhibit credible medicinal properties for the treatment of heart ailments and need to be explored to identify their potential application in the prevention and therapy of human ailments.

Foods obtained from plants contain a wide range of phytochemicals that are synthesized by plants for their defense and other biological functions. Functional foods rich in bioactive chemicals possess medicinal importance against cellular oxidative stress and, therefore, cardiovascular disease when added to the diet. Herbal medicines and other complementary therapies have been used for centuries by humans to reduce cardiometabolic risk factors.

14.2 HISTORY OF TRADITIONAL MEDICINE

Almost all ancient human civilizations developed their food habit patterns and medicine known as traditional foods and traditional medicines. According to social anthropologists/historians, it was perhaps a small band of a human community who, by chance, for the first time about 12,000 years ago discovered agriculture. For the first time in the history of Earth, one of its species was able to domesticate and ultimately cultivate plants to meet their primary food requirement. Barley, oats, wheat, and sesame were perhaps the first plants selected by humans for domestication and subsequent cultivation. The Western nations' 16th-century colonization of the biodiversity-rich Southern counties led to the introduction of many indigenous culinary plants, which later included species of industrial importance. The globalization of food and diet has led to the prevalence of numerous physiological ailments and diseases classified as lifestyle diseases today. The finest foods for humans are those that are adapted to their environment and climate, as scientific understanding of food and nutrition has grown.

Different established civilizations including the world such as Babylonian, Egyptian, Sumerian, Chinese, Indian, and South American cultures emerged around 6000 BC. A highly developed and well-organized city civilization had arisen in the Indian subcontinent at Mohenjo-Daro and Harappa around 3500 BC, constructed by agricultural societies. However, by the turn of the tenth century, more than 10,000 plant species were providing food for human populations all over the planet.

India is blessed with diverse agro-climatic conditions and rich in all levels of biodiversity species, genes, and habitat. It is rich in cultural diversity that has generated rich Traditional Knowledge. The search for novel genes, medicinal components, nutraceuticals, and other biologically active compounds and raw materials for the growing drug discovery and research industry endeavors a promising opportunity as we have accessed only a small portion of nature's enormous gene and traditional knowledge library. For India, the unexplored genetic potential is around 70–80%. Kerala is endowed with a rich and varied cultural heritage rooted in indigenous traditional knowledge systems. Apart from Ayurveda, there is a strong and vibrant oral healthcare tradition existing in the countryside, villages, and tribal habitats.

"Karkkidaka kanji" is a medicinal rice soup traditionally used to rejuvenate health in Kerala during the rainy season (Malayalam month – Karkkidakam). "Kerala Sadhya," another traditional food of Kerala, is a nutrition-dense vegetarian meal that has a great balance of antioxidants, anti-inflammatory, cardioprotective foods, vitamins, minerals, and all essential nutrients, making it a powerhouse of nutrients. Traditional foods rich in nutraceuticals have a central role in reducing the adverse biological effects exerted by many diseases such as cardiovascular diseases, as their systematic usage provides an excellent way to control the diseases in addition to their role as a source of nutrients.

14.2.1 KARKKIDAKA KANJI

'Karkkidaka kanji' is a medicinal gruel and a side dish prepared by 10 medicinal plants ('Dasapushpam') known as 'Marunnuthoran' which has much importance in the regulation of cardiac health. The ingredients of the gruel include 'Njavara' rice (*Oryza sativa* L.), broken wheat (*Triticum aestivum* L.), green gram (*Vigna radiata* (L) Wilczek), fenugreek seeds (*Trigonella foenum-graceum* L.), cumin seeds (*Cuminum cyminum* L.), dried ginger powder (*Zingiber officinale* Roscoe), garlic (*Allium sativum* L.), onion (*Allium cepa* L.), pepper (*Piper nigrum* L.), and coconut milk (*Cocos nucifera* L.). The side dish includes the leaves of 10 locally available medicinal plants. They are 'Cherula' (*Aerva lanata* (L.) Juss), 'Mukkutti' (*Biophytum sensitivum* (L.) DC), 'Uzhinja' (*Cardiospermum halicacabum* L.), 'Nilappana' (*Curculigo orchioides* Gaertn.), 'Karuka' (*Cynodon dactylon* (L.) Pers), 'Kayyonni' (*Eclipta prostata* (L.) L), 'Muyalcheviyan' (*Emilia sonchifolia* (L.) DC. ex DC), 'Vishnukranthi' (*Evolvulus alsinoides* (L.) L.), 'Thiruthali' (*Ipomoea obscura* (L.) Ker Gawl.), 'Poovamkurunnila' (*Vernonia cinerea* Less.).

14.2.2 ORYZA SATIVA L (NJAVARA RICE)

Cereals are essential in a balanced diet. Rice is considered one of the most popular grains consumed worldwide and is the staple diet for more than 3 billion people, especially in Asia, and is cultivated in more than 2000 different types on a commercial scale. The United Nations General Assembly proclaimed 2004 as the International Year of Rice with the theme "Rice is Life" (UN General Assembly session 57, 16/12/2002) in recognition of the significance of rice-based foods around the world. Since ancient times, traditional healers have employed rice as a medicine. Njavara (*Oryza sativa* L., variety 'njavara') is a unique indigenous rice variety grown in South India, especially in Kerala. The black glumed Njavara rice is used for Ayurvedic treatments during the monsoon season from the age of Charaka, i.e., 600 B.C. 'Najavara' rice has equal importance as food and as a curative folklore medicine and is reported to have the power to improve the immune function of the body (Sreejayan et al., 2003; Simi & Abraham, 2008).

Njavara is the only rice cultivar traditionally used effectively in the Ayurvedic system of medicine in certain specific treatments like Panchakarma (Sulochana & Bakiyalakshmi, 2011). This treatment in Ayurveda is now getting popular, not only in Kerala but also in other parts of the nation and even in other countries of the world. Several reports are available on the agronomic evaluation; lipid profile; thermal, starch, and genetic characteristics of Njavara grains (Deepa et al., 2008, 2009). Reports show that Njavara possesses antioxidant and anti-inflammatory properties, and the unsaponifiable component present in rice bran of 'njavara' – γ-oryzanol regulates hypercholesterolemia. The concentration of this compound is higher in black-glumed 'njavara' compared to other rice varieties available (Smitha et al., 2012; Shalini et al., 2011). Njavara has the properties to rectify the basic illnesses affecting the circulatory, respiratory, and digestive systems, and it is mainly used for the preparation of "Karkkidaka Kanji," "Njavarakizhi," and "Njavaratheppu" for monsoon treatment to enhance the body's immunity. "Njavarakizhi" and "Njavaratheppu" are regarded as the best treatments for rheumatic disorders, which are very popular in Ayurveda (Deepa et al., 2008).

Atherosclerosis, the initial stage of cardiovascular disease, has been characterized as a chronic inflammatory disease. Even though strict dietary modifications and other therapies, including lipid-lowering medications, atherosclerotic vascular disease continues to account for higher morbidity and mortality. Njavara rice bran oil is reported to have an effect on the lipid-lowering mechanism of the body by regulating the enzymes involved in cholesterol metabolism and possessing anti-inflammatory properties in hypercholesterolemic rats (Chithra et al., 2015, 2016).

14.2.3 TRITICUM AESTIVUM L (WHEAT)

The prevalence of lifestyle diseases such as atherosclerotic vascular disease, diabetes, obesity, hypertension, and cancer is attributed to the substantially reduced consumption of cereal grains by individuals around the world. To reduce these problems, a high intake of dietary fiber is suggested. Dietary fiber improves vascular health by reducing plasma cholesterol and blood pressure (Fardet, 2010). Wheat foods are the major source of dietary fiber, providing about one-fifth of the energy and one-third of the fiber. Wheat is the second most widely consumed staple food in the world after rice. Wheat (*Triticum aestivum* L.), with a global production of 763.1 million tons in 2019, is the most widely cultivated crop in the world (FAO-Statistic data 2020, http://www.fao.org/worldfoodsituation/csdb/en/).

The wheat kernel consists of three principal parts: the germ, the central endosperm, and the outer bran husk. Conventional milling of wheat grains produces white flour by separating the endosperm from the bran layers (Sakhare et al., 2015). The wheat bran (WB) fractions are rich sources of fiber, minerals, and phytochemicals that are known to possess health-promoting properties (Anderson et al., 2000). Broken wheat is used to prepare "Karkkidaka Kanji" because whole wheat grain is good for health as it contains all three principal parts and is a rich source of dietary fiber.

The consumption of whole wheat foods could lower the risk of many chronic diseases, including obesity, type 2 diabetes (T2D), cardiovascular diseases (CVD), and cancer, through anti-inflammatory, antioxidant, immunity improvement, and gut microbiota modulation. This is considered to be due to the effect of dietary fiber, nutraceuticals, and bioactive phytochemicals present in it. The bioactive phytochemicals found in whole grain wheat include alkylresorcinols (ARs), benzoxazinoids (BXs), phytosteroids, sphingolipids, lignans, flavonoids, phenolic acids, fatty acids, glycolipids, tocols, carotenoids, and other minor components (Anderson et al., 2000). Numerous epidemiological and experimental research studies have shown that the consumption of whole-grain wheat may help lower the risk of cardiovascular disease. Clinical studies have demonstrated that the ingestion of whole-grain wheat significantly reduces CVD risk, mainly through blood pressure-lowering mechanisms (Tighe et al., 2010; Harris & Kris-Etherton, 2010). A study involving 7,822 diabetic women in the US found that intake of whole grain wheat and its bran reduced CVD-specific mortality in women with diabetes mellitus (He et al., 2010). Studies have found that high dietary flavonoid consumption has been related to a reduced risk of CVD and mortality from coronary heart disease. Wheat flavonoids and their metabolites reduce endothelial oxidative stress and the pro-inflammatory process by decreasing eNOS and ROS levels and enhancing NO bioavailability (Yamagata et al., 2020). In an experimental study, whole wheat bread consumption significantly decreased plasma cholesterol and triglyceride levels, whereas total steroid excretion was markedly enhanced in rats, suggesting a beneficial effect of whole wheat food consumption in CVD prevention (Adam et al., 2003). Costabile et al. reported that intake of a wheat-based breakfast diet for 3 weeks significantly reduced total serum cholesterol by 21.4% in humans. The possible mechanism involved in the health-beneficial effects of whole wheat on CVD was modulating bacterial fermentation to increase the production of short-chain fatty acids in the human colon (Costabile et al., 2008). Arabinoxylans present in wheat were reported to significantly reduce plasma total cholesterol and LDL-cholesterol concentrations in hamsters (Tong et al., 2014). Diet supplemented with 0.4% alk(en)ylresorcinols (ARs) prepared from wheat significantly increased fecal cholesterol excretion by 39.6% and reduced the blood cholesterol concentrations by 30.4% in mice (Oishi et al., 2015). Alkyl resorcinols have been shown to inhibit platelet binding to fibrinogen, stimulate thromboxane production, and inhibit triglyceride formation, suggesting a potential role for phenolic compounds found in the bran fractions in CVD. ARs significantly decreased liver cholesterol while significantly increasing the levels of γ-tocopherol in the liver and lungs in rats (Ross et al., 2004), which are inversely associated with the incidence of coronary heart disease (Jiang et al., 2001). The phenolic antioxidants present in wheat bran inhibited LDL oxidation, possibly by binding with apolipoprotein-B (Yu et al., 2005; Liyana-Pathirana & Shahidi, 2007). The dietary fiber and phenolic compounds present in wheat grain may contribute to their effects in reducing the risk of CVD.

14.2.4 VIGNA RADIATA (L) WILCZEK

Mung bean, the seeds of *Vigna radiata* L., are popular food legumes in China, India, Korea, Japan, and other parts of Southeast Asian countries. They are well known for their detoxification activities and are used to refresh mentally, alleviate heat stroke, and reduce swelling in the summer. Mung beans are used as a staple in many diets worldwide and are essential to human nutrition, particularly as a good source of plant proteins (20.97–32.6%), which contain predominantly essential amino acids. As a food, *Vigna radiata* contains abundant nutrients with biological activities, including proteins, phenolic acids, fatty acids, and minerals that possess anti-inflammatory (Lee et al., 2011b), antibacterial (Yao et al., 2011), antitumor (Soucek et al., 2006), hypolipidemic (Wang et al., 1990), antidiabetic (Yao et al., 2008), detoxication (Gao et al., 2014), hepatoprotective effect (Liu et al., 2014), and antioxidant activity (Lee et al., 2011a; Li et al., 2012).

The main contributing factors to hyperlipidemia, hypertension, and atherosclerosis are cardiovascular illnesses and the fatalities they cause. A significant risk factor for the development of hyperlipidemia and coronary heart disease is thought to be an elevated serum cholesterol level. Therefore, it's critical to keep the body functioning normally by bringing the high serum cholesterol down to a safe level. There are reports that consumption of the *Vigna radiata* seed is associated with the regulation of cholesterol levels by modulating lipid metabolism. Mung bean protein has been reported to have a reducing effect on plasma lipid levels, such as serum total cholesterol

(TC), triglyceride (TG), Low-density Lipoprotein (LDL) cholesterol, and VLDL-cholesterol in high-cholesterol diet-fed hamsters, and this effect was partially mediated by the up-regulation of HMG CoA reductase and cholesterol-7-alpha-hydroxylase (CYP7A1), in both transcriptional and translational levels (Yao et al., 2014a, b). The mechanism underlying the cholesterol-lowering activity of mung bean protein was considered to increase the fecal bile acids and sterol excretion, as well as decrease the cholesterol absorption and biosynthesis. Reports have suggested that sprouted mung beans possess an anti-hypertensive effect on the systolic blood pressure of spontaneously hypertensive rats (Hsu et al., 2011).

14.2.5 TRIGONELLA FOENUM GRACEUM L.

Trigonella foenum-graecum L. (Fenugreek), a medicinal herb from the Fabaceae family, is one of the promising plants mentioned in the Indian system of medicine, with potent actions and is cultivated mostly in India and North African countries (Srinivasan, 2006). Fenugreek seeds have been used both as a spice and as therapeutic materials in traditional medicine (Krishnaswamy, 2008). Fenugreek seeds contain soluble and insoluble dietary fiber, alkaloids, steroidal saponins, and flavonoids (Khorshidian et al., 2016). Several reports revealed the therapeutic effects of the fenugreek plant, such as hypoglycemic, analgesic, anti-atherosclerotic, anti-inflammatory, anti-spasmodic, anticancer, cardioprotective, blood cholesterol-lowering, lipid-lowering, labor induction, promoting milk flow, antibacterial, and anti-worm properties (Bash et al., 2003; Yadav et al., 2014).

Rituraj et al have reported that fenugreek seed and trigonelline have a role in countering hepatic very low-density lipoprotein (VLDL) overproduction and insulin resistance by enhancing the insulin signaling pathways and ameliorating metabolic inflammatory stress in the liver (Rituraj et al., 2018). Soleyman et al. (2021) demonstrate that fenugreek seed extract may have high therapeutic potential in treating diabetic cardiac myopathy, one of the major complications associated with diabetes-induced cardiovascular disorders, through ameliorating metabolic abnormalities and oxidative stress (Soleyman et al., 2021). Pradeep and Srinivasan suggested that the combination of fenugreek seeds and onion offers a higher beneficial influence in ameliorating cardiac damage accompanying diabetes in experimental diabetic rats via blocking the Renin-Angiotensin system (Pradeep & Srinivasan, 2018). The seeds of fenugreek also contain lysine and L-tryptophan-rich proteins, mucilaginous fiber, and other rare chemical constituents, such as coumarin, fenugreekine, nicotinic acid, folic acid, sapogenins, phytic acid, scopoletin, and trigonelline, which are thought to account for many of the presumed therapeutic effects that may inhibit cholesterol absorption and decrease blood sugar concentrations (Ram et al., 2022).

14.2.6 CUMINUM CYMINUM L

Seeds of *Cuminum cyminum* (Apiaceae), commonly known as *jeera*, which is one of the culinary aromatic plants and are consumed as a condiment across the globe. It has been used as primary medicine for a long time. Cumin seeds play an important role in India's therapeutic medical system, especially for the treatment of digestive problems. Cumin seeds are reported to have diuretic, anti-inflammatory, and antispasmodic activities and are used to relieve the difficulties of flatus and toothache (Yarnell & Abascal, 2011). It can be used as additional nutritional support for the treatment of epilepsy, jaundice, and indigestion (Rebey et al., 2012).

Body weight, BMI, serum plasma lipids, and oxidative stress can all be reduced by consuming cumin seeds (Haslam & James, 2005). An animal experimental study proves that the plant *C. cyminum* L. has an anti-atherosclerotic effect due to its capacity to reduce ox-LDL and LDL concentration in serum. The plant also possesses antioxidant, hypoglycemic, anti-cancerous, and carminative effects (Harshlatha & Ashok, 2018). Amna and Nizwa reported that cumin seeds have enormous therapeutic potential for the treatment of obese people by lowering body fat percentages, therefore, reducing body weight, and can also be used as an alternative to other conventional chemicals for the treatment of certain bodily issues (Amna & Nizwa, 2019).

14.2.6 ZINGIBER OFFICIANALE ROSCOE

Ginger (*Zingiberaceae*) is one of the most popular spices in the world and has long been valued for its therapeutic properties and positive effects on health (Kiyama, 2020; Jafarzadeh et al., 2021). Ginger-derived terpenes are identified to have antioxidant, anti-inflammatory, antibacterial, antidiabetic, analgesic, gastroprotective, neuroprotective, and anti-carcinogenic properties (Kiyama, 2020). Of the 400 types of compounds present in ginger, four phenolic compounds are mainly responsible for their pharmacological effects: gingerols, shogaols, paradols, and zingerone (Prasad & Tyagi, 2015; Mao et al., 2019). There are also some derivative compounds of gingerol (6-gingerol, 8-gingerol, 10-gingerol, and 12-gingerol) and shogaol (1-dehydrogingerdione, 6-gingerdione, and 10-gingerdione) (Jafarzadeh et al., 2021).

6-gingerol, 8-gingerol, 10-gingerol, and 6-shogaol are the bioactive compounds isolated from ginger, and they possess good free radical scavenging activity. 6-gingerol is the compound having the highest antioxidant activity among different compounds from ginger and is reported to show a wide range of pharmacological actions, including its anti-inflammatory, analgesic, antipyretic, and chemopreventive characteristics (Dugasani et al., 2010; Ippoushi et al., 2003; Koo et al., 2001; Kundu & Surh, 2009; Suekawa et al., 1984). 6-gingerol is also reported to have a regulatory effect on the enzyme, Xanthine oxidase, which catalyzes the oxidation of hypoxanthine to xanthine and xanthine to uric acid in the final step of purine catabolism and results in the generation of reactive oxygen species (Rondanelli et al., 2020). Uric acid accumulation in the joints and other body parts leads to gout, which is also a risk factor for cardiovascular diseases. 6-gingerol is capable of increasing the antioxidant enzyme activity such as superoxide dismutase and catalase (Danwilai et al., 2017).

Different studies are reporting that ginger and its bioactive compounds possess potent anti-inflammatory activity by regulating the toll-like receptor (TLR) pathway and by inhibiting the transcription factors such as NF-κB, signal transducer, and activators of transcription (STAT), proteins of NOD-like receptor family (NLRP), mitogen-activated protein kinase (MAPK), and several proinflammatory cytokines such as interleukins IL-6, IL-8, TNF-α, inducible nitric oxide synthase (iNOS), and interferon-gamma (IFN-γ), PGE2, COX-2 (Jalali et al., 2020; Song et al., 2021; Zadorozhna & Mangieri, 2021; Unuofin et al., 2021; Chen et al., 2018; Han et al., 2017; Stevens et al., 2019). Many data have shown that ginger has an effect on ameliorating obesity, which is a main cause of cardiac diseases, by increasing thermogenesis through catecholamines and lipolysis of white adipose tissue (Tramontin et al., 2020). Gingerenone-A, a bioactive compound of ginger, is reported to activate the adenine monophosphate (AMP)-activated protein kinase (AMPK) pathway modulating fatty acid metabolism and thereby reducing adipogenesis and lipid accumulation and regulating obesity (Suk et al., 2017). Ginger and its bioactive compound 6-gingerol are reported to have a glucose tolerance effect on Type-2 diabetic patients, which is considered a major risk factor associated with cardiovascular diseases (Pourmasoumi et al., 2018;

Arablou et al., 2014). Epidemiological and experimental studies revealed the hypolipidemic effect, i.e., reducing the effect of serum total cholesterol, triglycerides, and LDL cholesterol, and the biochemical mechanism of action of this effect of ginger and its bioactive compounds (El Gayer et al., 2019; Arablou et al., 2018; Atashak et al., 2011; Attari et al., 2015; Mahluji et al., 2013; Jafarnejad et al., 2017; Mazidi et al., 2016; Gao et al., 2012). Clinical studies reported that ginger consumption significantly has a favorable effect on blood pressure (Wang et al., 2017; McEwen, 2014).

The crude extract of ginger is cardioprotective due to its antihypertensive, antiplatelet, and cardiotonic effects. Hsing et al. reported that ginger crude extract induces relaxant and vasoprotective effects on porcine coronary arteries, and may possess free radical-scavenging activities which may be considered a potential cardioprotective factor in the context of human diseases (Hsing et al., 2018).

14.2.7 ALLIUM SATIVUM L

Allium sativum L (garlic) has been utilized extensively as a culinary and medicinal ingredient for centuries. According to different sources, garlic has been utilized as medicine by people from all over the world since ancient times, especially heavy laborers, Greek Olympic athletes, ancient Chinese medicine, and old traditional medicine in India including Tibbi, Unani, and Ayurveda (Lawson, 1998; Moyers, 1996; Woodward, 1996). Allicin (diallyl thiosulfinate or allyl 2-propenethiosulfinate) is the chief bioactive component in aqueous garlic. When garlic is diced or crushed, the alliinase enzyme present in garlic converts the compound 'alliin,' which is present in intact garlic, to form allicin. Heat renders the enzyme allinase inactive. The heat-treated plant material's aqueous extract contains Allin. Several experimental studies revealed the hypolipidemic activity of different preparations of garlic including garlic paste, garlic oil, allicin, and ajoene via inhibiting HMG-CoA reductase, the rate-limiting enzyme involved in cholesterol metabolism in hepatocytes (Gebhardt & Beck, 1996; Yeh & Yeh, 1994; Yeh & Liu, 2001; Gebhardt, 1993; Liu & Yeh, 2002; Rajasree et al., 1998). Augusti et al. confirmed the inhibition of HMG-CoA reductase by garlic (Augusti et al., 2005).

Meta-analysis research conducted to study the hypolipidemic effect of garlic in humans demonstrated its anti-hyperlipidemic properties by lowering TC and LDL levels rather than HDL and TG. Consequently, it is advised to consume more garlic for those who have high blood lipid levels (Sun et al., 2018). Reports suggest that LDL is considerably more oxidation-resistant in human participants who were administered with AGE (Munday et al., 1999) and aqueous garlic extract (Lewin & Popov, 1994). These results proved that decreased LDL oxidation may be the potent mechanism responsible for the advantages of garlic in atherosclerosis. Augusti and Sheela reported that an isolated compound from garlic, namely S-allyl cysteine sulfoxide, has antioxidant properties that may also contribute to its positive effects on diabetes and thus revealed the insulin secretagogue function (Augusti & Sheela, 1996). The prostaglandin-like effects, nitric oxide-dependent relaxation of the pulmonary arteries, inhibition of the angiotensin-converting enzyme, and modulation of endothelium-derived relaxing and constrictory factors that may prevent hypoxic pulmonary vasoconstriction may contribute to the potential antihypertensive properties of garlic (Rashid & Khan, 1985; Sendl et al., 1992; Kim-Park & Ku, 2000). Epidemiological and experimental data suggest the potent antiplatelet aggregation activity and antifibrinolytic activity of garlic, which is considered a favorable mechanism in the prevention of cardiovascular disease. Ginter and Simko reported that garlic-derived organic polysulfides are converted by erythrocytes into hydrogen sulfide, which has a relaxing activity in vascular smooth muscle, induces vasodilation of blood vessels, and significantly decreases blood pressure (Ginter & Simko, 2010).

14.2.8 ALLIUM CEPA L.

Allium cepa L. (Onion) is widely used as a food and it contains many phytochemicals which possess health benefits. Onion is an important source of antioxidant phytochemicals such as organosulfur compounds, phenolic acids, flavonoids, thiosulfinates, and anthocyanins. The major components with cardioprotective effect present in onion are quercetin, quercetin glucosides, isorhamnetin glucosides, and kaempferol glucoside (Tedesco et al., 2015). Onion peel extract is an important ingredient for many nutraceuticals and functional foods, which contain p-coumaric acid, vanillic acid, epicatechin, and morin (Jaiswal et al., 2014).

Quercetin and other flavonoids present in onion are reported to have a beneficial effect on regulating cardiovascular disease by decreasing cholesterol levels and antioxidation ability (Lu et al., 2015). Quercetin isolated from onion skin reduces ambulatory blood pressure in hypertensive patients

(Brüll et al., 2015). Onion stalk extract can be used for decreasing atherosclerosis and proinflammatory response. Sekhon-Loodu et al reported that quercetin-3-O-glucoside isolated from onion combined with eicosapentaenoic acid possesses significant anti-inflammatory and hypolipidemic activity and can be used for the treatment of obesity (Sekhon-Loodu et al., 2015). Quercetin is reported to have a potent antiatherosclerotic effect by attenuating proinflammatory mechanisms and regulating inflammatory markers like iNOS, COX, LOX, MPO, etc., in experimental animals (Bhaskar et al., 2013). Quercetin from onion peel could attenuate flow-mediated dilation and circulating progenitor cells, reduce obesity by suppressing preadipocyte differentiation, inhibit adipogenesis, and ameliorate the genes regulating intracellular lipolysis (Choi et al., 2015; Bae et al., 2015; Moon et al., 2013). The flavonoids and S-methylcysteine present in onion have a regulatory effect on the phosphatidylinositol-4,5-bisphosphate 3-kinase/Akt-dependent pathway, thereby decreasing blood glucose, serum lipids, oxidative stress, and lipid peroxidation, increasing insulin secretion and antioxidant enzyme activity, and thus reducing the occurrence of cardiovascular diseases (Akash et al., 2014; Gautam et al., 2015).

14.2.9 PIPER NIGRUM L

Several spices have been used in folk medicine for the treatment of various diseases because of the presence of abundant bioactive compounds. Pepper (*Piper nigrum* L.) is one such spice known as 'the King of Spices' used worldwide. The bioactive compounds present in black pepper include alkaloids, terpenes, steroids, lignans, and flavones (Nusenga et al., 2007). The alkaloids present in black pepper include piperine, chavicine, piperidine, and piperitine (Shaikh et al., 2006).

Studies have identified that black pepper has a significant effect on lowering the serum cholesterol level, triglycerides, and LDL cholesterol, and increasing the good cholesterol HDL. Piperine-enriched extract reduced cholesterol-enriched proteins and scavenger receptor expression, thereby preventing intestinal cholesterol uptake and subsequently reducing serum cholesterol levels, one of the major risk factors of CVD (Tachakittirungrod, 2007). Vijayakumar et al. reported that consumption of black pepper/piperine reduced oxidative damage and regulated the enzyme systems functioning in the body (Vijayakumar & Nalini, 2006) and reduced low-density lipoprotein (LDL) oxidation by attenuating prostaglandins and leukotrienes synthesis

(Srinivasan, 2005). Piperine administration decreased the blood pressure caused by the blockage of voltage-dependent calcium channels (Hlavackova et al., 2010). Piperine inhibited platelet aggregation by ameliorating the enzymes involved in arachidonic acid metabolism such as phospholipase A2 and thromboxane A2 synthase activities in platelets (Son et al., 2014).

14.2.10 COCOS NUCIFERA L

Cocos nucifera L (Coconut), Coconut milk is used in the Karkkidaka kanji to enhance its taste. Coconut fruit is composed of about 38.5% shell, 51.7% kernel, and 9.8% water (Vigila & Baskaran, 2008). Arginine and glutamic acid were shown to be the two amino acids most prevalent in coconut kernel protein (CKP), which makes up 22.8% of the crude protein in the kernel (Salil et al., 2011). CKP isolated from coconut kernel possesses beneficial anti-peroxidative and cardioprotective effects on alcohol and isoproterenol-treated rats as well as on human volunteers (Nair et al., 1998a, b; Mini & Rajamohan, 2002, 2004). CKP is also reported to have an effect on maintaining glucose homeostasis by regulating NF-κB and RAGE in diabetic rats (Salil et al., 2014).

14.2.11 DASAPUSHPAM (HERBS IN MARUNNUTHORAN)

The herbs used to prepare Marunnuthoran are 'Cherula' (*Aerva lanata* (L.) Juss), 'Mukkutti' (*Biophytum sensitivum* (L.) DC), 'Uzhinja' (*Cardiospermum halicacabum* L.), 'Nilappana' (*Curculigo orchioides* Gaertn.), 'Karuka' (*Cynodon dactylon* (L.) Pers), 'Kayyonni' (*Eclipta prostata* (L.)), 'Muyalcheviyan' (*Emilia sonchifolia* (L.) DC. ex-DC), 'Vishnukranthi' (*Evolvulus alsinoides* (L.) L.), 'Thiruthali' (*Ipomoea obscura* (L.) Ker Gawl.), 'Poovamkurunnila' (*Vernonia cinerea* Less.).

Aerva lanata is reported to possess antidiabetic (Deshmukh, 2008) and hepatoprotective activity (Nevin & Vijayammal, 2005) and also act as a hypolipidemic agent in calcium oxalate urolithiasis (Soundararajan, 2007). Riya et al. reported that *Aerva lanata* has alpha-glucosidase inhibition, antiglycation, and adipogenic potential and thus possesses significant antidiabetic activity. Insulin sensitization and antioxidant activity may enhance its therapeutic potential (Riya et al., 2015). Aerva was also reported to have potent antioxidant activity and reduced Xanthine Oxidase enzyme activity and Lipoxygenase (LOX) activity proving its anti-inflammatory potential (Pieczykolan et al., 2021).

Biophytum sensitivum (L.) DC has health-beneficial effects as it improves parameters of lipid profile including VLDL and LDL cholesterol except HDL cholesterol and also reduces plasma glucose levels without any risk of causing severe hypoglycemia (Puri, 2003). *Biophytum* inhibits the production of nitric oxide (NO), proinflammatory cytokines like IL-1β, IL-6, and TNF-α and downregulates the gene expression of inducible NO synthase and COX-2 enzymes and thus possesses potent anti-inflammatory activity (Guruvayoorappan & Kuttan, 2008).

Cardiospermum halicacabum L. ethanol extract has anti-inflammatory activity against carrageenan-induced rat paw edema which has been established by Sadique et al. (1987). The ethanol extract of *Cardiospermum* suppresses the production of proinflammatory mediators like TNF-alpha and nitric oxide in human peripheral blood mononuclear cells (Venkatesh Babu, 2006).

Curculigo orchioides Gaertn possesses demulcent and diuretic properties and is used for the treatment of diarrhea, piles, jaundice, asthma, and some skin diseases (Yoganarasimhan, 2000). It is also reported to have hepatoprotective, antioxidant, and anti-inflammatory properties (Venukumar & Lathanm, 2002; Wu et al., 2005); and antidiabetic activity (Madhavan et al., 2007).

Cynodon dactylon (L.) Pers is reported to have many health benefits including antidiabetic (Annapurna et al., 2013; Karthik & Ravikumar, 2011; Jananie et al., 2012), antioxidant (Saroja et al., 2012; Albert-Baskar et al., 2012; Jananie et al., 2011), cardioprotective (Garjani et al., 2009; Shabi et al., 2012), and anti-inflammatory activities (Garg & Paliwal, 2011; Dhande, 2013; Sindhu et al., 2009).

Eclipta prostata (L.) L. has been used in the treatment of infective hepatitis (Wagner, 1986), and snake venom poisoning (Melo et al., 1994), and possesses anti-inflammatory, antifungal, antihepatotoxic, antibacterial, and antioxidant properties (Karthikumar et al., 2007).

Emilia sonchifolia (L.) DC. ex DC is used in ethnomedicine for the treatment of rheumatism, cut wounds, eye sores, convulsions, and insect bites (Agra et al., 2007; Shylesh et al., 2005). Different studies have demonstrated that certain substances isolated from *Emilia sonchifolia* have anti-tumor, anti-inflammatory, and antioxidant properties (Gayathri Devi et al., 2006; Kawaree & Chowwanapoonpoh, 2009).

Evolvulus alsinoides is reported to possess antioxidant properties (Purohit et al., 1996), immunomodulatory effects (Ganju et al., 2003), gastroprotective properties (Auddy et al., 2003), and antiulcer and anticatatonic activities (Retnasooriya et al., 2005).

Ipomoea obscura (L.) Ker Gawl seeds and fruits are used as cleansing agents to improve difficult breathing, relieve pain, and enhance vision. This plant is also included among plants affecting the central nervous system (Shahina, 1994) and is actively used as an antioxidant (Srinivasan et al., 2008). *Ipomoea obscura* is also reported to possess hepatoprotective (Aravind et al., 2010), anti-inflammatory, and anti-tumor activities (Hamsa & Girija, 2011).

Studies reported that Ayurvedic drugs containing *Vernonia cinerea* Less. is renoprotective and antiurolithiatic (Rao & Rao, 1998; Kumaram & Patki, 2011). It exerts anti-inflammatory (Mazumdar et al., 2003; Kumar & Kuttan, 2009; Latha et al., 1998), antitumor (Pratheeshkumar & Kuttan, 2010, 2011), antidiabetic (Choudhary et al., 2013; Sayeed & Ferdous, 2013), and antioxidant activities (Kumar & Kuttan, 2009).

14.3 KERALA SADHYA

The harvest festival of Kerala, "Onam," and other special occasions like Vishu, Hindu marriage functions, etc., are celebrated with a colorful vegetarian feast served on a banana leaf called traditional 'Kerala Sadhya.' It includes up to 28 different vegetarian dishes at a time. Traditionally, Kerala Sadhya is served on a banana leaf, which consists of parboiled red rice, side dishes, savories, pickles, and desserts, all served at different times during the meal. The first item served is boiled rice, followed by Parippu curry, which is a mashed gravy made from cooked green gram and ghee, then followed by Sambar, a vegetable stew made from a variety of vegetables boiled in a gravy of crushed lentils, onions, chilies, coriander, turmeric, and a pinch of asafetida. Avial is one of the main side dishes in Kerala Sadhya, prepared with different vegetables, coconut paste, green chilies blended with fresh coconut oil, and raw curry leaves. Sambar and Avial contain a large number of vegetables that are nutritious, and the nutraceuticals and dietary fibers present in these vegetables help with regulated digestion and absorption. Thoran is another important side dish that contains minced string beans, cabbage, radish, or grams mixed with grated coconut, blended with red chilies and turmeric powder. Olan is yet another side dish in Sadhya that contains red grams cooked in a thin gravy of coconut milk, with its main ingredient being pumpkin.

Sadhya also serves Payasam (Kheer), a popular dessert in Kerala that comes in a variety of flavors like Pal Payasam, usually prepared with rice/wheat cooked in cow's milk, Palada Pradhaman, which contains flat-shaped 'ada' prepared from rice flour cooked in jaggery and coconut milk, and Kadalaparippu Pradhaman which is prepared with broken black chickpeas cooked and smashed with jaggery and coconut milk. A payasam is a pudding decorated with spices, raisins, and cashew nuts fried in ghee and it is typically served with yellow plantains (pazham). The ingredients of payasam are rich in protein and micronutrients which are beneficial to the maintenance of good health.

Other significant savory items in the Sadhya include three to five pieces of Upperi (deep-fried banana chips), Pappadams (fried black gram flour wafers), different pickles including Ginger Pickle, Mango Pickle, lemon pickle, and Kichadi (sliced cucumber/ladies' finger (okra) in curd, seasoned with mustard, red chilies, and curry leaves in coconut oil). At the end of the feast, traditional Rasam and more rice are served. Rasam is a concoction of tomato, pepper, garlic, and chili powders cooked in watered-down tamarind juice. Kaalan, a concoction of sour buttermilk with salt and chopped green chilies along with seasoned buttermilk with turmeric powder and green chilies, would help in easy digestion.

14.3.1 HEALTH BENEFITS OF KERALA SADHYA

The Kerala Sadhya is well-known for its flavors and variety of meals, and it accentuates the advantages of several traditional eating habits that are also beneficial to health. Traditionally, Sadhya is served on fresh banana leaves that are rich in polyphenols, a type of natural antioxidant. The antioxidant is absorbed into the food when heated food is placed on the leaf, which also contains vitamin A, calcium, and beta-carotene, and possesses antimicrobial activities.

Sadhya is a nutrition-dense meal and a healthy mixture comprising a balance of antioxidants, cardioprotective, anti-inflammatory foods, high calcium, and gut-friendly foods. All of Kerala Sadhya's ingredients are rich in vitamins and plant proteins, which are beneficial to maintaining health. The traditional Sadhya includes kuthari rice (matta red rice), dal curry with ghee, pappad, plantain chips and sarkaravaratty, pickles, pachadi, kichadi, avail, thoran, sambar, olan, kalan, kootukari, rasam, and buttermilk. The order in which these dishes are served depends on the taste and flavor profile.

- **Rice:** The rice with bran is perfect for people with different lifestyle conditions because of its low glycemic index rate. It is rich in B complex vitamins like thiamine, riboflavin, and niacin. The bran of rice is rich in plant nutrients with fibers that reduce the fat content and provide 80% of the manganese.
- **Dal Curry, Ghee, and Pappad:** Dal curry is rich in iron, potassium, calcium, and magnesium, which helps in controlling blood pressure.
- **Ghee is Rich in Vitamins A, D, and E:** Ingi curry is rich in Vitamins A, D, and E, magnesium, phosphorus, potassium, and calcium. It flushes out toxins, and fights fungus, viruses, etc. It boosts immunity owing to the presence of antioxidants.
- **Pickles:** Mangoes and lime are storehouses of vitamin C, flavonoids, minerals, vitamin B, and potassium, and are good for digestion too.
- **Kichadi:** Kichadi is prepared with cucumbers and beetroots. Cucumbers have detoxification properties, and beetroot is rich in antioxidant compounds.
- **Pachadi:** Varieties of pachadi are made using ingredients like pineapple, beetroot, and pumpkin.

  Bromelain, an enzyme present in pineapple, enhances digestion. Beetroot contains carbohydrates, folic acid, and micronutrients like iron and zinc. Pumpkin is rich in vitamin C, dietary fibers, alpha-carotene, beta-carotene, potassium, and magnesium.
- **Avial:** Avial is prepared with lots of vegetables and coconut and is the main item in Kerala Sadhya, loaded with vitamins and minerals. Avial is one of the healthiest dishes in Kerala Sadhya platter. Meanwhile, the fibers in it help reduce body weight and fight malnutrition.
- **Sambar:** Sambar contains Dal, which is a vital ingredient rich in protein and is a nutritious food. The fibers in it reduce constipation.
- **Pulisssery, Buttermilk:** Pulisssery and Buttermilk are rich in calcium, vitamin D, potassium, phosphorus, zinc, iodine, and riboflavin.

- **Rasam:** It is a soup of spices traditionally prepared using tamarind juice as a base, with the addition of Indian sesame oil, turmeric, tomato, chili pepper, pepper, garlic, cumin, curry leaves, mustard, coriander, asafetida, sea salt, and water. All the ingredients used to prepare Rasam are medicinally claimed for various ailments.
- **Payasam:** Payasam is made with jaggery which contains micronutrients like zinc, potassium, and other minerals. Pal payasam is prepared with cow's milk and is rich in calcium and phosphorous.

14.4 CONCLUSION

With the advent of an increasing number of heart diseases in all age groups, it is time to explore various herbs and their preparations so that morbidity and mortality from heart diseases can be reduced to a minimum in our everyday lives. In Kerala, it is evident from the available literature that the ingredients used in the 'Karkkidaka kanji' are a rich source of beneficial phytochemicals with a vast number of effects in maintaining good health. The use of whole grains increases the availability of dietary fibers, which enhances the digestive process and helps in the excretion of excess lipids in the body. Other phytochemicals present in the porridge possess a cardioprotective effect by regulating different molecular mechanisms and reducing the adverse effects exerted by various risk factors leading to cardiovascular disease, including atherosclerosis, diabetes, oxidative stress, hypertension, hyperlipidemia, etc. Herbs in Dasapushpam, which are used for the preparation of 'Marunnuthoran,' also possess favorable effects like anti-inflammatory, cardioprotective, antioxidant, and antidiabetic activities. Thus, Kerala's traditional monsoon food is a good source of phytochemicals that have cardioprotective potential to protect from CVD. Kerala Sadhya includes a plethora of dishes enriched with carbohydrates, proteins, vitamins, and minerals. Rice and lentils are the sources of carbohydrates and proteins for our body. Vitamin requirements of the body are fulfilled to some extent by the Sambar, which is full of seasonal vegetables. Avial and thoran are enriched with different vegetables that are high in dietary fibers, which help in easy digestion as they comprise a variety of seasonal vegetables and coconut. Rasam, buttermilk, Kaalan, and pachadi have ingredients that pacify the stomach. The pappadams and pickles meet the sodium requirement, and Payasams are enriched with carbohydrates. Therefore, Kerala

Sadhya is nutritious and enriched with components that are responsible for maintaining good health.

There is an association between oxidative stress and cardiovascular diseases. From a dietary perspective, traditional foods are powerhouses of antioxidants as they are rich in dietary phytochemicals. Hence, consumption of traditional food is an innovative strategy that helps to reduce cardiovascular risk factors. As dietary and healthy lifestyles are integral parts of a practical approach to treating cardiovascular diseases, traditional medicinal foods devoid of side effects gain further attention. The preservation of traditional food knowledge and consumer awareness is urgently needed because these foods are vital to a person's diet, helping to improve their nutritional status, fostering good health, and maintaining food security. Overall, accepting the fact that traditional food has an indispensable role in the enhancement of health, livelihood, and well-being of the people, sustainable policy measures have to be undertaken.

ACKNOWLEDGMENT

The expertise and assistance of all the authors throughout the preparation of manuscript is acknowledged.

KEYWORDS

- **alkylresorcinols**
- **allium sativum**
- **benzoxazinoids**
- **cardiovascular diseases**
- **low-density lipoprotein**
- **medicinal foods**
- **Oryza sativa**
- **phytochemicals**
- **traditional foods**
- **World Health Organization**

REFERENCES

Adam, A., Lopez, H. W., Leuillet, M., Demigné, C., & Rémésy, C. (2003). Whole wheat flour exerts cholesterol-lowering in rats in its native form and after use in bread-making. *Food Chemistry, 80*, 337–344.

Agra, M. F., Freitas, P. F., & Barbosa-Filho, J. M. (2007). Synopsis of the plants known as medicinal and poisonous in Northeast of Brazil. *Brazilian Journal of Pharmacognosy, 17*, 114–140.

Akash, M. S. H., Rehman, K., & Chen, S. (2014). Spice plant Allium cepa: dietary supplement for treatment of type 2 diabetes mellitus. *Nutrition, 30*(10), 1128–1137.

Albert-Baskar, A., Numair, K. S., Alsaif, M. A., & Ignacimuthu, S. (2012). In vitro antioxidant and antiproliferative potential of medicinal plants used in traditional Indian medicine to treat cancer. *Redox Report, 17*(4), 145–156.

Amna, A., & Nizwa, I. (2019). Hypolipidemic and Antiobesity Impact of Cuminum Cyminum Powder in Overweight and Obese Females. *International Innovative Science and Research Technology, 4*(4), 396–402.

Anderson, J. W., Hanna, T. J., Peng, X., & Kryscio, R. J. (2000). Whole grain foods and heart disease risk. *Journal of the American College of Nutrition, 19*(3), 291S–299S.

Annapurna, H. V., Apoorva, B., Ravichandran, N., Purushothaman, K., Brindha, P., Swaminathan, S., Vijayalakshmi, M., & Nagarajan, A. (2013). Isolation and in silico evaluation of antidiabetic molecules of *Cynodondactylon* (L). *Journal of Molecular Graphics and Modelling, 39*, 87–97.

Anu, K., Zhao, D., Wang, Z., et al. (2016). Comparison of different drying methods on Chinese ginger (*Zingiber officinale* Roscoe): Changes in volatiles, chemical profile, antioxidant properties, and microstructure. *Food Chemistry, 197*, 1292–1300.

Arablou, T., & Aryaeian, N. (2018). The effect of ginger (*Zingiber officinale*) as an ancient medicinal plant on improving blood lipids. *Journal of Herbal Medicine, 12*, 11–15.

Arablou, T., Aryaeian, N., Valizadeh, M., et al. (2014). The effect of ginger consumption on glycemic status, lipid profile, and some inflammatory markers in patients with type 2 diabetes mellitus. *International Journal of Food Sciences and Nutrition, 65*, 515–520.

Aravind, J. M., Ravi, A., Alka, C., & Prakash, Z. (2010). Preliminary phytochemical screening of *Ipomoea obscura* (L.)- A hepatoprotective medicinal plant. *International Journal of PharmTech Research, 2*(4), 2307–2312.

Atashak, S., Peeri, M., Jafari, A., et al. (2011). Effects of ginger supplementation and resistance training on lipid profiles and body composition in obese men. *Journal of Medicinal Plant Research, 5*, 3827–3832.

Attari, V. E., Mahluji, S., Jafarabadi, M. A., et al. (2015). Effects of supplementation with ginger (*Zingiber officinale* Roscoe) on serum glucose, lipid profile, and oxidative stress in obese women: A randomized, placebo-controlled clinical trial. *Pharmaceutical Sciences, 21*, 184–191.

Auddy, B., et al. (2003). Screening of antioxidant activity of three Indian medicinal plants, traditionally used for the management of neurodegenerative diseases. *Journal of Ethnopharmacology, 84*, 131–138.

Augusti, K. T., & Sheela, C. G. (1996). Antiperoxide effect of S-allyl cysteine sulfoxide, a insulin secretagogue, in diabetic rats. *Experientia, 52*, 115–120.

Augusti, K. T., Chackery, J., Jacob, J., Kuriakose, S., George, S., & Nair, S. S. (2005). Beneficial effects of a polar fraction of garlic (*Allium sativum* Linn.) oil in rats fed with two different high-fat diets. *Indian Journal of Experimental Biology, 43*(1), 76–83.

Bae, C. R., Park, Y. K., & Cha, Y. S. (2014). Quercetin-rich onion peel extract suppresses adipogenesis by down-regulating adipogenic transcription factors and gene expression in 3T3-L1 adipocytes. *Journal of the Science of Food and Agriculture, 94*(13), 2655–2660.

Basch, E., Ulbricht, C., Kuo, G., Szapary, P., & Smith, M. (2003). Therapeutic applications of fenugreek. *Alternative Medicine Review, 8*(1), 20–27.

Bhaskar, S., Kumar, K. S., Krishnan, K., & Antony, H. (2013). Quercetin alleviates hypercholesterolemic diet induced inflammation during progression and regression of atherosclerosis in rabbits. *Nutrition, 29*, 219–229.

Brüll, V., Burak, C., Stoffel-Wagner, B., et al. (2015). Effects of a quercetin-rich onion skin extract on 24 h ambulatory blood pressure and endothelial function in overweight-to-obese patients with (pre-) hypertension: a randomized double-blinded placebo-controlled cross-over trial. *British Journal of Nutrition, 114*(8), 1263–1277.

Chen, C. Y., Kao, C. L., & Liu, C. M. (2018). The cancer prevention, anti-inflammatory, and anti-oxidation of bioactive phytochemicals targeting the TLR4 signaling pathway. *International Journal of Molecular Sciences, 19*, 2729.

Chithra, K. P., Shalini, V., Sindhu, G., Parvathy, R., Jayalekshmi, A., & Helen, A. (2016). Attenuation of atherosclerotic complications by modulating inflammatory responses in hypercholesterolemic rats with dietary Njavara rice bran oil. *Biomedicine & Pharmacotherapy, 83*, 1387–1397.

Chithra, K. P., Sindhu, G., Parvathy, R., Jayalekshmi, A., & Helen, A. (2015). Dietary Njavara rice bran oil reduces experimentally induced hypercholesterolemia by regulating genes involved in lipid metabolism. *British Journal of Nutrition, 113*(8), 1–13.

Choi, E. Y., Lee, H., Woo, J. S., et al. (2015). Effect of onion peel extract on endothelial function and endothelial progenitor cells in overweight and obese individuals. *Nutrition, 31*(9), 1131–1135.

Choudhary, S., Sharma, M., Tripathi, J., & Mishra, P. (2013). Antihyperglycemic activity of Vernonia cinerea L. on alloxan-induced diabetic mice. *International Journal of Advanced Research, 1*, 35–42.

Costabile, A., Klinder, A., Fava, F., Napolitano, A., et al. (2008). Whole-grain wheat breakfast cereal has a prebiotic effect on the human gut microbiota: a double-blind, placebo-controlled, crossover study. *British Journal of Nutrition, 99*, 110–120.

Danwilai, K., Konmun, J., Sripanidkulchai, B., & Subongkot, S. S. (2017). Antioxidant activity of ginger extract as a daily supplement in cancer patients receiving adjuvant chemotherapy: a pilot study. *Cancer Management and Research, 9*, 11–18.

Deepa, G., Singh, V., & Naidu, K. A. (2008). Nutrient composition and physicochemical properties of Indian medicinal rice-Njavara. *Food Chemistry, 106*, 165–171.

Deepa, G., Venkatachalam, L., Bhagyalakshmi, N., Shashidhar, H. E., Singh, V., & Naidu, K. A. (2009). Physicochemical and genetic analysis of an endemic rice variety, Njavara (*Oryza sativa* L.), in comparison to two popular south Indian cultivars, Jyothi (PTB 39) and IR 64. *Journal of Agricultural and Food Chemistry, 57*, 11476–11483.

Deshmukh, T. A., Yadav, B. V., Badole, S. L., Bodhankar, S. L., & Dhaneshwar, S. R. (2008). Antihyperglycaemic activity of alcoholic extract of *Aerva lanata* (L.) A. L. Juss. ex J. A. Schultes leaves in alloxan induced diabetic mice. *Journal of Applied Biomedicine, 6*, 81–87.

Dhande, S. R. (2013). Anti-inflammatory and analgesic properties of the 50% ethanolic extract of *Cynodon dactylon* Pers. *International Research Journal for Inventions in Pharmaceutical Sciences, 1*(2), 8–16.

Dugasani, S., Pichika, M. R., Nadarajah, V. D., et al. (2010). Comparative antioxidant and anti-inflammatory effects of [6]-gingerol, [8]-gingerol, [10]-gingerol, and [6]-shogaol. *Journal of Ethnopharmacology, 127*, 515–520.

El Gayar, M. H., Aboromia, M. M. M., Ibrahim, N. A., et al. (2019). Effects of ginger powder supplementation on glycemic status and lipid profile in newly diagnosed obese patients with type 2 diabetes mellitus. *Obesity Medicine; Endocrine Abstracts, 63*, 122.

Fardet, A. (2010). New hypotheses for the health-protective mechanisms of whole-grain cereals: What is beyond fiber? *Nutrition Research Reviews, 23*(1), 65–13.

Ganju, L., Karan, D., Chanda, S., Srivastava, K. K., Sawhney, R. C., & Selvamurthy, W. (2003). Immunomodulatory effects of agents of plant origin. *Biomedicine & Pharmacotherapy, 57*, 296–300.

Gao, E. Z., Yu, X. H., Liu, T., Li, H. L., Wang, P., Wei, Y. Q., Zhao, Y. L., & Yu, Z. G. (2014). Comparative study on effects of single and multiple oral administration of mungbean (*Phaseolus radiatus* L.) seed extract on the pharmacokinetics of aconitine by UHPLC-MS. *Biomedical Chromatography, 28*, 1313–1319.

Gao, H., Guan, T., Li, C., et al. (2012). Treatment with ginger ameliorates fructose-induced fatty liver and hypertriglyceridemia in rats: Modulation of the hepatic carbohydrate response element-binding protein-mediated pathway. *Evidence-Based Complementary and Alternative Medicine, 2012*, 570948.

Garg, V. K., & Paliwal, S. K. (2011). Anti-inflammatory activity of aqueous extract of *Cynodon dactylon. International Journal of Pharmacology, 7*(3), 370–375.

Garjani, A., Afrooziyan, A., Nazemiyeh, H., Najafi, M., Kharazmkia, A., & Maleki-Dizaji, N. (2009). Protective effects of hydroalcoholic extract from rhizomes of *Cynodon dactylon* (L) Pers on compensated right heart failure in rats. *BMC Complementary and Alternative Medicine, 9*, 28–36.

Gautam, S., Pal, Maurya, S. R., & Srivastava, A. K. (2015). Ethanolic extract of *Allium cepa* stimulates glucose transporter type 4-mediated glucose uptake by the activation of insulin signaling. *Planta Medica, 81*(3), 208–214.

Gayathri Devi, D., Lija, Y., Cibin, T. R., Biju, P. G., Gayathri Devi, V., & Abraham, A. (2006). Evaluation of the protective effects of *Emilia sonchifolia* Linn. (DC.) on perchlorate-induced oxidative damage. *Journal of Biological Sciences, 6*, 887–892.

Gebhardt, R. (1993). Multiple inhibitory effects of garlic extract on cholesterol biosynthesis in hepatocytes. *Lipids, 28*(7), 613–619.

Gebhardt, R., & Beck, H. (1996). Differential inhibitory effects of garlic-derived organosulfur compounds on cholesterol biosynthesis in primary rat hepatocyte cultures. *Lipids, 31*(12), 1269–1276.

Ginter, E., & Simko, V. (2010). Garlic (*Allium sativum* L.) and cardiovascular diseases. *Bratislava Medical Journal, 111*(8), 452–456.

Guruvayoorappan, C., & Kuttan, G. (2008). Methanol extract of *Biophytum sensitivum* alters the cytokine profiles and inhibits iNOS and COX-2 expression in LPS/Con A stimulated macrophages. *Drug and Chemical Toxicology, 31*, 175–188.

Hamsa, T. P., & Girija, K. (2011). Evaluation of anti-inflammatory and anti-tumor effect of *Ipomoea obscura* (L.) and its mode of action through the inhibition of proinflammatory cytokines, NO and COX-2. *Inflammation, 34*, 171–183.

Han, Q., Yuan, Q., Meng, X., et al. (2017). 6-Shogaol attenuates LPS-induced inflammation in BV2 microglia cells by activating PPAR-γ. *Oncotarget, 8*, 42001–42006.

Harris, K. A., & Kris-Etherton, P. M. (2010). Effects of whole grains on coronary heart disease risk. *Current Atherosclerosis Reports, 12*, 368–376.

Harshlatha, C., & Ashok, P. (2018). Protective effect of cumin (*Cuminum cyminum* L.) seed extract on cardiovascular system, toxicity, and hematology on hyperlipidemic rabbits: an experimental study. *Asian Journal of Pharmaceutical and Clinical Research, 11*(10), 353–356.

Haslam, D. W., & James, W. P. (2005). Obesity. *The Lancet, 366*, 1197–1209.

He, M., van Dam, R., Rimm, E., Hu, F., & Qi, L. (2010). Whole-grain, cereal fiber, bran, and germ intake and the risks of all-cause and cardiovascular disease-specific mortality among women with Type 2 Diabetes Mellitus. *Circulation, 121*(20), 2162–2168.

Hlavackova, L., Urbanova, A., Ulicna, O., Janega, P., Cerna, A., & Babal, P. (2010). Piperine, active substance of black pepper, alleviates hypertension induced by NO synthase inhibition. *Bratislava Medical Journal, 111*, 426–431.

Hsing, C. W., Chi, T. H., Shih, C. T., You, L. L., Shou, C. H., Yi, J. T., Fuu, J. T., & Jo, H. C. (2018). Relaxant and Vaso protective effects of ginger extracts on porcine coronary arteries. *International Journal of Molecular Medicine, 41*, 2420–2428.

Hsu, G., Lu, Y., Chang, S., & Hsu, S. (2011). Antihypertensive effect of mung bean sprout extract in spontaneously hypertensive rats. *Journal of Food Biochemistry, 35*, 278–288.

Ippoushi, K., Azuma, K., Ito, H., et al. (2003). [6]-Gingerol inhibits nitric oxide synthesis in activated J774.1 mouse macrophages and prevents peroxynitrite-induced oxidation and nitration reactions. *Life Sciences, 73*, 3427–3437.

Jafarzadeh, A., Jafarzadeh, S., & Nemati, M. (2021). Therapeutic potential of ginger against COVID-19: Is there enough evidence? *Journal of Traditional Chinese Medical Sciences, 8*, 267–279.

Jaiswal, N., & Rizvi, S. I. (2014). Onion extract (*Allium cepa* L.), quercetin and catechin up-regulate paraoxonase 1 activity with concomitant protection against low-density lipoprotein oxidation in male Wistar rats subjected to oxidative stress. *Journal of the Science of Food and Agriculture, 94*(13), 2752–2757.

Jalali, M., Mahmoodi, M., Moosavian, S. P., et al. (2020). The effects of ginger supplementation on markers of inflammatory and oxidative stress: A systematic review and meta-analysis of clinical trials. *Phytotherapy Research, 34*, 1723–1733.

Jananie, R. K., Priya, V., & Vijayalakshmi, K. (2011). In vitro assessment of free radical scavenging activity of *Cynodon dactylon*. *Journal of Chemical and Pharmaceutical Research, 3*(4), 647–654.

Jananie, R. K., Priya, V., & Vijayalakshmi, K. (2012). Secondary metabolites of *Cynodon dactylon* as an antagonist to angiotensin II type 1 receptor: Novel in silico drug targeting approach for diabetic retinopathy. *Journal of Pharmacology & Pharmacotherapeutics, 3*(1), 20–25.

Jiang, Q., Christen, S., Shigenaga, M. K., & Ames, B. N. (2001). Gamma-tocopherol, the major form of vitamin E in the US diet, deserves more attention. *American Journal of Clinical Nutrition, 74*, 714–722.

Karthik, D., & Ravikumar, S. (2011). A study on the protective effect of *Cynodon dactylon* leaves extract in diabetic rats. *Biomedical and Environmental Sciences, 24*(2), 190–199.

Karthikumar, S., Vigneswari, K., & Jagatheesan, K. (2007). Screening of antibacterial and antioxidant activities of leaves of *Eclipta prostrata* (L.). *Scientific Research and Essays, 2*(4), 101–104.

Kawaree, R., & Chowwanapoonpoh, S. (2009). Stability of chemical components and antioxidant activity of volatile oils from some medicinal plants in Thailand. *Chiang Mai University Journal of Natural Science, 8*, 23–35.

Khorshidian, N., Yousefi Asli, M., Arab, M., Adeli Mirzaie, A., & Mortazavian, A. M. (2016). Fenugreek: Potential applications as a functional food and nutraceutical. *Nutrition and Food Sciences Research, 3*(1), 5–16.

Kim-Park, S., & Ku, D. D. (2000). Garlic elicits a nitric oxide-dependent relaxation and inhibits hypoxic pulmonary vasoconstriction in rats. *Clinical and Experimental Pharmacology and Physiology, 27*, 780–786.

Kiyama, R. (2020). Nutritional implications of ginger: Chemistry, biological activities and signaling pathways. *Journal of Nutritional Biochemistry, 86*, 108486.

Koo, K. L., Ammit, A. J., Tran, V. H., et al. (2001). Gingerols and related analogues inhibit arachidonic acid-induced human platelet serotonin release and aggregation. *Thrombosis Research, 103*, 387–397.

Krishnaswamy, K. (2008). Traditional Indian spices and their health significance. *Asia Pacific Journal of Clinical Nutrition, 17*, 265–268.

Kumar, P. P., & Kuttan, G. (2009). Vernonia cinerea L. scavenges free radicals and regulates nitric oxide and proinflammatory cytokines profile in carrageenan induced paw edema model. *Immunopharmacology and Immunotoxicology, 31*, 94–102.

Kumaran, M. G. S., & Patki, P. S. (2011). Evaluation of an ayurvedic formulation (cystone), in urolithiasis: A double blind, placebo-controlled study. *European Journal of Integrative Medicine, 3*, 23–28.

Kundu, J., & Surh, Y. J. (2009). Molecular basis of chemoprevention with dietary phytochemicals: Redox-regulated transcription factors as relevant targets. *Phytochemistry Reviews, 8*, 333–347.

Latha, R. M., Geetha, T., & Varalakshmi, P. (1998). Effect of *Vernonia cinerea* Less flower extract in adjuvant-induced arthritis. *General Pharmacology, 31*, 601–606.

Lau, B. H. S. (2001). Suppression of LDL oxidation by garlic. *Journal of Nutrition, 131*(3S), 958S–988S.

Lawson, L. D. (1998). Garlic: A review of its medicinal effects and indicated active compounds. In: L. D. Lawson & R. Bauer (Eds.), *Phytomedicines of Europe: Chemistry and Biological Activity* (pp. 176–209). Washington, DC: American Chemical Society.

Lee, J. H., Jeon, J. K., Kim, S. G., Kim, S. H., Chun, T., & Imm, J. Y. (2011a). Comparative analyses of total phenols, flavonoids, saponins and antioxidant activity in yellow soy beans and mung beans. *International Journal of Food Science and Technology, 46*, 2513–2519.

Lee, S. J., Lee, J. H., Lee, H. H., Lee, S., Kim, S. H., Chun, T., & Imm, J. Y. (2011b). Effect of mung bean ethanol extract on pro-inflammatory cytokines in LPS stimulated macrophages. *Food Science and Biotechnology, 20*, 519–524.

Lewin, G., & Popov, I. (1994). Antioxidant effects of aqueous garlic extract. 2nd communication: Inhibition of the Cu (2+)-initiated oxidation of low-density lipoproteins. *Arzneimittelforschung, 44*, 604–607.

Li, H., Cao, D. D., Yi, J. Y., Cao, J. K., & Jiang, W. B. (2012). Identification of the flavonoids in mungbean (*Phaseolus radiatus* L.) soup and their antioxidant activities. *Food Chemistry, 135*, 2942–2946.

Liu, L., & Yeh, Y. Y. (2002). S-alk(en)yl cysteines of garlic inhibit cholesterol synthesis by deactivating HMG-CoA reductase in cultured rat hepatocytes. *Journal of Nutrition, 132*(6), 1129–1134.

Liu, T., Yu, X. H., Gao, E. Z., Liu, X. N., Sun, L. J., Li, H. L., Wang, P., Zhao, Y. L., & Yu, Z. G. (2014). Hepatoprotective effect of active constituents isolated from mung beans (Phaseolus radiatus L.) in an alcohol-induced liver injury mouse model. *Journal of Food Biochemistry, 38*, 453–459.

Liyana-Pathirana, C. M., & Shahidi, F. (2007). The antioxidant potential of milling fractions from bread, wheat and durum. *Journal of Cereal Science, 45*, 238–247.

Lu, T. M., Chiu, H. F., Shen, C. Y., Chung, C. C., Venkatakrishnan, K., & Wang, C. K. (2015). Hypocholesterolemic efficacy of quercetin rich onion juice in healthy mild hypercholesterolemic adults: A pilot study. *Plant Foods for Human Nutrition, 70*(4), 395–400.

Madhavan, V., Richa, J., Anita, M., & Yoganarasimhan, S. N. (2007). Antidiabetic activity of *Curculigo orchioides* root tuber. *Pharmacology and Biology, 45*(1), 18–21.

Mahluji, S., Attari, V. E., Mobasseri, M., et al. (2013). Effects of ginger (*Zingiber officinale*) on plasma glucose level, HbA1c and insulin sensitivity in type 2 diabetic patients. *International Journal of Food Sciences and Nutrition, 64*, 682–686.

Mao, Q. Q., Xu, X. Y., Cao, S. Y., et al. (2019). Bioactive compounds and bioactivities of ginger (*Zingiber officinale* Roscoe). *Foods, 8*, 185.

Mazidi, M., Gao, H. K., Rezaie, P., et al. (2016). The effect of ginger supplementation on serum C-reactive protein, lipid profile and glycaemia: A systematic review and meta-analysis. *Food & Nutrition Research, 60*, 2613.

Mazumder, U. K., Gupta, M., Manikandan, L., Bhattacharya, S., Haldar, P. K., & Roy, S. (2003). Evaluation of anti-inflammatory activity of *Vernonia cinerea* Less. extract in rats. *Phytomedicine, 10*, 185–188.

McEwen, B. J. (2014). The influence of diet and nutrients on platelet function. *Seminars in Thrombosis and Hemostasis, 40*, 214–226.

Melo, P. A., Nascimento, M. C., Mors, W. B., & Suarez-Kurtz, G. (1994). Inhibition of the myotoxic and hemorrhagic activities of crotalid venoms by *Eclipta prostrata* (Astraceae) extracts and constituents. *Toxicon, 32*, 595–603.

Mini, S., & Rajamohan, T. (2002). Cardioprotective effect of coconut kernel protein in isoproterenol administered rats. *Indian Journal of Biochemistry and Biophysics, 39*, 197–200.

Mini, S., & Rajamohan, T. (2004). Influence of coconut kernel protein on lipid metabolism in alcohol fed rats. *Indian Journal of Experimental Biology, 42*, 53–57.

Mohanlal, S., Parvathy, R., Shalini, V., et al. (2012). Chemical indices, antioxidant activity and anti-inflammatory effect of extracts of the medicinal rice njavara and staple varieties: A comparative study. *Journal of Food Biochemistry, 37*, 369–380.

Moon, J., Do, H. J., Kim, O. Y., & Shin, M. J. (2013). Antiobesity effects of quercetin-rich onion peel extract on the differentiation of 3T3-L1 preadipocytes and the adipogenesis in high fat-fed rats. *Food and Chemical Toxicology, 58*, 347–354.

Moyers, S. (1996). *Garlic in Health, History and World Cuisine*. St. Petersburg, FL: Suncoast Press.

Muko, K. N., & Ohiri, F. C. (1999). A preliminary study on the anti-inflammatory properties of *Emilia sonchifolia* leaf extract. *Fitoterapia, 71*, 65–68.

Munday, J. S., James, K. A., Fray, L. M., Kirkwood, S. W., & Thompson, K. G. (1999). Daily supplementation with aged garlic extract, but not raw garlic, protects low density lipoprotein against in vitro oxidation. *Atherosclerosis, 143*, 399–404.

Musenga, A., Mandrioli, R., Ferranti, A., D'Orazio, G., Fanali, S., & Raggi, M. A. (2007). Analysis of aromatic and terpenic constituents of pepper extracts by capillary electrochromatography. *Journal of Separation Science, 30*, 612–619.

Nair, K. G. P., Rajamohan, T., & Kurup, P. A. (1998a). Changes in the metabolism of lipoproteins in rats fed coconut kernel protein. *Journal of Clinical Biochemistry and Nutrition, 25*, 159–168.

Nair, K. G. P., Rajamohan, T., & Kurup, P. A. (1998b). Coconut kernel protein modifies the effect of coconut oil on serum lipids. *Plant Foods for Human Nutrition, 53*, 133–144.

Nevin, K. G., & Vijayammal, P. L. (2005). Effect of *Aerva lanata* against hepatotoxicity of carbon tetrachloride in rats. *Environmental Toxicology and Pharmacology, 20*, 471–477.

Oishi, K., Yamamoto, S., Itoh, N., Nakao, R., et al. (2015). Wheat alkylresorcinols suppress high-fat, high-sucrose diet-induced obesity and glucose intolerance by increasing insulin sensitivity and cholesterol excretion in male mice. *Journal of Nutrition, 145*, 199–206.

Pieczykolan, A., Pietrzak, W., Gawlik-Dziki, U., & Nowak, R. (2021). Antioxidant, anti-inflammatory and antidiabetic activity of phenolic acids fractions obtained from *Aerva lanata* (L.) Juss. *Molecules, 26*, 2486.

Pourmasoumi, M., Hadi, A., Rafie, N., et al. (2018). The effect of ginger supplementation on lipid profile: A systematic review and meta-analysis of clinical trials. *Phytomedicine, 43*, 28–36.

Pradeep, S. R., & Srinivasan, K. (2018). Alleviation of cardiac damage by dietary fenugreek (*Trigonella foenum*-graecum) seeds is potentiated by onion (*Allium cepa*) in experimental diabetic rats via blocking Renin-Angiotensin system. *Cardiovascular Toxicology, 18*(3), 221–231.

Prasad, S., & Tyagi, A. K. (2015). Ginger and its constituents: Role in prevention and treatment of gastrointestinal cancer. *Gastroenterology Research and Practice, 2015*, 142979.

Pratheeshkumar, P., & Kuttan, G. (2010). Ameliorative action of *Vernonia cinerea* L. on cyclophosphamide-induced immunosuppression and oxidative stress in mice. *Inflammopharmacology, 18*, 197–207.

Pratheeshkumar, P., & Kuttan, G. (2011). Vernonia cinerea Less. inhibits tumor cell invasion and pulmonary metastasis in C57BL/6 mice. *Integrative Cancer Therapies, 10*, 178–191.

Puri, D. (2003). Hypocholesterolemic effect of *Biophytum sensitivum* leaf water extract. *Pharmaceutical Biology, 41*, 253–258.

Purohit, M. G., Shanthaveerappa, B. K., Badami, S., Swamy, H. K. S., & Shrishailappa, B. (1996). Antiulcer and anticatatonic activity of alcoholic extract of *Evolvulus alsinoides* (Convolvulaceae). *Indian Journal of Pharmaceutical Sciences, 58*, 110–112.

Rajasree, C. R., Rajamohan, T., & Agusti, K. T. (1999). Biochemical effects of garlic on lipid metabolism in alcohol-fed rats. *Indian Journal of Experimental Biology, 37*, 243–247.

Ram, B. S., Manal, M. A. S., Richa, H. R., Anuj, M., Narsingh, V., & Adrianlsaza. (2022). Effects of fenugreek seeds on cardiovascular diseases and other chronic diseases. In *Functional Foods and Nutraceuticals in Metabolic and Non-Communicable Diseases* (pp. 399–410).

Rao, K. S., & Mishra, S. H. (1997). Antihepatotoxic principles from the rhizomes of *Curculigo orchioides*. *Indian Drugs, 34*, 68–71.

Rao, M., & Rao, M. N. A. (1998). Protective effects of cystone, a polyherbal ayurvedic preparation, on cisplatin-induced renal toxicity in rats. *Journal of Ethnopharmacology, 62*, 1–6.

Rashid, A., & Khan, H. H. (1985). The mechanism of hypotensive effect of garlic extract. *Journal of the Pakistan Medical Association, 35*, 357–362.

Ratnasooriya, W. D., Hewageegana, H. G. S. P., Jayakody, J. R. A. C., Ariyawansa, H. A. S., & Kulatunga, R. D. H. (2005). Gastroprotective activity of *Evolvulus alsinoides* L. powder. *Australian Journal of Medical Herbalism, 17*, 55–60.

Rebey, I. B., Jabri-Karoui, I., Hamrouni-Sellami, I., Bourgou, S., Limam, F., & Marzouk, B. (2012). Effect of drought on the biochemical composition and antioxidant activities of cumin (*Cuminum cyminum* L.) seeds. *Industrial Crops and Products, 36*, 238–245.

Registrar General of India. (2019). Report on Medical Certification of Cause of Death 2019. New Delhi, India: Office of the Registrar General. https://dc.crsorgi.gov.in/assets/download/Annual-Reports/mccd/2019.pdf.

Rituraj, K., Jing, S., Yongyan, S., Dipak, S., & Qiaozhu, S. (2018). Phytoceuticals in fenugreek ameliorate VLDL overproduction and insulin resistance via the Insig signaling pathway. *Molecular Nutrition & Food Research, 62*(5), 1–7.

Riya, M. P., Antu, K. A., Pal, S., Chandrakanth, K. C., Anilkumar, K. S., Tamrakar, A. K., Srivasthava, A. K., & Raghu, K. G. (2015). Antidiabetic property of *Aerva lanata* (L.) Juss. Ex Schult. is mediated by inhibition of alpha glucosidase, protein glycation and stimulation of adipogenesis. *Journal of Diabetes, 7*(4), 548–561.

Rodenelli, M., Fossari, F., Vecchio, V., Gasparri, C., Peroni, G., Spadaccini, D., Riva, A., Petrangolini, G., Lanello, G., Nichetti, M., Infantino, V., & Perna, S. (2020). Clinical trials on pain lowering effect of ginger – A narrative review. *Phytotherapy Research, 34*(11), 2843–2856.

Ross, A. B., Chen, Y., Frank, J., Swanson, J. E., et al. (2004). Cereal alkylresorcinols elevate gamma-tocopherol levels in rats and inhibit gamma-tocopherol metabolism in vitro. *Journal of Nutrition, 134*, 506–510.

Sadique, J., Chandra, T., Thenmozhi, V., & Elango, V. (1987). Biochemical modes of action of *Cassia occidentalis* and *Cardiospermum halicacabum* in inflammation. *Journal of Ethnopharmacology, 19*, 201–212.

Saji, N., Francis, N., Schwarz, L. J., Blanchard, C. L., & Santhakumar, A. B. (2019). Rice bran derived bioactive compounds modulate risk factors of cardiovascular disease and Type-2 diabetes mellitus: An updated review. *Nutrients, 11*, 2736.

Sakhare, S. D., Inamdar, A. A., Indrani, D., Madhu Kiran, M. H., & Venkateswara Rao, G. (2015). Physicochemical and microstructure analysis of flour mill streams and milled products. *Journal of Food Science and Technology, 52*(1), 407–414.

Salil, G., Nevin, K. G., & Rajamohan, T. (2011). Arginine rich coconut kernel protein modulates diabetes in alloxan treated rats. *Chemico-Biological Interactions, 189*, 107–111.

Salil, G., Nithya, R., Nevin, K. G., & Rajmohan, T. (2014). Dietary coconut kernel protein beneficially modulates NFκB and RAGE expression in streptozotocin-induced diabetes in rats. *Journal of Food Science and Technology, 51*(9), 2141–2147.

Saroja, M., Santhi, R., & Annapoorani, S. (2012). Antioxidant potential of ethyl acetate fraction of *Cynodon dactylon* against ELA implanted Swiss albino mice. *International Journal of Pharmacy and Biological Sciences, 3*(2), 415–419.

Sayeed, M. S. B., & Ferdous, F. M. T. I. (2013). A randomized, placebo-controlled, crossover study of an herbal preparation containing Vernonia cinerea in the treatment of Type 2 diabetes. *Journal of Alternative and Complementary Medicine, 19*, 767–771.

Sekhon-Loodu, S., Ziaullah, Z., Rupasinghe, H. P. V., Wang, Y., Kulka, M., & Shahidi, F. (2015). Novel quercetin-3-O-glucoside eicosapentaenoic acid ester ameliorates inflammation and hyperlipidemia. *Inflammopharmacology, 23*(4), 173–185.

Sendl, A., Elbl, G., Steinke, B., Redl, K., Breu, W., & Wagner, H. (1992). Comparative pharmacological investigations of *Allium ursinum* and *Allium sativum*. *Planta Medica, 58*, 1–7.

Shabi, M. M., Raj David, C., Sasikala, C., Gayathri, K., & Joseph, J. (2012). Negative inotropic and chronotropic effects of phenolic fraction from *Cynodon dactylon* (Linn) on isolated perfused frog heart. *Journal of Scientific Research, 4*(3), 657–663.

Shaikh, J., Bhosale, R., & Singhal, R. (2006). Microencapsulation of black pepper oleoresin. *Food Chemistry, 94*, 105–110.

Shalini, V., Shobha, B., & Helen, A. (2011). Anti-inflammatory activity of Njavara (*Oryza sativa* Linn.). *Journal of Natural Remedies, 11*(1), 24–30.

Shylesh, B. S., Nair, S. A., & Subramoniam, A. (2005). Induction of cell-specific apoptosis and protection from Dalton's lymphoma challenge in mice by an active fraction from *Emilia sonchifolia*. *Indian Journal of Pharmacology, 37*, 232–237.

Simi, C. K., & Abraham, T. E. (2008). Physicochemical, rheological and thermal properties of Njavara rice (*Oryza sativa*) starch. *Journal of Agricultural and Food Chemistry, 56*, 12105–12111.

Sindhu, G., Ratheesh, M., Shyni, J. L., & Helen, A. (2009). Inhibitory effects of *Cynodon dactylon* L. on inflammation and oxidative stress in adjuvant-treated rats. *Immunopharmacology and Immunotoxicology, 31*(4), 647–653.

Soleyman, B., Maryam, M., Saeed, N., Seyed, A. R., & Mohammad, S. (2021). Cardioprotective effects of Fenugreek (*Trigonella foenum*-graceum) seed extract in streptozotocin induced diabetic rats. *Journal of Cardiovascular and Thoracic Research, 13*(1), 28–36.

Son, D. J., Akhiba, S., Hong, J. T., Yun, Y. P., Hwang, S. Y., Park, Y. H., & Lee, S. E. (2014). Piperine inhibits the activities of platelet cytosolic phospholipase A2 and thromboxane A2 synthase without affecting cyclooxygenase-1 activity: Different mechanisms of action are involved in the inhibition of platelet aggregation and macrophage inflammatory response. *Nutrients, 6*(8), 3336–3352.

Song, M. Y., Lee, D. Y., Park, S. Y., et al. (2021). Steamed ginger extract exerts anti-inflammatory effects in Helicobacter pylori-infected gastric epithelial cells through inhibition of NF-κB. *Journal of Cancer Prevention, 26*, 289.

Soucek, J., Skvor, J., Pouckova, P., Matougek, J., Slavik, T., & Matousek, J. (2006). Mung bean sprouts (*Phaseolus aureus*) nuclease and its biological and antitumor effects. *Neoplasma, 53*, 402–409.

Soundararajan, P., Mahesh, R., Ramesh, T., & Begum, V. H. (2007). Hypolipidemic activity of *Aerva lanata* on ethylene glycol induced calcium oxalate urolithiasis in rats. *Pharmacologyonline, 1*, 557–563.

Sreejayan., Kumar, V. R., & Thomas, G. (2003). Collecting and morphological evaluation of "Njavara," a traditional medicinal rice (*Oryza sativa* L.), in Kerala, India. *Plant Genetic Resources Newsletter, 135*, 12–17.

Srinivasan, K. (2005). Spices as influencers of body metabolism: An overview of three decades of research. *Food Research International, 38*, 77–86.

Srinivasan, K. (2006). Fenugreek (*Trigonella foenum*-graecum): A review of health beneficial physiological effects. *Food Reviews International, 22*(2), 203–224.
Srinivasan, R., Chandrasekar, M. J. N., Nanjan, M. J., & Suresh, B. (2008). Free radical scavenging activity of *Ipomoea obscura* (L) Ker-Gawl. *Journal of Natural Remedies, 7*(2), 184–188.
Stevens, S., Frenis, K., Oelze, M., et al. (2019). Vascular inflammation and oxidative stress: Major triggers for cardiovascular disease. *Oxidative Medicine and Cellular Longevity, 2019*, 7092151.
Suekawa, M., Ishige, A., Yuasa, K., et al. (1984). Pharmacological studies on ginger. I. Pharmacological actions of pungent constituents, (6)-gingerol and (6)-shogaol. *Journal of Pharmacobiodynamics, 7*, 836–848.
Sulochana, S., & Bakiyalakshmi, S. V. (2011). Effect of neutraceutical dosa on antimicrobial activity. *International Journal of Environmental Sciences, 5*, 727–735.
Sun, Y. E., Wang, W., & Quin, J. (2018). Anti-hyperlipidemia of garlic by reducing the level of total cholesterol and low-density lipoprotein – A meta-analysis. *Medicine, 97*(18), 1–8.
Tachakittirungrod, S., Okonogi, S., & Chowwanapoonpohn, S. (2007). Study on antioxidant activity of certain plants in Thailand: Mechanism of antioxidant action of guava leaf extract. *Food Chemistry, 103*, 381–388.
Tedesco, I., Carbone, V., Spagnuolo, C., Minasi, P., & Russo, G. L. (2015). Identification and quantification of flavonoids from two southern Italian cultivars of *Allium cepa* L., Tropea (Red Onion) and Montoro (Copper Onion), and their capacity to protect human erythrocytes from oxidative stress. *Journal of Agricultural and Food Chemistry, 63*(21), 5229–5238.
Tighe, P., Duthie, G., Vaughan, N., Brittenden, J., et al. (2010). Effect of increased consumption of whole-grain foods on blood pressure and other cardiovascular risk markers in healthy middle-aged persons: A randomized controlled trial. *American Journal of Clinical Nutrition, 92*, 733–740.
Tong, L. T., Zhong, K., Liu, L., Qiu, J., et al. (2014). Effects of dietary wheat bran arabinoxylans on cholesterol metabolism of hypercholesterolemic hamsters. *Carbohydrate Polymers, 112*, 1–5.
Tramontin, N. D. S., Luciano, T. F., de Marques, O., et al. (2020). Ginger and avocado as nutraceuticals for obesity and its comorbidities. *Phytotherapy Research, 34*, 1282–1290.
United Nations General Assembly. (2002). International Year of Rice, 2004, https://press.un.org/en/2002/ga10112.doc.htm.
Unuofin, J. O., Masuku, N. P., Paimo, O. K., et al. (2021). Ginger from farmyard to town: Nutritional and pharmacological applications. *Frontiers in Pharmacology, 12*, 779352.
Upadhyay, R. K. (2015). Emerging risk biomarkers in cardiovascular diseases and disorders. *Journal of Lipids, 2015*, pp. 1–50.
Venkatesh Babu, K. C. (2006). *Cardiospermum halicacabum* suppresses the production of TNF-α and NO by human peripheral blood mononuclear cells. *African Journal of Biomedical Research, 9*, 95–99.
Venukumar, M. R., & Lathan, M. R. (2002). Antioxidant activity of *Curculigo orchioides* in CCl4 induced hepatopathy in rats. *Indian Journal of Clinical Biochemistry, 17*, 80–87.
Vigila, A. G., & Baskaran, X. (2008). Immunomodulatory effect of coconut protein on cyclophosphamide-induced immune-suppressed Swiss albino mice. *Ethnobotanical Leaflets, 12*, 1206–1212.

Vijayakumar, R. S., & Nalini, N. (2006). Efficacy of piperine, an alkaloidal constituent from *Piper nigrum* on erythrocyte antioxidant status in high-fat diet and antithyroid drug-induced hyperlipidemic rats. *Cell Biochemistry and Function, 24*, 491–498.

Wagner, H., Geyer, B., Kiso, Y., Hikino, H., & Rao, G. S. (1986). Coumestans as the main active principles of the liver drugs *Eclipta alba* and *Wedelia calendulacea. Planta Medica, 52*, 370–374.

Wang, P., Song, Q. Y., Zhou, Z., Li, X. C., Han, Y. Z., & Wang, W. L. (1990). Hypocholesteremic effect of mung bean (*Phaseolus radiates* L.) in animal tests. *Journal of Shenyang Pharmaceutical University, 7*, 42–44.

Wang, Y., Yu, H., Zhang, X., et al. (2017). Evaluation of daily ginger consumption for the prevention of chronic diseases in adults: A cross-sectional study. *Nutrition, 36*, 79–84.

Woodward, P. W. (1996). *Garlic and Friends: The History, Growth and Use of Edible Alliums*, pp.1–248. Hyland House, Melbourne, Australia.

Wu, Q., Fu, D. X., Hou, A. J., Lei, G. Q., & Liu, Z. J. (2005). Antioxidative phenols and phenolic glycosides from *Curculigo orchioides. Chemical and Pharmaceutical Bulletin, 53*, 1065–1067.

Yadav, U. C., & Baquer, N. Z. (2014). Pharmacological effects of *Trigonella foenum*-graecum L. in health and disease. *Pharmaceutical Biology, 52*(2), 243–254.

Yamagata, K., & Yamori, Y. (2020). Inhibition of endothelial dysfunction by dietary flavonoids and preventive effects against cardiovascular disease. *Journal of Cardiovascular Pharmacology, 75*(1), 1–9.

Yao, Y., Chen, F., Wang, M., Wang, J., & Ren, G. (2008). Antidiabetic activity of mung bean extracts in diabetic KK-Ay 403 mice. *Journal of Agricultural and Food Chemistry, 56*, 8869–8873.

Yao, Y., Cheng, X. Z., & Ren, G. X. (2011). Contents of D-chiro-inositol, vitexin, and isovitexin in various varieties of mung bean and its products. *Agricultural Sciences in China, 10*, 1710–1715.

Yao, Y., Hao, L., Shi, Z., Wang, L., Cheng, X., Wang, S., & Ren, G. (2014a). Mung bean decreases plasma cholesterol by up-regulation of cyp7a1. *Plant Foods for Human Nutrition, 69*, 134–136.

Yao, Y., Zhu, Y., & Ren, G. (2014b). Mung bean protein increases plasma cholesterol by up-regulation of hepatic HMG-CoA reductase, and cyp7a1 in mRNA levels. *Journal of Food and Nutrition Research, 2*, 770–775.

Yarnell, E., & Abascal, K. (2011). Nigella sativa: holy herb of the Middle East. *Alternative and Complementary Therapies, 17*, 99–10.

Yeh, Y. Y., & Liu, L. (2001). Cholesterol-lowering effect of garlic extracts and organosulfur compounds: Human and animal studies. *Journal of Nutrition, 131*(3s), 989S–993S.

Yeh, Y. Y., & Yeh, S. M. (1994). Garlic reduces plasma lipids by inhibiting hepatic cholesterol and triacylglycerol synthesis. *Lipids, 29*(3), 189–193.

Yoganarasimhan, S. N. (2000). *Medicinal Plants of India, Vol. 2.* Tamil Nadu, Bangalore, Cyber Media, 169.

Yu, L., Zhou, K., & Parry, J. W. (2005). Inhibitory effect of wheat bran extracts on human LDL oxidation and free radicals. *LWT – Food Science and Technology, 38*, 463–470.

Zadorozhna, M., & Mangieri, D. (2021). Mechanisms of chemopreventive and therapeutic properties of ginger extracts in cancer. *International Journal of Molecular Sciences, 22*(12), 6599.

PART IV

MARINE-DERIVED NUTRIENTS IN CARDIOVASCULAR

CHAPTER 15

ROLE OF SPIRULINA SUPPLEMENTATION AND OTHER NUTRACEUTICALS IN CARDIOVASCULAR DISEASE

CHARU GUPTA

Amity Institute of Herbal Research and Studies, Amity University, Noida, Uttar Pradesh, India

ABSTRACT

Cardiovascular disease (CVD) stands amongst the most shared health-related and fiscal problems globally. Nutritional aspects are significant contributors to cardiovascular danger, either directly or through their special effects on other cardiovascular risk factors including high blood pressure, unhealthy levels of one or more types of lipids in the blood (dyslipidemia), and high blood sugar (diabetes mellitus). Nutrient-rich foods (nutraceuticals) are usual nourishing combinations that have been shown to be effective in preventive therapy or the management of disease. Numerous diets and dietary supplements have been shown to protect against the development of CVD. *Spirulina* (*Arthrospira platensis*) is an extremely nourishing nutraceutical that has not been adequately studied. This establishes functional foods with potential beneficial effects on numerous cardiovascular diseases, but there is little convincing medical evidence to support their use in human patients. Similarly, other nutrients/phytochemicals such as vitamins, allicin in garlic, polyphenols and flavonoids in fruits and vegetables, resveratrol in grapes, lycopene in tomatoes, and phytosterols in nuts and oils have been shown to be effective against cardiovascular diseases and to reduce blood pressure.

Antioxidants as Nutraceuticals. Nayan A. Gujarathi, Raj K. Keservani, Rajesh K. Kesharwani, Bhushan R. Rane, Yogeeta Sameer Goyal (Eds.)

However, further studies are needed to confirm their effects, especially regarding their supplementation in humans. The present study provides an overview of the existing data on the health-promoting functions of *Spirulina* and other nutraceuticals against cardiovascular disease, which are major health concerns in advanced nations.

15.1 INTRODUCTION

These days, many illnesses and biological and morphological sicknesses, such as diabetes, obesity, oxidative stress, cancer, cardiovascular diseases, and severe infections, are growing and disturbing the value of the lifecycle. Several of these ailments are associated with the abuse of synthetic additives, unbalanced diets, radiation exposure, and powerful viruses (Saadi et al., 2015). In agreement with the World Health Organization (WHO), India accounts for one-fifth of these demises globally, particularly in the newer populace. The consequences of Global Burden of Disease learning portray an age-standardized CVD death ratio of 272 per 1,00,000 populations in India, which is far greater than the worldwide average of 235. CVDs attack Indians in an era prior to the Western populace (Prabhakaran et al., 2016). Coronary Artery Disease (CAD), a kind of atherosclerotic cardiovascular sickness, is the greatest sort of CVD, which is described by endothelial dysfunction resulting from atherosclerosis and blocking by oily commemoration. High blood pressure is the most common and insidious type of modifiable CVD. Individuals at high risk for CVD can improve their health outcomes by exercising, quitting smoking, managing high blood pressure and blood sugar levels, and making dietary changes. Dietary modifications have always been a key preventive measure for individuals with chronic cardiovascular conditions. Therefore, in recent years, the search for new medications and functional food products capable of combating worsening conditions has increased. Natural sources are particularly appealing in this context. Some of these new products are small molecules, such as peptides, that have beneficial bioactivities and unique properties for the development of new medications, nutraceuticals, and functional food ingredients (Nooshkam & Madadlou, 2016).

Nutraceuticals are nutrients or food by-products that deliver remedial and well-being benefits, including the prevention, control, and/or cure of an illness. They comprise a class of isolated nutrients, concentrated dietary supplements, herbal products, and processed nutrients, such as mueslis, broths, and drinks. Most nutraceuticals still require support from large clinical trials to prove their effectiveness and safety profile before their use in cardiovascular prevention and management (Keservani et al., 2010a, b, 2017, 2020; Zuchi et al., 2010).

There are numerous modifications in broadcasting regimen and decrease of lifeblood heaviness mend cardiac fitness, though the connotation between diverse nutrients and high blood pressure is uncertain. This is primarily because there are numerous biases and inadequate, unpredictable studies, which have led to incomplete rules for the safe and active use of nutrients for controlling high blood pressure when related to a regular diet plot and management with medicine (Turner & Spatz, 2016).

Blue-green algae (BGA) are amongst the greatest primeval living systems on earth and have been used as foodstuff or medication by people for periods. BGA comprises many bioactive constituents, such as phycocyanin, carotenoids, γ-linolenic acid, fibers, and plant sterols, which can encourage ideal fitness in people. Studies have confirmed that numerous BGA types or their active mechanisms have plasma total cholesterol and triglyceride-lowering effects due to their inflection of abdominal cholesterol absorption and hepatic lipogenic gene expression. BGA can also decrease inflammation by impeding the nuclear factor κB activity, subsequently decreasing the construction of pro-inflammatory cytokines. Moreover, BGA hinders lipid peroxidation and has free radical scavenging activity, which can be favorable for defense against oxidative stress. The above-mentioned benefits of BGA can contribute to the prevention of metabolic and inflammatory diseases (Ku et al., 2013). Spirulina, the cyanobacterium known for its high protein content and healing properties, has been investigated as a potential source of bioactive peptides. Several biologically active peptides derived from *Spirulina* are being studied for their ability to provide specific health benefits, such as antimicrobial, anti-allergic, antihypertensive, antitumor, and immunomodulatory properties. It is possible that peptide fractions derived from *Spirulina* could be valuable as nutraceutical components in foods and pharmaceuticals.

This analysis aims to examine the effects and mechanisms of action of many of the most well-known nutrients used in the treatment of heart diseases, particularly hypertension.

15.2 SPIRULINA

Aquatic creatures are noble bases of fundamentally varied bioactive complexes with several biological activities (Fan et al., 2014). *Spirulina*, essentially categorized as a cyanobacterium, is an exceptional basis of bioactive constituents. *Spirulina* is a type of blue-green algae that is developed into two types – *maxima* and *plantensis* and has been broadly cultured due to its immense nutritive importance, comprising 70% vitamins such as B12 and pro-vitamin A), minerals, and fatty acids. This organism possesses a rich protein variety covering all vital amino acids and has a whole nutritive conformation in vitamins, carotenoids, fatty acids, and minerals (Becker, 2007). *Spirulina* is presently promoted as an addition for its high antioxidant, anti-inflammatory, immunomodulatory, and hyperlipidemia activities. Research shows spirulina's manifold activities have proven favorable in the avoidance and cure of heart-related disorders (Lietstianty et al., 2019). Numerous biotic activities, such as antimicrobial, anti-allergic, antihypertensive, and immunomodulatory activities, have been reported for *Spirulina* peptides (Gibbs et al., 2004 Bioactive peptides are usually small and composed of 2–20 amino acids and have small molecular weight, i.e., less than 6,000 Da (Fan et al., 2014). With this magnitude, bioactive peptides have an additional chance of surpassing the intestinal barrier and exhibiting potent bioactivities (Sayari et al., 2016). Furthermore, in addition to its nutritive significance, *Spirulina* has also been applied in beauty uses (Kim et al., 2008) and has been considered a generally recognized safe ingredient since 2003 by the FDA. It is imperative to assess the existing investigations on peptides resulting from *Spirulina* in order to recognize designs, styles, and research gaps.

15.2.1 SPIRULINA AS BASIS OF UNIQUE BIOACTIVE PEPTIDES AND PHYTO-CONSTITUENTS

Spirulina is a prokaryotic cyanobacteria derivative of *Arthrospira.* It is a viable and environmentally approachable organic material of herbal origin that is equally extremely nourishing and cost-effective. Spirulina contains several biopolymers, fats, crystals, steroids, vital elements, and polypeptides (Wu et al., 2016). It comprises numerous useful complexes that are responsible for its antioxidant, anti-inflammatory, and immune-stimulant potential, such as flavones, flavanones, polyphenols, and sugars (Keservani & Sharma, 2014; Park et al., 2018). The three essential active ingredients are phycocyanin, phycocyanobilin, and β-carotene. Spirulina does not possess any lethal or teratogenic properties. Phycocyanin belongs to a set of so-called phycobiliproteins that are a type of polypeptides existing in cyanobacteria and capture sunlight to be delivered to the chlorophylls in photosynthesis.

The structure is similar to bilirubin, imparting its antioxidant properties (Romay et al., 2003). Bilirubin is a pigment originating in bile from the breakdown of hemoglobin that gives bile its orange-yellow color (Sticova & Jirsa, 2013). Bilirubin possesses effective antioxidant activity by inhibiting oxidation and radical by-products in plasma proteins and aromatic amino acid residues.

Phycocyanobilin is an isomer of mesobiliverdin (Liwa et al., 2017). It is currently used as a food coloring and is present in the chromophore of phycocyanin. It binds to the non-protein part of phycocyanin with its exposed tetrapyrrole ring. Structurally, phycocyanin is similar to biliverdin, which is another pigment but for bile instead. Due to the structural similarities, phycocyanobilin can be converted by biliverdin reductase into its reduced form, phycocyanobilin. Phycocyanobilin also exhibits strong antioxidant and anti-inflammatory properties by actively inhibiting the NADPH oxidase enzyme, which is a major cause of oxidative stress (Sosnowska et al., 2017).

15.2.2 RESEARCH EVIDENCE OF SPIRULINA AGAINST CVD

There are several scientific studies that support the role of *Spirulina* against cardiovascular disease. Vo & Kim (2013) assessed the defensive effects of similar *Spirulina* peptides against initial atherosclerosis by responses prompted by histamine in endothelial cells. Histamine prompts endothelial cells to yield pro-inflammatory cytokines (IL-6), monocyte chemoattractant protein-1 (MCP-1), adherent and adhesion molecules, and vascular cells, but this stimulates the growth and advancement of atherosclerosis. The consequences of this study advocated that *Spirulina* peptides are operational in overpowering (downregulation) inflammatory responses (Aneiros & Garateix, 2004).

The antihypertensive outcome of the five bioactive peptides derived from *S. platensis* was measured by spectrophotometric ACE inhibition (angiotensin I-converting enzyme) using a modification of Cheung & Cushman (1973) assay. The antihypertensive effects were also assessed in spontaneously hypertensive rats (SHRs) (Suetsuna & Chen, 2001).

In yet another study, the ACE inhibition activity of *Spirulina* peptides was measured by a fluorescence resonance energy transfer assay. In order to measure the hypertensive effect *in vivo*, spontaneously hypertensive rats were used: the oral delivery of the isolated peptide from *S. platensis* displayed a decrease in the systolic and diastolic BP in the animals (Lu et al., 2011).

Furthermore, in a recent study, a unique strong decameric peptide of *Spirulina platensis* was found to decrease blood pressure intensities through a PI3K/AKT/eNOS-dependent mechanism. Considered a superfood of the future, *Spirulina platensis* has been extensively used because of its beneficial effects on the control of cardiovascular diseases. It is well known that hypertensive patients have a dysfunction in the endothelium-dependent NO system; this significantly contributes to increased vascular resistance in the basal situation and to impairment of endothelium-dependent vasorelaxation. Furthermore, oral administration of SP6 to SHRs, one of the best animal models replicating the modifications seen in human hypertension, increased serum nitrite levels and exerted an antihypertensive effect. It was revealed that GID-spirulina directly induces vasodilation of mouse resistance arteries, an important vascular region involved in blood pressure regulation. This action was dependent on the stimulation of eNOS in the endothelium as vascular effects were completely abolished in eNOS-knockout mice. Additionally, effects observed *in vivo* on the inhibition of eNOS clearly demonstrated that the hemodynamic action of SP6 is mediated by NO. Therefore, the antihypertensive effect observed in hypertensive rats could be attributed to SP6 directly promoting the improvement of endothelial function and, thus, vasorelaxation (Carrizzo et al., 2018).

15.2.3 PATHOPHYSIOLOGY/MOLECULAR TARGETS OF SPIRULINA

Preclinical trials established an important escalation in lipase activity after consumption of spirulina, which is hypothesized to aid with hyperlipidemia (Deng & Chow, 2010). However, the precise mechanism of action for this outcome is still being explored. One stimulating assumption is that spirulina fixes fatty acid metabolites and bile acids, initiating an upsurge in fecal elimination of these end-products. This, in principle, will decrease blood lipid points. Few studies also advocate that the lipid things may have originated from C-phycocyanin actions (Romay et al., 2003).

One potential target that spirulina aims for is Tumor Necrosis Factor-alpha (TNF-α), which is a well-known pro-inflammatory signaling protein. In addition, the C-phycocyanin aims and obstructs the nuclear factor-kappa B (NF-kB) pathway in specific (Ku et al., 2013). As a result, TNF-α along with other inflammatory signaling proteins (IL-6, IL-8, IL-1B) are not produced, thereby stumbling the concluding phases that result in inflammation. Innate immunity was not exaggerated as research disclosed that the macrophage activity was unobstructed with spirulina ingesting. This contributes to spirulina its inflammation-reducing effects.

C-phycocyanin also displays antioxidant activity. It hinders enzymes such as cyclooxygenase-2 (COX-2) and inducible nitric oxide synthase (iNOS) in a similar manner to resveratrol (O'Leary et al., 2004). COX-2 is a pro-oxidant enzyme that aids in increasing the oxygenation of arachidonic acid, which results in natural reactions including pain, unease, and tenderness. Nevertheless, by hindering COX-2, spirulina aids in decreasing these natural reactions.

15.2.4 SPIRULINA IN CVD WITH MEDICAL DATA

The cardio-protective effect of *Spirulina* can be maintained with numerous clinical trials that discover its prospective in the management of CVD. Cardiovascular protective capacities of *Spirulina* are inspected through their efficacy as a healing involvement of hypertension, hyperlipidemia, and metabolic disease in medical tribunals.

In Caucasian persons with a history of heart attack and heart, illness detected through angiography, everyday oral administration of 10 milligrams of resveratrol for three months revealed an upsurge in flow-mediated vasodilation and left ventricular diastolic function while dropping LDL-cholesterol levels related to placebo (Agarwal et al., 2013).

In additional research by Martinez-Samano et al., an experimental medical test with about 16 persons, with eight in each treatment group, was performed to determine if *Spirulina maxima* have valuable blood pressure regulating properties in persons affected with systemic arterial hypertension (SAH) who are undergoing angiotensin-converting enzyme inhibitor (ACE-I) treatment (Martínez-Sámano et al., 2018). According to the outcomes, systolic blood pressure variations were only statistically noteworthy after 12 weeks post-start, and no statistically noteworthy consequences were perceived in the diastolic blood pressure changes. The only inference established was the add-on properties of spirulina for the treatment of SAH. No additional reports were made on the prevention or single treatment for SAH with spirulina.

In an initial report, 36 patients (between 18 and 65 years old) were cured with 4.5 g/day by an oral dose of *Spirulina maxima* for 6 weeks without any alterations to food or routine (Torres-Duran et al., 2007). Statistically important changes were seen in lipids, high-density lipoprotein-cholesterol, and low-density lipoprotein-cholesterol levels. The researchers established that *Spirulina maxima* had beneficial effects on hyperlipidemia; however, *Spirulina maxima* presented secondary effects on high-density lipoprotein-cholesterol and total cholesterol levels. Nevertheless, the researchers considered *Spirulina maxima* as a treatment for patients with a milder case of hypercholesterolemia. Clinical implications were not conclusive for *Spirulina maxima* for lowering properties, as it is not as harmful as pharmacological options.

Instead, New Zealand White bunnies were used in studying *Spirulina platensis* in preventing atherosclerosis (Cheong et al., 2010). After 8 weeks of treatment with spirulina, the atherosclerotic lesions induced by the hypercholesterolemic diets were significantly reduced. The findings indicated *Spirulina platensis* has protective effects against atherosclerosis and can be used as a functional food to improve and recover from elevated cholesterol levels and prevent atherosclerosis from developing. It remains uncertain the exact mechanism of how Spirulina platensis is capable of such effects.

15.2.5 DIETARY SUGGESTIONS FOR SPIRULINA

Research varied about dosage for spirulina. Numerous medical readings used between 1 and 4 grams per day; however, some even went as high as 10 g. Maximum over-the-counter supplementations endorse 500 mg to 4 g per bottle tag (Joventino et al., 2012; Miczke et al., 2016). The arrays of suggested dosages vary amongst the usage of the nutraceutical (blood sugar control vs. high blood pressure); therefore, it is suggested to refer to a pharmacist or primary care physician to strive for all suitable choices. There are no studies reported to date about the dosages of Spirulina and the frequency of its intake in a day (Cho et al., 2017). The safety and efficiency of both supplements have been tested only for the adult population, while the efficacy of both supplements if consumed consecutively has not been researched sufficiently (Jeong et al., 2019).

15.3 OTHER PHYTOCHEMICALS AS NUTRACEUTICALS FOR CARDIOVASCULAR DISEASES (CVD)

15.3.1 POLYPHENOLS

Polyphenols are phytochemicals with extensive circulation in foodstuffs from vegetal sources. They are present in fruits, vegetables, cereals, and legumes. Furthermore, they are present in beverages formed from plant harvests such as infusions, brunets, wine, and cocoa. Polyphenols are physically varied, and more than 8,000 types have been recognized. These comprise flavonoids, phenolic acids, stilbenes, and lignans (Pandey & Rizvi, 2009). Polyphenols present in grapes and grape derivatives, cocoa, and tea are of importance in the avoidance of CVD. Phenolic compounds are present in grapes and contain anthocyanins, flavonols, stilbenes, and phenolic acids (Spácil et al., 2008). Resveratrol (3,5,4′-trihydroxy-trans-stilbene) is the most widely considered grape-derived stilbene existing mostly in grapes. However, resveratrol is collected in a range of types containing various types of berries such as cranberries, blueberries, groundnuts, and Japanese knotweed (Burns et al., 2002).

The end product of cocoa beans (*Theobroma cacao*) is broadly used in cocoa and chocolate. A range of polyphenols has been identified in cocoa and its derivatives. These include catechins, flavonol glycosides, anthocyanins, and procyanidins. Coco-containing foods offer a larger quantity of flavonoids per serving than other beverages such as red wine and tea (Andres-Lacueva et al., 2008).

Polyphenols found in tea include catechins, theaflavins, tannins, and flavonoids. The degree of fermentation of tea leaves affects the biochemical composition. Green tea, which is minimally fermented, contains more catechins such as epigallocatechin gallate, epicatechin-3-gallate, and epicatechin, whereas the more extensively fermented black tea is rich in flavonoids and thearubigins (Khan & Mukhtar, 2007).

Grape seeds and red wine residues are also known to contain high levels of polyphenols, and the beneficial health properties have been attributed to the consumption of these compounds. Grape and wine polyphenols may help reduce high blood pressure and have beneficial effects on heart diseases by preventing platelet aggregation, reducing oxidative stress, and decreasing LDL oxidation (Rasines-Perea & Teissedre, 2017).

Although the exact mechanism of action of grape seeds is not fully understood, their extract possesses antioxidant activity, which reduces the amount of reactive oxygen species (ROS). Due to this capability, grape seed oil has potential in cardiovascular diseases as high ROS levels are often observed in cardiovascular and metabolic diseases (Carlson et al., 2008).

It has been recommended that ingesting flavonoid-rich fruits and vegetables may lower blood pressure (Wang et al., 2014a). Research on the effect of polyphenols on blood pressure is very varied and has included a wide variety of polyphenol-containing foods, including grapes, berries, cocoa products, tea, etc. Some studies have established a significant beneficial effect of grape-derived polyphenols on blood pressure (Draijer et al., 2015). On the other hand, there are numerous studies that did not find such a correlation (Vaisman & Niv, 2015). The contradictory results may result from the heterogeneity of study design, polyphenol source, and population characteristics. A recently published randomized controlled trial showed that grape seed extract significantly decreased systolic blood pressure by 5.6% and diastolic blood pressure by 4.7% after 6 weeks of supplementation in subjects with slightly elevated blood pressure. Furthermore, the blood pressure-lowering properties seemed to be dependent on baseline blood pressure, with the greatest decrease observed in subjects with higher baseline blood pressure (Park et al., 2016).

The effects of resveratrol on blood pressure have also been considered. A meta-analysis of 6 randomized controlled trials (247 subjects) seemed to display a dose-response association; only higher dosages ($\geq$150 mg day^{-1}) of resveratrol considerably decreased systolic blood pressure, while there were no noteworthy effects on diastolic blood pressure (Liu et al., 2015). An additional meta-analysis, which comprised data from 10 randomized controlled trials, showed that resveratrol supplementation did not affect systolic and diastolic blood pressure (Sahebkar et al., 2015). Alterations in the reference line blood pressure of participants in the study may be responsible for some of these differences.

Cocoa flavanols are the most considered polyphenols in the clinical setting. A meta-analysis of 20 randomized controlled trials comprising fit participants showed that ingesting polyphenol-rich cocoa products was related to a decrease in blood pressure (Ried et al., 2012). Another meta-analysis of 42 randomized controlled trials showed that chocolate or cocoa was associated with reduced diastolic blood pressure and mean arterial pressure (Hooper et al., 2012). Very new medical research also endorses that cocoa flavanols have a beneficial effect on blood pressure in patients with type 2 diabetes and hypertension and elderly subjects. Additionally, new research has shown similar outcomes after consuming cocoa in healthy individuals. This was associated with a dose-dependent improvement in flow-mediated dilation, reduced endothelin-1, and pulse wave velocity. These results allow for further investigation into the potential uses of cocoa in preventing CVD (Grassi et al., 2015).

Similarly, other research found no evidence of an effect of regular consumption of dark chocolate (49 g/day) on blood pressure or arterial stiffness in patients with mild hypertension (Koli et al., 2015). The Flaviola Health Study found that cocoa flavanol intake (450 mg) for 1 month reduced systolic and diastolic blood pressure by 4.4 and 3.9 mmHg, pulse wave velocity by 0.4 m/s, and helped improve endothelial function in a healthy, primary prevention population, indicating potential benefits of cocoa in maintaining cardiovascular health (Sansone et al., 2015).

Studies on tea polyphenols have also demonstrated blood pressure-lowering properties (Khalesi et al., 2014). A meta-analysis of 10 trials (834 participants) established that a statistically significant decrease in systolic blood pressure was associated with diastolic blood pressure with black or green tea consumption (Yarmolinsky et al., 2015). Additionally, a recent meta-analysis on the effects of green tea consumption on the risk of CVD showed that consuming green tea is linked to a reduced risk of myocardial infarction and stroke (Pang et al., 2016).

Numerous medical studies have confirmed the antihypertensive effects of pomegranate juice. A recent meta-analysis, which included the results of eight randomized controlled trials investigating the effects of pomegranate juice on blood pressure, demonstrated that consuming this polyphenol-rich juice significantly reduced both systolic and diastolic blood pressure. Furthermore, the lipid-lowering, antioxidant, and anti-atherosclerotic properties of pomegranate juice have been described, making it a promising candidate as a nutraceutical with the potential to improve cardiovascular health (Sahebkar et al., 2017).

The commercially available nutraceutical product, Armolipid Plus, comprising red yeast rice, policosanol, berberine, folic acid, astaxanthin, and coenzyme Q10, is well-tolerated and helps in decreasing average 24-hour systolic and 24-hour pulse pressure in patients with high blood pressure and high cholesterol levels at low cardiovascular risk (Mazza et al., 2015).

In overweight adult patients with a history of angina pectoris on continuous treatment for at least one month, oral administration of 20 mg of resveratrol daily for two months significantly reduced Hs-CRP and NT-proBNP levels compared to calcium fructoborate, with a favorable change in the lipid profile (Militaru et al., 2013).

In adult patients with type 2 diabetes who have been on anti-diabetic treatment for at least 6 months and are not taking any antioxidant supplements, consistent oral intake of 1,000 mg of resveratrol for a total of 45 days significantly reduced systolic blood pressure and LDL while increasing HDL compared to placebo. Another study with similar inclusion criteria for participants involved consistent oral intake of 250 mg of resveratrol. After three months, the group taking resveratrol showed a decrease in systolic blood pressure, LDL, and total cholesterol levels compared to the placebo group (Movahed et al., 2013).

15.3.2 FLAVONOIDS

Flavonoids are a cluster of phenolic compounds occurring certainly in fruits, vegetables, tea, and red wine that have cardio-protective and anti-carcinogenic properties (Hollman & Katan, 1999). Numerous studies have confirmed that the properties of flavonoids, including antioxidants and anti-inflammatory effects, may also improve vascular functions. Additionally, a higher consumption of tea and flavonoids may contribute to the primary prevention of ischemic heart disease, as well as a reduced risk of coronary heart disease death, supported by a high dietary intake of flavonols (Alves et al., 2019).

Although many studies have established the heart-protective properties of flavonoids, there is also contradictory data. The link between flavonoid consumption and overall heart disease is not definitive, while studies have not ruled out the possibility that flavonoids may have a protective effect on traditional heart disease. The consistent and regular intake of flavonoids in foods has been shown to help improve endothelial function in patients with coronary artery disease, after heart surgery, or in healthy volunteers with or without heart risk factors (Zuchi et al., 2010).

Research readings in both fauna and hominids advocate that vascular activities of flavonoids happen, no less than in part, as a result of the augmented action of nitric oxide synthase. Soy isoflavones are one subtype of flavonoids, and so a food rich in these constituents will help to stimulate vasodilation, improve endothelial function, and decrease blood pressure in animal models (Mahn et al., 2005). In human trials, the outcomes have not been reliable due to investigational bias (Alves et al., 2019).

To authenticate and confirm the effect of food with soy isoflavones on blood pressure, a meta-analysis of randomized controlled trials was conducted, which established that soy-derived isoflavones lower blood pressure in individuals with high blood pressure but not in normotensive individuals; further studies are required to confirm these effects.

A systematic review with meta-analysis determined that the dietary consumption of subclasses of flavonoids is inversely related to heart risks; thus, the consumption of flavonoids reduces the risk of heart diseases. However, this meta-analysis was based on observational studies, and among other biases, potential errors in nutritional grouping and the presence of unmeasured/uncontrolled risk factors were identified (Wang et al., 2014b).

An additional flavonoid-rich diet includes extra virgin olive oil. The consumption of extra virgin olive oil is inversely related to an increase in systolic and diastolic blood pressure (Psaltopoulou et al., 2004). Blood pressure decrease was also observed in hypertensive twins treated with an olive leaf extract, at 500–1000 mg per day for 1–8 weeks, compared to a placebo (Perrinjaquet-Moccetti et al., 2008). Extra virgin olive oil may also help to lower blood pressure by increasing plasma nitrite/nitrate levels and reducing serum asymmetric dimethylarginine (ADMA) (Moreno-Luna et al., 2012), which is an endogenously formed molecule capable of inhibiting the synthesis of nitric oxide (NO) (Blackwell, 2010). Taken together, a diet rich in polyphenols may contribute to improving endothelial function by enhancing the bioavailability of NO.

A significant amount of evidence exists regarding the effects of flavonoids on the cardiovascular system; however, further research is needed to better understand the appropriate dietary intake that leads to significant and safe results. Additionally, it is important to determine which specific subclasses of flavonoids contribute to these specific outcomes and in which exact disease conditions they would be beneficial.

15.3.3 VITAMINS

High blood pressure subjects generally possess the ability for greater production of ROS and hence present a larger than normal response to oxidative stress. Furthermore, the endogenous and exogenous antioxidant defense mechanisms of the high blood pressure subjects are lessened. Numerous epidemiological studies have revealed that antioxidant deficiency has been involved in high blood pressure and heart diseases. Considering the epidemiological progress of chronic non-communicable diseases, such as diabetes mellitus and cardiovascular trials, a variety of foods rich in antioxidants should be consumed, for instance, ascorbic acid (vitamin C) (Zimmermann & Kirsten, 2016).

The significance of vitamin consumption is well known and acknowledged, but the extent to which vitamins affect fitness and heart function remains poorly explained. Several studies have shown that decreased levels of plasma vitamin E were linked to an increased risk of heart disease. Similarly, lower plasma levels of ascorbic acid or vitamin C were associated with a higher risk of cardiovascular events (Song et al., 2009).

Greater blood amounts of ascorbic acid in persons are linked with lower blood pressure. This finding was confirmed in a 17-week controlled-diet depletion-repletion of vitamin C study. The research established an opposite connection between plasma ascorbate levels, and diastolic and systolic blood pressures, and admitted that the effectiveness of berries and spuds in dropping blood pressure may be associated with ascorbic acid. In addition, the vitamin C level in tissues may be significant in upholding low blood pressure. Therefore, in order to get a positive result on blood pressure, it is suggested to uphold a serum level of plasma vitamin C of at least 100 mc mol/L. Still, further long-term intervention research should be made to approve this result (Sherman et al., 2000). Ascorbic acid reduces the binding attraction of the AT1 receptor, without altering its greatest binding capability and without changing the binding capability of the AT2 receptor for angiotensin II. These outcomes offer a mechanical explanation for the stated blood pressure-dropping result of ascorbic acid, as most of the angiotensin II-induced heart properties, such as vascular contraction, aldosterone secretion, heart cell growth, and propagation, among others, are facilitated by AT1 receptor. This decrease of the AT1 receptor attraction for angiotensin II seems to happen by disturbing the ATR1 disulfide bridges (Leclerc et al., 2008).

A randomized, double-blind, placebo-controlled factorial trial of vitamin E and vitamin C performed between 1997 and 2007, which included 14641 US male physicians, who were primarily aged 50 years or older and included 754 men with established cardiovascular disease at randomization, was conducted to address studies suggesting that vitamin E or vitamin C may reduce the risk of cardiovascular disease. According to the authors of this study, few long-term trials have evaluated men at initially low risk of cardiovascular disease, and no previous trial in men has examined vitamin C alone in the prevention of cardiovascular disease. Therefore, in this large, long-term study of male doctors, neither vitamin E nor vitamin C supplementation reduced the risk of major cardiovascular events. In middle-aged and older men, these findings provided no support for the use of these supplements in the prevention of cardiovascular disease (Sesso et al., 2008). Furthermore, additional research has shown that vitamin C properties lead to a decrease in blood pressure with an increase in nitric oxide, resulting in an improvement in endothelial function and arterial compliance (Song et al., 2009).

The opposite association between plasma vitamin C and blood pressure was perceived in the reduction of growth in blood pressure in fit young adults which decreased the danger of related vascular trials. This reading advocates that ascorbic acid may be a significant reason in blood pressure regulation, even among fit fresh grown-ups (Block et al., 2008). Consumption of foodstuffs rich in vitamin C appears to be vital for dropping blood pressure, yet more long-term readings in patients of diverse age groups, as well as altered phases of high blood pressure, need to be made to explain which patients may benefit.

Another significant vitamin involved in heart disease is vitamin D. This vitamin is manufactured in the skin after exposure to sunlight, is also consumed with food, and is found in a few types of fish (Lu et al., 2007). Upon ingestion of vitamin D, it is quickly changed to 25-hydroxyvitamin D (25 (OH) D), its chief circulating form (Judd & Tangpricha, 2009). Vitamin D has a conventional part in regulating calcium-phosphate homeostasis and also performs to apply immune-regulatory and anti-inflammatory effects (Dozio et al., 2015).

Several study results display that there is a firm relation between vitamin D shortage and heart ailments (Zuchi et al., 2010; Martins et al., 2007) and define opposite relations amid little sun contact, i.e., low serum 25(OH)D intensities, and bigger dangers of stroke, myocardial infarction, peripheral vascular diseases, and heart failure (Young et al., 2011). Also, complete and indigenous vitamin D shortage in coronary artery disease (CAD) patients is related to an enlarged stimulation of inflammatory pathways at the epicardial adipose tissue (EAT) level (Dozio et al., 2015), and its accumulation may lead to cardiac illness. By means of a visceral model, Gunasekar & co-workers (2018) proved that vitamin D shortage upsurges both the employment of M1 macrophages, as the pro-inflammatory expression of adipokine in the EAT; furthermore, it recommends that vitamin D supplementation drops inflammatory processes and encourages anti-inflammatory responses in EAT. The shortage of vitamin D is also proficient for stimulating the growth of atherosclerosis and lessening plasma HDL-C levels, and the supplementation of vitamin D3 in the food can significantly upsurge the level of HDL-C, as macrophage pro-inflammatory polarization, in the visceral model, resulting in defense against the expansion of atherosclerosis (Yin et al., 2015).

Vitamin D plays a vital part in cardiovascular protective effects over several mechanisms, such as inflection of vascular nature, ruling of blood pressure, vascular smooth muscle cell purposes, and maintenance of fit endothelium. The anti-inflammatory and anti-mitotic actions of vitamin D assist in the balance of the endothelium, which validates, at least in part, its heart properties (Venkatesh & Nair, 2014).

Although numerous facts recommend a connection between vitamin D shortage and endothelial malfunction and heart diseases, there is no proof of randomized clinical trials demonstrating that heart diseases are prevented with vitamin D supplementation. There remains a great necessity to know the mechanism of cardiovascular role to improve treatment goals, as well as potential medical interventions to enhance the evidence of the effectiveness of vitamin D repletion on heart health (Wimalawansa, 2018).

15.3.4 LYCOPENE

Lycopene is a carotenoid originating in red fruits and vegetables like papayas, tomatoes, red peppers, watermelons, and others. Tomatoes are well known for their culinary usefulness and also contribute to nutritional value. Nearly 90% of all carotenoids that make up the tomato are composed of lycopene, although it also includes carotene, folate, phenolic compounds, and vitamins C and E. The association between tomato and lycopene consumption with a reduction in heart disease risk has sparked research interest (Burton-Freeman & Sesso, 2014).

As per the Framingham Heart Offspring Study, there is a strong inverse relationship between the consumption of lycopene and the occurrence of myocardial infarction, coronary insufficiency, and angina pectoris. Furthermore, plasma levels of lycopene in high blood pressure, acute myocardial infarction, stroke, and atherosclerosis were described as low (Jacques et al., 2013).

Among the major carotenoids, lycopene is the most potent antioxidant and plays a significant role in preventing heart disease in individuals. The bioavailability of lycopene in supplements has not been widely studied and remains an important area for research (Burton-Freeman & Sesso, 2014).

An experimental study using Wistar rats showed that tomato consumption for three months led to changes in miRNA expression and reduced oxidative stress. Additionally, these changes appear to be responsible for the reduction in the cross-sectional area of left ventricular myocytes and the improvement in diastolic function. However, more studies need to be conducted to explore the potential roles of tomato and lycopene in the prevention and treatment of heart diseases and to elucidate their beneficial effects on the heart, which have not yet been fully understood (Pereira et al., 2015).

It is well known that endothelial function reflects vascular health. Additionally, endothelial dysfunction is involved in the development of atherosclerosis and coronary or peripheral vascular endothelial dysfunction appears to be an independent predictor of cardiovascular events. Increased oxidative stress may be a causative mechanism for endothelial dysfunction (Bonetti et al., 2003).

Remarkably, in a randomized, double-blind, placebo-controlled study, the eight-week intake of lycopene has been shown to promote positive effects on oxidative stress biomarkers (by reducing oxidative DNA damage and increasing plasma superoxide dismutase enzymatic activity). Additionally, its antioxidant effects may play a significant role in improving endothelial function, which is closely linked to inflammatory markers. These findings demonstrate the beneficial impact of regular lycopene consumption (Kim et al., 2011).

Several studies have associated tomatoes and lycopene with lower rates of heart disease (Wolak & Paran, 2013), but the effectiveness of lycopene supplementation remains uncertain and unconfirmed. While lycopene accounts for nearly 90% of the total carotenoids present in tomatoes, the other bioactive compounds present should also be taken into consideration to fully understand its beneficial effects. Furthermore, until further research clarifies and confirms the significant benefits of lycopene supplementation in humans, it is recommended to consume fruits and vegetables rich in natural carotenoids (Chen et al., 2013).

15.3.5 ALLICIN

Garlic (*Allium sativum*) is a significant and momentous part of both food and therapeutic reputation. Garlic commonly contains water (65%), carbohydrates such as fructose, sulfur compounds, proteins, and free amino acids. The sulfur compounds existing or produced from garlic are accountable for their nutritional and remedial roles. It has lately been proven that part of the heart benefits of garlic is due to the existence of allicin, also known as diallelic thiosulfinate (Bradley et al., 2016).

When the cellular arrangement of garlic is injured, C-S-lyase (alliinase) acts on alliin (S-allyl-L-Cysteine sulfoxide) and alters it into allicin (allylthiosulfinate). Allicin makes numerous sulfides through non-enzymatic responses such as diallyl sulfide (DAS), diallyl disulfide (DADS), diallyl trisulfide (DATS), or methyl allyl trisulfide (MATS) (Ariga & Seki, 2006), all of which perform with strong antiplatelet activity. Garlic ingestion can prevent platelet aggregation in human persons, and enhance vasodilatation, and fibrinolysis in animals and individuals (Benavides et al., 2007).

A significant and well-studied garlic research is ripened garlic extract (AGE), which is made by keeping cut fresh garlic in an ethanol solution for 20 months, at room temperature. More studies are essential to evaluate the benefits of this garlic preparation. In order to further examine the properties of AGE, future studies could investigate a variety of antioxidants over a longer period and examine a diabetic group with higher heart risk, such as those with established heart disease (Atkin et al., 2016).

In addition to AGE, there are other formulations of garlic, such as garlic oil, garlic powder, and garlic extract that may present beneficial effects (Bradley et al., 2016). In addition to the aforementioned heart properties, garlic was found to act in a heart-protective manner as induced by H_2S, which can be produced by the metabolism of garlic components in human red blood cells, protecting the heart through antioxidant, anti-apoptotic, and anti-inflammatory actions. H_2S is a cardio-protective gas-signaling molecule and is responsible for a wide range of biological functions in mammalian tissues. It is crucial for cell function and protects the cell against apoptosis, oxidative stress, and necrosis (Donnarumma et al., 2017).

Treatment with exogenous hydrogen sulfide is likely and may be accountable for a significant decrease in the extent of myocardial infarction in rats with murine abrasions and ischemia/reperfusion. A large body of technical work supports the suggestion that garlic ingestion yields a notable heart-protective effect. Clinical trials to assess the effects of garlic on heart ailments were very promising after positive *in vitro* findings indicating the beneficial effects of garlic, although some of these clinical trials were inconclusive (Sivarajah et al., 2009).

A systematic review and meta-analysis concluded that in patients with high blood pressure treated with garlic-only preparations, there was a reduction in blood pressure in individuals with hypertension compared to placebo. A recent study found that garlic has the potential to lower blood pressure in hypertensive individuals, similar to conventional blood pressure medications such as angiotensin-converting enzyme inhibitors, angiotensin II receptor blockers, calcium-channel blockers, and diuretics (Ried & Fakler, 2014).

Furthermore, the supplementation with garlic formulations may be a balancing cure selection for hypertension, and research should be made to explore whether garlic possesses any anti-hypertensive outcome in pre-hypertensive persons, which would be vital in the stoppage of hypertension progress. In a meta-analysis, garlic presented significant outcomes in subjects with minor hypertension; still, inadequate proof was collected to endorse clinical therapy, and regardless of readings of blood pressure, garlic preparations have been indecisive (Pittler & Ernst, 2007). Further trials should be done to elucidate the aids of garlic in the management of high blood pressure and heart ailments. Even though there is solid proof of its useful cardiac effects, carefulness should be applied in the use of garlic due to the arrival of gastrointestinal glitches (Hoshino et al., 2001). Taken together, the clinical trials recommend that garlic plays a part in averting or deferring heart illness, but more readings are required to check its properties.

15.3.6 PHYTO-STEROLS/STANOLS

Phytosterols, phytostanols, and their esters are a collection of steroid alcohols and esters that are naturally present in plants as a non-saponifiable fraction of plant oils. Humans cannot manufacture phytosterols, which comprise plant sterols and stanols, and all plant sterols and stanols in human form thus originate from the diet (De Jong et al., 2008). They are known to have several bioactive potentials with likely consequences for human well-being. Their abilities to lower blood lipid levels, as well as their other valuable health properties, have been recognized for several ages. Since high cholesterol levels are a major predisposing factor leading to cardiovascular diseases, it is imperative to mention these phytochemicals. Phytosterols are sterols that are fundamentally similar to cholesterol but are produced in plants and phytoplankton. Typically, they are characterized by alkyl groups (methyl or ethyl group) at C-24, by side-chain double bonds at C-22 or C-24, and/or by nuclear double bonds at locations other than C-5 (Morreau et al., 2002). The proposed mechanisms for the cholesterol-lowering properties of phytosterols have centered on pathways in which cholesterol is directly involved, including intestinal solubility, interaction with digestive enzymes, protein-mediated absorption, and gene regulation.

The precise mode by which phytosterols lessen serum cholesterol levels is not entirely clear, but numerous concepts have been proposed. One of them suggests that cholesterol in the abdomen, previously slightly soluble, is precipitated into a non-absorbable form in the presence of supplementary phytosterols and stanols (Rozner & Garti, 2006). An alternative concept is based on the fact that phytosterols when ingested, may decrease cholesterol absorption by competing with cholesterol for integration into the bile salts micelles or uptake of cholesterol by enterocytes through the Niemann-Pick C1 Like 1 (NPC1L1) transporter. Furthermore, phytosterols may improve cholesterol elimination back into the intestinal lumen through the ATP-binding cassette G5 (ABCG5) and G8 (ABCG8) transporters. Phytosterols could also prevent the esterification of free cholesterol into cholesterol esters, thus preventing its accumulation in the chylomicrons. As a result of reducing cholesterol absorption by phytosterols, the amount of cholesterol produced may rise, but the net effect is a decrease in LDL-cholesterol levels (Jones & AbuMweis, 2009).

Cholesterol assimilation is a very significant biological mechanism that controls cholesterol metabolism. A new study has shown that the effectiveness of phytosterols is not influenced by dietary cholesterol intake in hypercholesterolemic individuals (Kassis et al., 2008). Both dietary cholesterol and recirculating biliary cholesterol mixed in the intestine are moderately absorbed. Failure to reabsorb intestinal cholesterol is the standard means of eliminating cholesterol from the body.

In distinction to the sound calculated properties of sterols and stanols upon fats, there is a comparative scarcity of data connecting to their effects on blood pressure. Research has failed to validate the antihypertensive effects of sterols/stanols regardless of lasting treatment for a year or more. One recent study, which aimed to analyze the result of plant stanol esters on artery rigidity and endothelial function in adults similarly found no effect on measured blood pressure (Gylling et al., 2013). Although the findings are partial, there seem to be no anti-hypertensive properties of these compounds in individuals, nor is there any sign of adverse effects on blood pressure.

Some studies show that phytosterols compete with and displace cholesterol from bile salt/phospholipid micelles, the form from which cholesterol absorption occurs. In one trial, nine adults were fed a meal containing 500 mg of cholesterol and 1 g beta-sitosterol or 2 g beta-sitosterol oleate (Mattson et al., 1982). The addition of beta-sitosterol resulted in a 42% decrease in cholesterol absorption, and the beta-sitosterol oleate caused a 33% reduction compared to the control group, resulting in a subsequent decrease in plasma cholesterol. Sitosterol has an increased affinity for biliary micelles associated with cholesterol, so sitosterol acceptance by micelles is actively favored.

Phytosterols are present at broadly variable concentrations in the fat-soluble fractions of kernels, root shoots, twigs, foliage, and flowers. They are components of both edible and decorative plants, comprising herbs, shrubs, and trees (Clifton, 2002). As natural components of the human diet, phytosterols naturally occur in all food items of plant origin, mainly oils, pulses, and dried fruits. Their amount is highest in edible oils, seeds, and nuts. The total contents are variable and differ from nearly 8 g/kg in corn oil to 0.5 g/kg in palm oil, with transitional levels being found in commonly used oils. Tall oil comprises a greater quantity of plant stanols than vegetable oils do (Anon, 2005).

Phytosterol ingestion of 2 grams per day is suggested by the National Cholesterol Education Program to decrease LDL cholesterol (Racette et al., 2010). However, the effects of diverse types of phytosterol ingestion on cholesterol metabolism are uncertain. In a study, the effects of three phytosterol ingestions on whole-body cholesterol metabolism were assessed. In this placebo-controlled, crossover trial, 18 adults were given a phytosterol-lacking diet (50 mg phytosterols/2000 kcal) plus beverages enhanced with 0, 400, or 2,000 mg phytosterols/day for 4 weeks each, in random order. All mealtimes were arranged in a metabolic kitchenette; feasts and banquets on weekdays were held on-site. The principal results included fecal cholesterol elimination and abdominal cholesterol immersion calculated with stable-isotope tracers, as well as serum lipoprotein levels. It was finally established that nutritive phytosterols in moderate and high amounts favorably modify whole-body cholesterol absorption in a quantity-dependent manner. A reasonable phytosterol intake (459 mg/day) can be achieved through a healthy diet without supplementation. This experiment was registered at clinicaltrials.gov as NCT00860054 (Racette et al., 2010).

15.4 CONCLUSION

The control, prevention, and treatment of heart conditions such as high blood pressure are based on lifestyle, genetic factors, and physical activity. Nutritional supplements represent a promising approach for controlling and preventing high blood pressure and other heart conditions. Nutraceuticals function not only directly through antioxidant or anti-inflammatory properties but also indirectly, by affecting various functional pathways. A variety of nutraceuticals discussed in the previous chapter, such as oils, extracts, fruits, vegetables, and plant extracts, have shown beneficial effects on heart health through compounds like phenolic complexes or polyphenols, lycopene, and flavonoids. Dietary functional components and their consumption can improve blood pressure management and should be considered as part of a well-planned approach aimed at preventing hypertension, given their benefits and low cost.

Studies have confirmed the varied effects of numerous phytochemicals to have beneficial effects in many diverse illness states with numerous molecular targets. They help prevent inflammation, oxidation reactions, and also diabetic effects. It is probable to predict that many phytochemicals will play a greater role in the prevention and management of CVD after additional studies. Preclinical data on spirulina, resveratrol, and other phytochemicals have been debatable, with both hopeful and dispiriting results. This variation may be attributed to different research strategies and populations, as well as low absorption and bioavailability.

Nevertheless, more widespread and procedural studies are necessary if we want to exploit the apparent astounding benefits of these phytochemicals. Studies should focus on using these phytochemicals and their equivalents as support complexes for the potential development of synthetic medicines. Similarly, not enough work has been done to show spirulina's full potential. Although some experimental studies exist, their small population size along with limited data delegitimizes their results. As mentioned earlier, research using Spirulina had varying amounts of Spirulina, making it difficult to determine the appropriate quantity to achieve clinically significant outcomes. Therefore, spirulina has been suggested to be taken in different quantities for different indications. Through additional data-based studies, clinicians will feel more comfortable recommending Spirulina to confirm the safety and efficacy of the patient. Further investigation on human and animal models is required to fully explore these potential targets.

CONFLICT OF INTEREST

The author endorses that this editorial content has not at all a conflict of interest.

ACKNOWLEDGMENTS

The authors are grateful to DST-SERB, New Delhi, India for the financial support. The writers are also thankful to Dr. Ashok K. Chauhan, Founder President, Dr. Atul Chauhan, Chancellor, and Prof. Dr. Balvinder Shukla, Vice-Chancellor, Amity University–UP, Noida, for their motivation and research facilities.

ETHICAL ISSUES

There is none to be declared.

KEYWORDS

- **blue-green algae**
- **cardiovascular disease**
- **coronary artery disease**
- **hypertension**
- **nutraceuticals**
- **phytosterols**
- **polyphenols**
- **reactive oxygen species**
- **spirulina**
- **systemic arterial hypertension**
- **World Health Organization**

REFERENCES

Agarwal, B., Campen, M. J., Channell, M. M., Wherry, S. J., Varamini, B., & Davis, J. G. (2013). Resveratrol for primary prevention of atherosclerosis: Clinical trial evidence for improved gene expression in vascular endothelium. *International Journal of Cardiology, 166*, 246–248. https://doi.org/10.1016/j.ijcard.2012.03.155.

Alves, Q. L., Camargo, S. B., & Silva, D. F. (2019). Role of nutraceuticals in the prevention and treatment of hypertension and cardiovascular diseases. *Journal of Hypertension Management, 5*, 037.

Andres-Lacueva, C., Monagas, M., Khan, N., et al. (2008). Flavanol and flavanol contents of cocoa powder products: Influence of the manufacturing process. *Journal of Agricultural and Food Chemistry, 56*, 3111–3117. https://doi.org/10.1021/jf073398f.

Aneiros, A., & Garateix, A. (2004). Bioactive peptides from marine sources: Pharmacological properties and isolation procedures. *Journal of Chromatography B: Analytical Technologies in the Biomedical and Life Sciences, 803*(1), 41–53. https://doi.org/10.1016/j.jchromb.2003.10.011.

Anon. (2005). Phytosterol esters (Plant sterols and stenols esters). https://www.ifst.org/resources/information-statements/phytosterol-esters-plant-sterol-and-stanol-esters.

Ariga, T., & Seki, T. (2006). Antithrombotic and anticancer effects of garlic-derived sulfur compounds: A review. *BioFactors, 26*, 93–103. https://doi.org/10.1002/biof.5520260109.

Atkin, M., Laight, D., & Cummings, M. H. (2016). The effects of garlic extract upon endothelial function, vascular inflammation, oxidative stress and insulin resistance in adults with type 2 diabetes at high cardiovascular risk: A pilot double blind randomized placebo-controlled trial. *Journal of Diabetes and its Complications, 30*, 723–727. https://doi.org/10.1016/j.jdiacomp.2016.02.002.

Becker, E. (2007). Micro-algae as a source of protein. *Biotechnology Advances, 25*, 207–210. https://doi.org/10.1016/j.biotechadv.2006.11.002.

Benavides, G. A., Squadrito, G. L., Mills, R. W., Patel, H. D., Isbell, T. S., et al. (2007). Hydrogen sulphide mediates the vaso-activity of garlic. *Proceedings of the National Academy of Sciences of the United States of America, 104*, 17977–17982. https://doi.org/10.1073/pnas.0705710104.

Blackwell, S. (2010). The biochemistry, measurement and current clinical significance of asymmetric dimethylarginine. *Annals of Clinical Biochemistry, 47*, 17–28. https://doi.org/10.1258/acb.2009.009194.

Block, G., Jensen, C. D., Norkus, E. P., Hudes, M., & Crawford, P. B. (2008). Vitamin C in plasma is inversely related to blood pressure and change in blood pressure during the previous year in young Black and White women. *Nutrition Journal, 7*, 35. https://doi.org/10.1186/1475-2891-7-35.

Bonetti, P. O., Lerman, L. O., & Lerman, A. (2003). Endothelial dysfunction: A marker of atherosclerotic risk. *Arteriosclerosis, Thrombosis, and Vascular Biology, 23*, 168–175. https://doi.org/10.1161/01.ATV.0000051384.43104.FC.

Bradley, J. M., Organ, C. L., & Lefer, D. J. (2016). Garlic-derived organic polysulfides and myocardial protection. *Journal of Nutrition, 146*(2), 403S–409S. https://doi.org/10.3945/jn.114.202333.

Burns, J., Yokota, T., Ashihara, H., et al. (2002). Plant foods and herbal sources of resveratrol. *Journal of Agricultural and Food Chemistry, 50*, 3337–3340. https://doi.org/10.1021/jf0112973.

Burton-Freeman, B., & Sesso, H. D. (2014). Whole food versus supplement: Comparing the clinical evidence of tomato intake and lycopene supplementation on cardiovascular risk factors. *Advances in Nutrition, 5*, 457–485. https://doi.org/10.3945/an.113.005518.

Carlson, S., Peng, N., Prasain, J. K., & Wyss, J. M. (2008). Effects of botanical dietary supplements on cardiovascular, cognitive, and metabolic function in males and females. *Gender Medicine, 5*, S76–S90. https://doi.org/10.1016/j.genm.2008.03.004.

Carrizzo, A., Conte, G. M., Sommella, E., Damato, A., Ambrosio, M., Sala, M., Scala, M. C., Aquino, R. P., et al. (2019). Novel potent decameric peptide of Spirulina platensis reduces blood pressure levels through a PI3K/AKT/eNOS-Dependent Mechanism. *Hypertension, 73*, 449–457. https://doi.org/10.1161/HYPERTENSIONAHA.118.11952.

Chen, J., Song, Y., & Zhang, L. (2013). Effect of lycopene supplementation on oxidative stress: An exploratory systematic review and meta-analysis of randomized controlled trials. *Journal of Medicinal Food, 16*, 361–374. https://doi.org/10.1089/jmf.2012.2664.

Cheong, S., Kim, M., Sok, D., Hwang, S., Kim, J., et al. (2010). Spirulina prevents atherosclerosis by reducing hypercholesterolemia in rabbits fed a high-cholesterol diet. *Journal of Nutrition Science and Vitaminology, 56*, 34–40. https://doi.org/10.3177/jnsv.56.34.

Cheung, H. S., & Cushman, D. W. (1973). Inhibition of homogeneous angiotensin converting enzyme of rabbit lung by synthetic venom peptides of Bothrops jararaca. *Biochimica et Biophysica Acta, 293*(2), 451–463. https://doi.org/10.1016/0005-2795(73)90224-2.

Cho, S., Namkoong, K., Shin, M., Park, J., Yang, E., et al. (2017). Cardiovascular protective effects and clinical applications of resveratrol. *Journal of Medicinal Food, 20*, 323–334. https://doi.org/10.1089/jmf.2016.0053.

Clifton, P. (2002). Plant sterol and stanols-comparison and contrasts. Sterol versus stanols in cholesterol lowering: Is there a difference? *Atherosclerosis, 3*, 5–9.

De Jong, A., Plat, J., Bast, A., Godschalk, R. W., Basu, S., & Mensink, R. P. (2008). Effects of plant sterol and stanol ester consumption on lipid metabolism, antioxidant status and markers of oxidative stress, endothelial function and low-grade inflammation in patients on current statin treatment. *European Journal of Clinical Nutrition, 62*, 263–273. https://doi.org/10.1038/sj.ejcn.1602717.

Deng, R., & Chow, T. J. (2010). Hypolipidemic, antioxidant, and anti-inflammatory activities of microalgae Spirulina. *Cardiovascular Therapy, 28*, e33–e45. https://doi.org/10.3109/17530250903455971.

Donnarumma, E., Trivedi, R. K., & Lefer, D. J. (2017). Protective actions of H2S in acute myocardial infarction and heart failure. *Comprehensive Physiology, 7*, 583–602. https://doi.org/10.1002/cphy.c160017.

Dozio, E., Briganti, S., Vianello, E., Dogliotti, G., Barassi, A., et al. (2015). Epicardial adipose tissue inflammation is related to vitamin D deficiency in patients affected by coronary artery disease. *Nutrition, Metabolism, and Cardiovascular Diseases, 25*, 267–273. https://doi.org/10.1016/j.numecd.2014.11.003.

Draijer, R., de Graaf, Y., Slettenaar, M., et al. (2015). Consumption of a polyphenol-rich grape-wine extract lowers ambulatory blood pressure in mildly hypertensive subjects. *Nutrients, 7*, 3138–3153. https://doi.org/10.3390/nu7053138.

Fan, X., Bai, L., Zhu, L., Yang, L., & Zhang, X. (2014). Marine algae-derived bioactive peptides for human nutrition and health. *Journal of Agricultural and Food Chemistry, 62*, 9211–9222. https://doi.org/10.1021/jf5025073.

Gibbs, B. F., Zougman, A., Masse, R., & Mulligan, C. (2004). Production and characterization of bioactive peptides from soy hydrolysate and soy-fermented food. *Food Research International, 37*, 123–131. https://doi.org/10.1016/j.foodres.2003.10.009.

Grassi, D., Desideri, G., Necozione, S., et al. (2015). Cocoa consumption dose-dependently improves flow-mediated dilation and arterial stiffness decreasing blood pressure in healthy individuals. *Journal of Hypertension, 33*, 294–303. https://doi.org/10.1097/HJH.0000000000000418.

Gunasekar, P., Swier, V. J., Fleegel, J. P., Boosani, C. S., Radwan, M. M., et al. (2018). Vitamin D and macrophage polarization in epicardial adipose tissue of atherosclerotic swine. *PLoS One, 13*(4), e0197479. https://doi.org/10.1371/journal.pone.0197479.

Gylling, H., Halonen, J., Lindholm, H., et al. (2013). The effects of plant stanol ester consumption on arterial stiffness and endothelial function in adults: A randomized controlled clinical trial. *BMC Cardiovascular Disorders, 13*, 50. https://doi.org/10.1186/1471-2261-13-50.

Hollman, P. H., & Katan, M. B. (1999). Dietary flavonoids: Intake, health effects and bioavailability. *Food and Chemical Toxicology, 37*, 937–942. https://doi.org/10.1016/S0278-6915(99)00081-6.

Hooper, L., Kay, C., Abdelhamid, A., et al. (2012). Effects of chocolate, cocoa, and flavan-3-ols on cardiovascular health: A systematic review and meta-analysis of randomized trials. *American Journal of Clinical Nutrition, 95*, 740–751. https://doi.org/10.3945/ajcn.111.023457.

Hoshino, T., Kashimoto, N., & Kasuga, S. (2001). Effects of garlic preparations on the gastrointestinal mucosa. *The Journal of Nutrition, 131*(3), 1109S–1113S. https://doi.org/10.1093/jn/131.3.1109S.

Jacques, P. F., Lyass, A., Massaro, J. M., Vasan, R. S., & D'Agostino, R. B., Sr. (2013). Relationship of lycopene intake and consumption of tomato products to incident CVD. *The British Journal of Nutrition, 110*, 545–551. https://doi.org/10.1017/S0007114512005455.

Jeong, S. J., Choi, J. W., Lee, M. K., Choi, Y. H., & Nam, T. J. (2019). Spirulina crude protein promotes the migration and proliferation in IEC-6 cells by activating EGFR/MAPK signaling pathway. *Marine Drugs, 17*(4), 205. https://doi.org/10.3390/md17040205.

Jones, P. J. H., & AbuMweis, S. S. (2009). Phytosterols as functional food ingredients: Linkages to cardiovascular disease and cancer. *Current Opinion in Clinical Nutrition and Metabolic Care, 12*, 147–151. https://doi.org/10.1097/MCO.0b013e328322f94b.

Joventino, I. P., Alves, H. G. R., Neves, N. C., Pinheiro-Joventino, F., Leal, L. K. A. M., et al. (2012). The microalga Spirulina platensis presents anti-inflammatory action as well as hypoglycemic and hypolipidemic properties in diabetic rats. *Journal of Complementary and Integrative Medicine, 9*, 1–5. Retrieved from: https://bit.ly/3c0EqEp (accessed on 12 June 2024).

Judd, S. E., & Tangpricha, V. (2009). Vitamin D deficiency and risk for cardiovascular disease. *The American Journal of the Medical Sciences, 338*, 40–44. https://doi.org/10.1097/MAJ.0b013e3181aaee91.

Kassis, A. N., Vanstone, C. A., AbuMweis, S. S., & Jones, P. J. H. (2008). Efficacy of plant sterol is not influenced by dietary cholesterol intake in hypercholesterolemic individuals. *Metabolism, 57*, 339–346. https://doi.org/10.1016/j.metabol.2007.10.004.

Keservani, R. K., Kesharwani, R. K., Sharma, A. K., Vyas, N., & Chadoker, A. (2010). Nutritional supplements: An overview. *International Journal of Current Pharmaceutical Review and Research, 1*(1), 59–75.

Khalesi, S., Sun, J., Buys, N., et al. (2014). Green tea catechins and blood pressure: A systematic review and meta-analysis of randomized controlled trials. *European Journal of Nutrition, 53*, 1299–1311.

Khan, N., & Mukhtar, H. (2007). Tea polyphenols for health promotion. *Life Sciences, 81*, 519–533.

Kim, J. Y., Paik, J. K., Kim, O. Y., Park, H. W., Lee, J. H., et al. (2011). Effects of lycopene supplementation on oxidative stress and markers of endothelial function in healthy men. *Atherosclerosis, 215*, 189–195.

Kim, S. K., Ravichandran, Y. D., Khan, S. B., & Kim, Y. T. (2008). Prospective of the cosmeceuticals derived from marine organisms. *Biotechnology and Bioprocess Engineering, 13*(5), 511–523.

Koli, R., Köhler, K., Tonteri, E., et al. (2015). Dark chocolate and reduced snack consumption in mildly hypertensive adults: An intervention study. *Nutrition Journal, 14*, 84.

Ku, C. S., Pham, T. X., Park, Y., Kim, B., Shin, M. S., et al. (2013). Edible blue-green algae reduce the production of pro-inflammatory cytokines by inhibiting NF-κB pathway in macrophages and splenocytes. *Biochimica et Biophysica Acta (BBA) – General Subjects, 1830*, 2981–2988.

Leclerc, P. C., Proulx, C. D., Arguin, G., Bélanger, S., Gobeil, Jr F., et al. (2008). Ascorbic acid decreases the binding affinity of the AT1 receptor for angiotensin II. *American Journal of Hypertension, 21*, 67–71.

Lietstianty, D., Rodianawati, I., Arfah, R. A., Assa, A., Patimah, et al. (2019). Nutritional analysis of Spirulina sp. to promote as superfood candidate. *Materials Science and Engineering,* 1–6.

Liu, Y., Ma, W., Zhang, P., et al. (2015). Effect of resveratrol on blood pressure: A meta-analysis of randomized controlled trials. *Clinical Nutrition, 34*, 27–34.

Liwa, A. C., Barton, E. N., & Cole, W. C. (2017). Bioactive plant molecules, sources and mechanism of action in the treatment of cardiovascular disease. In *Pharmacognosy: Fundamentals, Applied Strategies* (pp. 315–336).

Lu, J., Yang, Y., Lin, C., Di-Feng, R., Mu-Yi, C., Jian-Zhong, W., & Masaru, T. (2011). In vivo antihypertensive effect of Val-Glu-Pro in spontaneously hypertensive rats. *ShengwuHuaxue Yu ShengwuWuliJinzhan, 38*(4), 353–360.

Lu, Z., Chen, T. C., Zhang, A., Persons, K. S., Kohn, N., et al. (2007). An evaluation of the vitamin D3 content in fish: Is the vitamin D content adequate to satisfy the dietary requirement for vitamin D? *Journal of Steroid Biochemistry and Molecular Biology, 103*, 642–644.

Mahn, K., Borrás, C., Knock, G. A., Taylor, P., Khan, I. Y., et al. (2005). Dietary soy isoflavone induced increases in antioxidant and eNOS gene expression led to improved endothelial function and reduced blood pressure in vivo. *The FASEB Journal, 19*, 1755–1757.

Martínez-Sámano, J., Torres-Montes de Oca, A., Luqueño-Bocardo, O. I., Torres-Durán, P. V., & Juárez-Oropeza, M. A. (2018). Spirulina maxima decrease endothelial damage and oxidative stress indicators in patients with systemic arterial hypertension: Results from exploratory controlled clinical trial. *Marine Drugs, 16*, 496.

Martins, D., Wolf, M., Pan, D., Zadshir, A., Tareen, N., et al. (2007). Prevalence of cardiovascular risk factors and the serum levels of 25-hydroxyvitamin D in the United States: Data from the third national health and nutrition examination survey. *Archives of Internal Medicine, 167*, 1159–1165.

Mattson, F. H., Grundy, S. M., & Crouse, J. R. (1982). Optimizing the effect of plant sterols on cholesterol absorption in man. *The American Journal of Clinical Nutrition, 35*, 697–700.

Mazza, A., Lenti, S., Schiavon, L., et al. (2015). Nutraceuticals for serum lipid and blood pressure control in hypertensive and hypercholesterolemic subjects at low cardiovascular risk. *Advances in Therapy, 32*, 680–690.

Miczke, A., Szulińska, M., Hansdorfer-Korzon, R., Kręgielska-Narożna, M., Suliburska, J., et al. (2016). Effects of Spirulina consumption on body weight, blood pressure, and endothelial function in overweight hypertensive Caucasians: A double-blind, placebo-controlled, randomized trial. *European Review for Medical and Pharmacological Sciences, 20*, 150–156.

Militaru, C., Donoiu, I., Craciun, A., Scorei, I. D., Bulearca, A. M., et al. (2013). Oral resveratrol and calcium fructoborate supplementation in subjects with stable angina pectoris: Effects on lipid profiles, inflammation markers, and quality of life. *Nutrition, 29*, 178–183.

Moreno-Luna, R., Muñoz-Hernandez, R., Miranda, M. L., Costa, A. F., Jimenez-Jimenez, L., et al. (2012). Olive oil polyphenols decrease blood pressure and improve endothelial function in young women with mild hypertension. *American Journal of Hypertension, 25*, 1299–1304.

Morreau, R. A., Whitaker, B. D., & Hicks, K. B. (2002). Phytosterols, phytostanols, and their conjugates in foods: Structural diversity, quantitative analysis, and health-promoting uses. *Progress in Lipid Research, 41*, 457–500.

Movahed, A., Nabipour, I., Lieben Louis, X., Thandapilly, S. J., Yu, L., et al. (2013). Antihyperglycemic effects of short-term resveratrol supplementation in type 2 diabetic patients. *Evidence-Based Complementary and Alternative Medicine, 2013*, 11.

Nooshkam, M., & Madadlou, A. (2016). Maillard conjugation of lactulose with potentially bioactive peptides. *Food Chemistry, 192*, 831–836.

O'Leary, K. A., de Pascual-Teresa, S., Needs, P. W., Bao, Y. P., O'Brien, N. M., et al. (2004). Effect of flavonoids and vitamin E on cyclooxygenase-2 (COX-2) transcription. *Mutation Research, 551*, 245–254.

Pandey, K. B., & Rizvi, S. I. (2009). Plant polyphenols as dietary antioxidants in human health and disease. *Oxidative Medicine and Cellular Longevity, 2*, 270–278.

Pang, J., Zhang, Z., Zheng, T., et al. (2016). Green tea consumption and risk of cardiovascular and ischemic related diseases: A meta-analysis. *International Journal of Cardiology, 202*, 967–974.

Park, E., Edirisinghe, I., Choy, Y. Y., et al. (2016). Effects of grape seed extract beverage on blood pressure and metabolic indices in individuals with pre-hypertension: A randomized, double-blinded, two-arm, parallel, placebo-controlled trial. *British Journal of Nutrition, 115*, 226–238.

Park, W. S., Kim, H. J., Li, M., Lim, D. H., Kim, J., et al. (2018). Two classes of pigments, carotenoids and C-phycocyanin, in Spirulina powder and their antioxidant activities. *Molecules, 23*, 2065.

Pereira, B. L., Arruda, F. C., Reis, P. P., Felix, T. F., Santos, P. P., et al. (2015). Tomato (*Lycopersicon esculentum*) supplementation induces changes in cardiac miRNA expression, reduces oxidative stress and left ventricular mass, and improves diastolic function. *Nutrients, 7*, 9640–9649.

Perrinjaquet-Moccetti, T., Busjahn, A., Schmidlin, C., Schmidt, A., Bradl, B., et al. (2008). Food supplementation with an olive (*Olea europaea* L.) leaf extract reduces blood pressure in borderline hypertensive monozygotic twins. *Phytotherapy Research, 22*, 1239–1242.

Pittler, M. H., & Ernst, E. (2007). Clinical effectiveness of garlic (*Allium sativum*). *Molecular Nutrition & Food Research, 51*, 1382–1385.

Prabhakaran, D., Jeemon, P., & Roy, A. (2016). Cardiovascular diseases in India. *Circulation, 133*, 1605–1620.

Psaltopoulou, T., Naska, A., Orfanos, P., Trichopoulos, D., Mountokalakis, T., et al. (2004). Olive oil, the Mediterranean diet, and arterial blood pressure: The Greek European Prospective Investigation into Cancer and Nutrition (EPIC) study. *The American Journal of Clinical Nutrition, 80*, 1012–1018.

Racette, S. B., Lin, X., Lefevre, M., Spearie, C. A., Most, M. M., Ma, L., & Ostlund, R. E. (2010). Dose effects of dietary phytosterols on cholesterol metabolism: A controlled feeding study. *The American Journal of Clinical Nutrition, 91*(1), 32–38.

Rasines-Perea, Z., & Teissedre, P. L. (2017). Grape polyphenols' effects in human cardiovascular diseases and diabetes. *Molecules, 22*(1), Article 68.

Ried, K., & Fakler, P. (2014). Potential of garlic (*Allium sativum*) in lowering high blood pressure: Mechanisms of action and clinical relevance. *Integrated Blood Pressure Control, 7*, 71.

Ried, K., Sullivan, T. R., Fakler, P., et al. (2012). Effect of cocoa on blood pressure. *Cochrane Database of Systematic Reviews, 2012*(8), CD008893.

Romay, C., González, R., Ledón, N., Remirez, D., & Rimbau, V. (2003). C-phycocyanin: A biliprotein with antioxidant, anti-inflammatory and neuroprotective effects. *Current Protein & Peptide Science, 4*, 207–216.

Rozner, S., & Garti, N. (2006). The activity and absorption relationship of cholesterol and phytosterols. *Colloids and Surfaces A: Physicochemical and Engineering Aspects, 282*, 435–456.

Saadi, S., Saari, N., Anwar, F., Abdul Hamid, A., & Ghazali, H. M. (2015). Recent advances in food biopeptides: Production, biological functionalities and therapeutic applications. *Biotechnology Advances, 33*(1), 80–116.

Sahebkar, A., Ferri, C., Giorgini, P., et al. (2017). Effects of pomegranate juice on blood pressure: A systematic review and meta-analysis of randomized controlled trials. *Pharmacological Research, 115*, 149–161.

Sahebkar, A., Serban, C., Ursoniu, S., et al. (2015). Lipid and Blood Pressure Meta-Analysis Collaboration Group. Lack of efficacy of resveratrol on C-reactive protein and selected cardiovascular risk factors–Results from a systematic review and meta-analysis of randomized controlled trials. *International Journal of Cardiology, 189*, 47–55.

Sansone, R., Rodriguez-Mateos, A., Heuel, J., et al. (2015). Cocoa flavanol intake improves endothelial function and Framingham Risk Score in healthy men and women: A randomized, controlled, double-masked trial: The Faviola Health Study. *British Journal of Nutrition, 114*, 1246–1255.

Sayari, N., Sila, A., Haddar, A., Balti, R., Ellouz-Chaabouni, S., & Bougatef, A. (2016). Valorization of smooth hound (*Mustelus mustelus*) waste biomass through recovery of functional, antioxidative and antihypertensive bioactive peptides. *Environmental Science and Pollution Research, 23*, 366–376.

Sesso, H. D., Buring, J. E., Christen, W. G., Kurth, T., Belanger, C., et al. (2008). Vitamins E and C in the prevention of cardiovascular disease in men: The Physicians' Health Study II randomized controlled trial. *JAMA, 300*, 2123–2133.

Sherman, D. L., Keaney, J. F., Biegelsen, E. S., Duffy, S. J., Coffman, J. D., et al. (2000). Pharmacological concentrations of ascorbic acid are required for the beneficial effect on endothelial vasomotor function in hypertension. *Hypertension, 35*, 936–941.

Sivarajah, A., Collino, M., Yasin, M., Benetti, E., Gallicchio, M., et al. (2009). Anti-apoptotic and anti-inflammatory effects of hydrogen sulfide in a rat model of regional myocardial I/R. *Shock, 31*(3), 267–274.

Song, Y., Cook, N. R., Albert, C. M., Van Denburgh, M., & Manson, J. E. (2009). Effects of vitamins C and E and β-carotene on the risk of type 2 diabetes in women at high risk of cardiovascular disease: A randomized controlled trial. *The American Journal of Clinical Nutrition, 90*(2), 429–437.

Sosnowska, B., Penson, P., & Banach, M. (2017). The role of nutraceuticals in the prevention of cardiovascular disease. *Cardiovascular Diagnosis and Therapy, 7*(Suppl 1), S21–S31.

Spácil, Z., Nováková, L., & Solich, P. (2008). Analysis of phenolic compounds by high performance liquid chromatography and ultra-performance liquid chromatography. *Talanta, 76*(1), 189–199.

Sticová, E., & Jirsa, M. (2013). New insights in bilirubin metabolism and their clinical implications. *World Journal of Gastroenterology, 19*(40), 6398–6407.

Suetsuna, K., & Chen, J. R. (2001). Identification of antihypertensive peptides from peptic digest of two microalgae, Chlorella vulgaris and Spirulina platensis. *Marine Biotechnology (New York, N.Y.), 3*(4), 305–309.

Torres-Durán, P. V., Ferreira-Hermosillo, A., & Juárez-Oropeza, M. A. (2007). Antihyperlipemic and antihypertensive effects of Spirulina maxima in an open sample of Mexican population: A preliminary report. *Lipids in Health and Disease, 6*, 33.

Turner, J. M., & Spatz, E. S. (2016). Nutritional supplements for the treatment of hypertension: A practical guide for clinicians. *Current Cardiology Reports, 18*(12), 126.

Vaisman, N., & Niv, E. (2015). Daily consumption of red grape cell powder in a dietary dose improves cardiovascular parameters: A double blind, placebo-controlled, randomized study. *International Journal of Food Sciences and Nutrition, 66*(3), 342–349.

Venkatesh, B., & Nair, P. (2014). Hypovitaminosis D and morbidity in critical illness: Is there proof beyond reasonable doubt? *Critical Care, 18*(2), 138.

Vo, T.-S., & Kim, S.-K. (2013). Down-regulation of histamine-induced endothelial cell activation as potential anti-atherosclerotic activity of peptides from Spirulina maxima. *European Journal of Pharmaceutical Sciences, 50*(2), 198–207.

Wang, X., Ouyang, Y. -Y., Liu, J., & Zhao, G. (2014b). Flavonoid intake and risk of CVD: A systematic review and meta-analysis of prospective cohort studies. *British Journal of Nutrition, 111*(1), 1–11.

Wang, X., Ouyang, Y., Liu, J., et al. (2014a). Fruit and vegetable consumption and mortality from all causes, cardiovascular disease, and cancer: Systematic review and dose-response meta-analysis of prospective cohort studies. *The BMJ, 349*, g4490.

Wimalawansa, S. J. (2018). Vitamin D and cardiovascular diseases: Causality. *The Journal of Steroid Biochemistry and Molecular Biology, 175*, 29–43.

Wolak, T., & Paran, E. (2013). Can carotenoids attenuate vascular aging? *Vascular Pharmacology, 59*(2–3), 63–66.

Wu, Q., Liu, L., Miron, A., Klímová, B., Wan, D., et al. (2016). The antioxidant, immunomodulatory, and anti-inflammatory activities of Spirulina: An overview. *Archives of Toxicology, 90*(8), 1817–1840.

Yarmolinsky, J., Gon, G., & Edwards, P. (2015). Effect of tea on blood pressure for secondary prevention of cardiovascular disease: A systematic review and meta-analysis of randomized controlled trials. *Nutrition Reviews, 73*(4), 236–246.

Yin, K., You, Y., Swier, V., Tang, L., Radwan, M. M., et al. (2015). Vitamin D protects against atherosclerosis via regulation of cholesterol efflux and macrophage polarization in hypercholesterolemic swine. *Arteriosclerosis, Thrombosis, and Vascular Biology, 35*(11), 2432–2442.

Young, K. A., Snell-Bergeon, J. K., Naik, R. G., Hokanson, J. E., Tarullo, D., et al. (2011). Vitamin D deficiency and coronary artery calcification in subjects with type 1 diabetes. *Diabetes Care, 34*(2), 454–458.

Zimmermann, A. M., & Kirsten, V. R. (2016). Alimentos com função antioxidante em doenças crônicas: Uma abordagem clínica. *Disciplinarum Scientia, 8*, 51–68.

Zuchi, C., Ambrosio, G., Lüscher, T. F., & Landmesser, U. (2010). Nutraceuticals in cardiovascular prevention: Lessons from studies on endothelial function. *Cardiovascular Therapy, 28*(3), 187–201.

CHAPTER 16

ENDOTHELIAL EFFECTS OF MARINE AND PLANT-DERIVED OMEGA-3 FATTY ACIDS

DEEPANSHU RANA[1] and VIKASH SINGH JADON[2]

[1]Department of Microbiology, School of Life Sciences, Sardar Bhagwan Singh University, Balawala, Dehradun, Uttarakhand, India

[2]Department of Biochemistry and Biotechnology, School of Life Sciences, Sardar Bhagwan Singh University, Balawala, Dehradun, Uttarakhand, India

ABSTRACT

Human beings evolved with a diet that contained roughly equal amounts of omega-6 fatty acids and polyunsaturated essential fatty acids. Over the past 100–150 years, there has been a colossal increase in the consumption of omega-6 fatty acids due to the increased intake of vegetable oils from seeds of corn, sunflower, safflower, cotton, and soybeans. Omega-3 fatty acids possess anti-inflammatory, anti-thrombotic, anti-arrhythmic, hypolipidemic, and vasodilatory properties. These beneficial effects of omega-3 fatty acids have been shown in the secondary prevention of coronary heart disease, anti-inflammatory actions, and some other endothelial dysfunctions. The present review discusses the potential effect of plant- and marine-derived omega-3 fatty acids as a source for ALA, which further elongates into EPA and DHA.

Antioxidants as Nutraceuticals. Nayan A. Gujarathi, Raj K. Keservani, Rajesh K. Kesharwani, Bhushan R. Rane, Yogeeta Sameer Goyal (Eds.)

16.1 INTRODUCTION

The triumphs of treating nutritional deficiencies to improve health and disease prevention throughout medical history have and continue to abound. Some of the common examples are folic acid, other Vitamins-B to prevent neural tube defects (Keogh, 2003; Stevenson et al., 2000), and calcium and vitamin D supplements for osteoporosis (Moyad, 2002; Dawson-Hughes et al., 1997). A potential dietary manipulation that is beginning to emerge is the potential impact of correcting low levels of omega-3 fatty acids to prevent a variety of medical conditions from occurring or progressing, such as arthritis, some cancers, cardiovascular disease, depression, maternal/fetal well-being, and neurologic disease (Moyad, 2005; Harris, 2004).

Fatty acids consist of organic compound chains with a radical at one end and an alkyl radical group at the opposite. The radical is reactive and promptly forms organic compound links with alcohol groups, as an example those on glycerin or sterol alcohol, successively forming acylglycerols (e.g., triacylglycerols, phospholipids) and cholesteryl esters (Calder & Yakoob, 2009). Currently, fatty acids (FAs) may be classified into 3 classes based on the presence of double bonds, i.e., saturated fatty acids FAs (SFAs, no double bonds), monounsaturated FAs (MUFAs, one double bond), and unsaturated FAs (PUFAs, ≥2 double bonds) (Saini & Keum, 2018; Calder & Yakoob, 2009).

Omega-6 (n–6) and omega-3 (n–3) are the two major families of polyunsaturated fatty acids (PUFAs) (Sprecher, 2004). Omega-3 fatty acids are so called because the first double bond is on carbon number 3, counting the methyl carbon as carbon number 1 (Calder & Yakoob, 2009). The simplest omega-3 fatty acid is alpha-linolenic acid (ALA) (18:3ω–3). Alpha-linolenic acid is synthesized from linoleic acid (18:2ω–6) by desaturation, catalyzed by delta-15 desaturase (Calder & Yakoob, 2009). They can be of plant or animal origin. Plants synthesize linoleic acid (18:2n–6) and alpha-linolenic acid (18:3n–3), and consequently, these two fatty acids are found in many seeds, nuts, seed oils, and products produced from seed oils like margarine (Calder, 2017). Although animals cannot synthesize ALA, they can metabolize it by more desaturation and elongation; desaturation happens at carbon atoms below carbon number 9 (counting from the carboxyl carbon) and mainly occurs in the liver. Alpha-linolenic acid may be regenerated to stearidonic acid (18:4ω–3) by delta-6 desaturase, and so stearidonic acid may be elongated to 20:4ω–3 (Calder & Yakoob, 2009). This fatty acid can be further desaturated by delta-5 desaturase to yield eicosapentaenoic acid (EPA) (20:5ω–3). EPA, DPA, and DHA are found in vital quantities in fish and other foods, and they can collectively be referred to as marine n–3 fatty acids. These fatty acids are present in the flesh of both lean and oily fish, with much larger amounts in the latter, and in the livers of some lean fish (Calder, 2015).

This review encompasses not only the basic introduction to omega-3 fatty acids but also their potential benefits in preventing a variety of medical conditions from occurring or progressing, such as arthritis, cancers, cardiovascular disease, depression, maternal/fetal well-being, and neurological disease.

16.2 RISK RELATED TO ENDOTHELIAL DYSFUNCTION

For a very long time, the endothelium – a functional barrier between blood vessels and the bloodstream – was thought of as a relatively inert reservoir of blood (Stenvinkel, 2001). But over the past 20 years, scientists have discovered a remarkable diversity of endothelial functions, including the regulation of coagulation, fibrinolysis, vascular tone, growth, and immune response (Stenvinkel, 2001). Reduced dilatation, a proinflammatory state, and prothrombotic characteristics are associated with endothelial dysfunction. Reduced nitric oxide generation, oxidative stress, and decreased hyperpolarizing factor production are some of the mechanisms involved in the reduced vasodilatory responses in endothelial dysfunction (Endemann & Schiffrin, 2004).

Endothelial dysfunction was initially delineated in human hypertension in the forearm vasculature in 1990 (Panza et al., 1990). Impaired vasodilation in high blood pressure has been confirmed by several studies in different vascular beds, including small resistance vessels (Park et al., 2001; Schiffrin et al., 2000). Impairment of dilatation has also been described in type 1 (Beckman et al., 2003) and type 2 diabetes (Rizzoni et al., 2001; Schofield et al., 2000; Endemann et al., 2004), coronary artery disease (Monnink et al., 2002), congestive heart failure (Landmesser et al., 2002), and chronic renal failure (Bolton et al., 2001; Thambyrajah et al., 2005;). Further, a study of children with hypertensive patients revealed that this epithelial dysfunction manifestation may also precede the onset of the disorder in addition to being related to it (Taddei et al., 1996). Recent epidemiological studies have found a strong link between infection and inflammation with endothelial dysfunction in the chronic stage of inflammation acting as a sign of damaged arterial walls (Ross, 1999). Additionally, pro-inflammatory cytokines cause endothelial cells to express cell surface adhesion molecules which aid in monocyte adhesion (Stenvinkel, 2001; Alexander, 1995).

16.3 PLANT AND MARINE-BASED SOURCES OF OMEGA-3

Numerous studies and clinical investigations on the metabolism of polyunsaturated fatty acids (PUFA) in general and omega-3 fatty acids in particular have been conducted over the past 200 years. Today, everyone is aware of the importance of polyunsaturated fatty acids for growth and development as well as for the prevention and treatment of cancer, diabetes, heart diseases, arthritis, other inflammatory and immune disorders, and arterial coronary diseases (Simopoulos, 2002; Hamazaki & Okuyama, 2001; Lagarde et al., 1999; Simopoulos et al., 1997; Salem et al., 1996; Galli et al., 1994; Simopoulos, 1986, 1991; Galli & Simopoulos, 1989). Omega-6 fatty acid consumption has significantly increased over the past 100–150 years as a result of people consuming more vegetable oils made from the seeds of corn, sunflower, safflower, cotton, and soybeans. In contrast to the typical range of 1–2:1 for the omega-6 fatty acid to omega-3 fatty acid ratio, it has been varying from 10–20:1 in most Western countries (Djuricic & Calder, 2021).

The majority of crop seeds and vegetable oils, such as canola, soybean, corn, and sunflower oils, are a significant source of n–6 FAs in the form of LA with low n–3 FAs (ALA). Contrary to n–6 FAs, the intake of n–3 FAs is typically insufficient due to their constrained sources (Moghadasian, 2008). Numerous studies show that 18:3ω3 (ALA) is converted to EPA and DHA in people. It's critical to take into account terrestrial sources of omega-3 fatty acids in the food supply, firstly isolated from hempseed oil in 1887 (Deuel, 1951). A large amount of 18:3ω3, a crucial component of the polar lipid that makes up the chloroplast membrane, is typically present in the lipids found in the leaves of plants (Simopoulos, 2002). In the carcasses of wild animals and birds, only 3.9% of fat content is available and they have about fivefold more polyunsaturated fat per gram than is found in domestic livestock as they feed on plants only (Ledger, 1968; Wei & Draper, 1975; Crawford, 1968). According to the US Department of Agriculture (USDA), the highest content of omega-3 fatty acids was found to be in purslane, a good non-aquatic source comprising 4 mg/g wet weight of 18:3ω3. The amount of 18:3ω3 that is present in various terrestrial sources is listed in Table 16.1. Data related to the fat content of some commonly used food items is given in Figure 16.1.

TABLE 16.1 Fatty Acid Content of Different Terrestrial Sources

Terrestrial Sources	18:3 (g)
Plants	
Purslane	4.06
Spinach	0.89
Buttercrunch lettuce	0.26
Red Leaf lettuce	0.31
Mustard	0.48
Fruits	
Avocados, raw, California	0.1
Raspberries, raw	0.1
Strawberries	0.1
Grains	
Barley, bran	0.3
Corn, germ	0.3
Oats, germ	1.4
Wheat, bran	0.2
Legumes	
Beans, common, dry	0.6
Chickpeas, dry	0.1
Cowpeas, dry	0.3
Soybeans, dry	1.6
Vegetables	
Cauliflower, raw	0.1
Radish seeds, sprouted, raw	0.7
Broccoli, raw	0.1
Nuts	
Walnuts, English/Persian	6.8
Chia seeds dried	3.9
Butternuts, dried	8.7

The long-chain omega-3 fatty acids are also obtained from different marine sources. Fish and fish oil are sources of omega-3 fatty acids, specifically eicosapentaenoic acid (EPA) and docosahexaenoic acid (DHA), that are present in fatty fish (Covington, 2004). Fatty fish, such as salmon and tuna, are rich sources of omega-3 fatty acids. The consumption of fish and fish oil provides EPA and DHA directly, avoiding the need for enzymes to convert alpha-linolenic acid (ALA) to EPA (Covington, 2004). A diet based

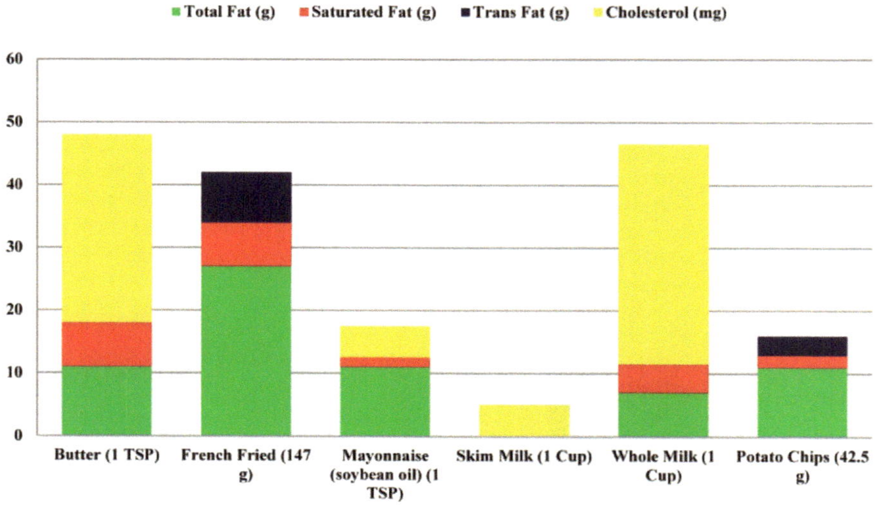

FIGURE 16.1 The fat content of some common food items.

Source: Adapted from White, 2009.

on fish, fish oil, beef, and lamb can also supply EPA, DPA, DHA, and ARA that can be directly utilized for normal physiological functions in the body (Table 16.2). Wild (marine) fishes contain more n–3 PUFAs than cultivated (farmed) fishes since most marine fishes prey on plant life and animals that are rich in n–3 PUFAs, while farmed fishes consume feed products made of cereal and vegetable oils that contain higher proportions of n–6 FAs. Similarly, cold-water fishes accumulate higher proportions of LC n–3 PUFAs that help them adapt to cold environments compared to warm-water fishes (Saini & Keum, 2018). The amount of fish consumption required to provide approximately 1 g of EPA plus DHA per day is provided in Figure 16.2 (Covington, 2004).

16.4 PHARMACOLOGICAL ASPECT OF OMEGA-3 RELATED TO ENDOTHELIAL FUNCTIONS

The essentiality of Omega-3 fatty acids is established because they can only be obtained through diet or supplementation since they are not synthesized by the body. Recent reports suggest that intake of omega-3 fatty acids significantly improves endothelial functions and other functions related to the endothelium. Through an inefficient desaturation method (the rate of

TABLE 16.2 Omega-3 Fatty Acid Contents in Selected Animal-Based Foods

Food	Omega-3 (g/100 g)		
	ALA	EPA	DHA
Fish Oil			
Menhaden	–	13.17	8.56
Salmon	–	13.20	18.23
Sardine	–	10.14	10.66
Cod liver	–	9.90	10.97
Herring	–	6.27	4.21
Fish			
Caviar, black and red, granular	–	2.74	3.80
Shad, American, raw	–	1.09	1.32
Salmon, Chinook, raw	–	1.01	0.94
Herring, Atlantic, kippered	–	0.97	1.18
Salmon, Atlantic, farmed, raw	0.15	0.86	1.10

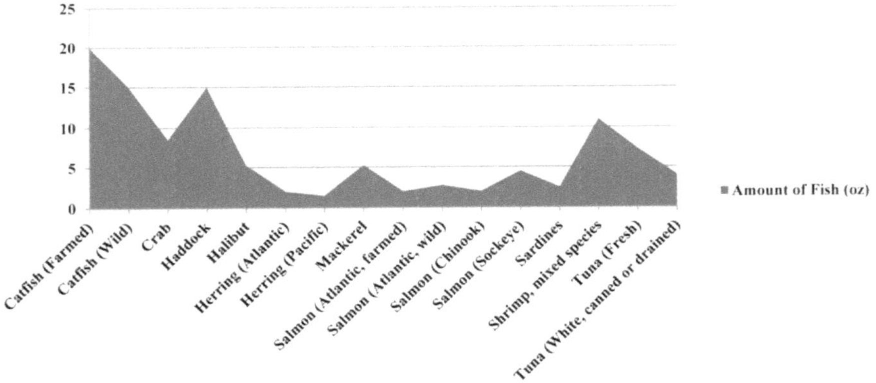

FIGURE 16.2 Amount of fish required providing 1 g of EPA plus DHA.

conversion is less than 1%), ALA produces EPA (20 carbons) and DHA (22 carbons), precursors to a variety of eicosanoids (prostaglandins, thromboxanes, and leukotrienes) that are medication, antithrombotic, antiarrhythmic, and vasodilatory (Covington, 2004). Effects of n–3 PUFAs are mediated by alterations in the properties of cancer cells by decreasing their proliferation, invasion, and metastasis while increasing their apoptosis. In addition, they affect host cells by regulating inflammation, immune response, and angiogenesis. Some of the above are shown in Figure 16.3 (Berquin et al., 2008).

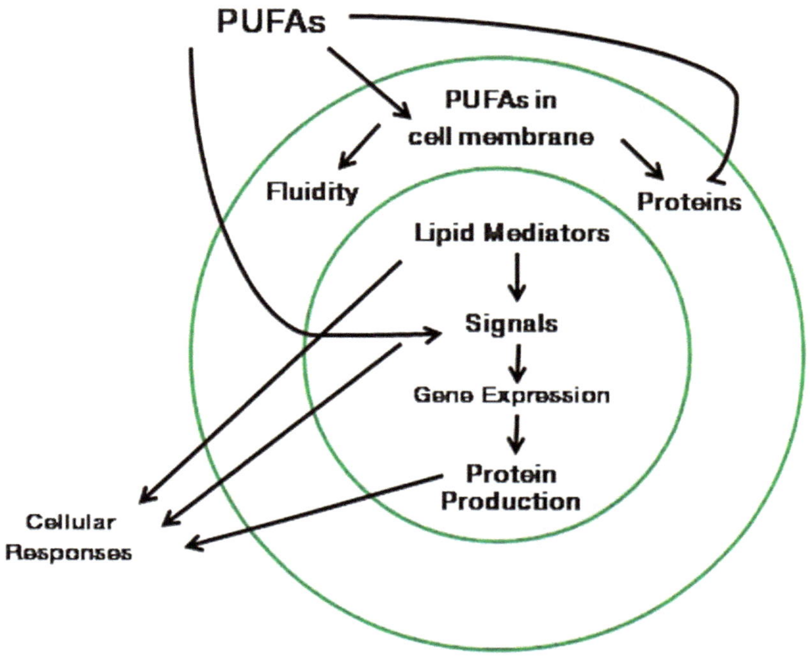

FIGURE 16.3 Schematic overview of PUFAs.
Source: Adapted from Djuricic & Calder (2021).

In hypertriglyceridemia conditions, Omega-3 fatty acids were found to help lower the blood plasma triglyceride levels (Harris et al., 1997) because they restrain the production of very-low-density lipoprotein (VLDL) cholesterol and triglycerides in the liver, thus reducing endothelial dysfunction by reducing oxidative stress and inflammatory responses. A review of human studies found that roughly four grams per day of omega-3 fatty acids reduced blood lipid concentrations by 25 to 30%, lowered blood beta-lipoprotein (LDL) cholesterol levels by 5 to 10%, and increased high-density lipoprotein (HDL) cholesterol levels by one to 3%. Total cholesterol levels were not significantly affected (Harris, 1997).

Fatty acids are generally incorporated into cell membrane phospholipids, which influence not only the inflammatory cell response but also the inflammation process (Calder, 2008). Therefore, the fatty acid composition of inflamed cells is always of interest, and how the intake of marine n–3 fatty acids might change the composition (Calder, 2015). Eicosanoids, which include PGs, thromboxanes (TXs), LTs, and lipoxins (LXs), are considered oxidative derivatives of 20-carbon fatty acids. The synthesis process starts with membrane phospholipids, but ARA is also considered the major substrate for its synthesis, and due to its high frequency, cells may get involved in inflammatory processes. The free ARA then acts as a substrate for cyclooxygenase (COX), lipoxygenase (LOX), or cytochrome P450 enzymes. COX enzymes lead to PGs and TXs, LOX enzymes to LTs and LXs, and cytochrome P450 enzymes to hydroxyeicosatetraenoic and epoxyeicosatrienoic acids. ARA metabolism results in 2-series PGs and TXs and 4-series LTs and LXs. While COX-1 is said to be involved in cellular housekeeping functions, COX-2 is induced in inflammatory cells by classical inflammatory stimuli such as bacterial endotoxin, resulting in a large increase in PG generation. PGE2, other 2-series PGs, and the 4-series LTs are among the best-known mediators and regulators of inflammation (Kroetz & Zeldin, 2002; Tilley et al., 2001; Lewis et al., 1990). Since increased intake of marine n–3 fatty acids decreases the amount of ARA in the membrane phospholipids of cells involved in inflammation, it might be expected that production of ARA-derived mediators would be decreased simply because of a reduced amount of substrate available and thus help in the maintenance of endothelial function. Furthermore, EPA has been shown to inhibit ARA metabolism and decrease the expression of the COX-2 gene.

16.5 FINAL COMMENT

Fatty acid exposure and the carboxylic acid composition of human inflammatory cells influence the performance of these cells associated with epithelial tissue pathology. The contents of ARA, EPA, and DHA seem to be particularly necessary. Dose-dependent actions of marine n–3 PUFAs on inflammatory responses haven't been well delineated, but it seems that a dose of a minimum of 2 g per day is critical to achieving a medication result. As a result of their medication actions, marine n–3 fatty acids may have therapeutic effectiveness in inflammatory diseases. Work with animal models of RA, IBD, and respiratory illness has demonstrated the effectiveness of marine-derived fatty acid fish oil and mediators derived from EPA and DHA, such as some of the resolvins. Due to the different interaction mechanisms of omega-6 fatty acids and omega-3 fatty acids, they lower the risk of CVDs. The omega-6 fatty acid PUFA LA acts mainly by lowering LDL-cholesterol, while blood flow is promoted by both the omega-3 fatty acid PUFAs EPA and DHA, lowering triglycerides and improving the functioning of the internal organs and blood vessels, as well as controlling clotting and inflammation. However, the link between omega-6 fatty acid and omega-3 fatty acid PUFAs and their bioactive supermolecule mediators within the context of inflammation isn't yet fully understood. Thus, there's a need to know more about the actions of marine n–3 fatty acids in patients with inflammatory disorders in order to optimize the strategy for their therapeutic use. Above all, a better understanding of dose-response relationships in various patient groups, of the relative importance of EPA and DHA, and of the factors that limit the effectiveness of EPA and DHA is required.

KEYWORDS

- **eicosapentaenoic Acid**
- **endothelial dysfunctions**
- **marine omega-3**
- **plant omega-3**
- **polyunsaturated fatty acids**

REFERENCES

Alexander, R. W. (1995). Hypertension and the pathogenesis of atherosclerosis: oxidative stress and the mediation of arterial inflammatory response: A new perspective. *Hypertension, 25*(2), 155–161.

Beckman, J. A., Goldfine, A. B., Gordon, M. B., Garrett, L. A., Keaney Jr, J. F., & Creager, M. A. (2003). Oral antioxidant therapy improves endothelial function in Type 1 but not Type 2 diabetes mellitus. *American Journal of Physiology – Heart and Circulatory Physiology, 285*(6), H2392–H2398.

Berquin, I. M., Edwards, I. J., & Chen, Y. Q. (2008). Multi-targeted therapy of cancer by omega-3 fatty acids. *Cancer Letters, 269*(2), 363–377.

Bolton, C. H., Downs, L. G., Victory, J. G., Dwight, J. F., Tomson, C. R., Mackness, M. I., & Pinkney, J. H. (2001). Endothelial dysfunction in chronic renal failure: roles of lipoprotein oxidation and proinflammatory cytokines. *Nephrology Dialysis Transplantation, 16*(6), 1189–1197.

Calder, P. C. (2008). The relationship between the fatty acid composition of immune cells and their function. *Prostaglandins, Leukotrienes, and Essential Fatty Acids, 79*(3–5), 101–108.

Calder, P. C. (2015). Marine omega-3 fatty acids and inflammatory processes: Effects, mechanisms and clinical relevance. *Biochimica et Biophysica Acta, 1851*(4), 469–484.

Calder, P. C. (2017). Omega-3 fatty acids and inflammatory processes: from molecules to man. *Biochemical Society Transactions, 45*(5), 1105–1115.
Calder, P. C., & Yaqoob, P. (2009). Understanding omega-3 polyunsaturated fatty acids. *Postgraduate Medicine, 121*(6), 148–157.
Crawford, M. A. (1968). Fatty-acid ratios in free-living and domestic animals: possible implications for atheroma. *The Lancet, 291*(7556), 1329–1333.
Dawson-Hughes, B., Harris, S. S., Krall, E. A., & Dallal, G. E. (1997). Effect of calcium and vitamin D supplementation on bone density in men and women 65 years of age or older. *New England Journal of Medicine, 337*(10), 670–676.
Deuel Jr, H. J. (1952). The Lipids: Their Chemistry and Biochemistry. Volume I: Chemistry. *Journal of the American Medical Association, 150*(12), 1262.
Djuricic, I., & Calder, P. C. (2021). Beneficial outcomes of omega-6 and omega-3 polyunsaturated fatty acids on human health: An update for 2021. *Nutrients, 13*(7), 2421.
Endemann, D. H., & Schiffrin, E. L. (2004). Endothelial dysfunction. *Journal of the American Society of Nephrology, 15*(8), 1983–1992.
Endemann, D. H., Pu, Q., De Ciuceis, C., Savoia, C., Virdis, A., Neves, M. F., & Schiffrin, E. L. (2004). Persistent remodeling of resistance arteries in type 2 diabetic patients on antihypertensive treatment. *Hypertension, 43*(2), 399–404.
Galli, C., Simopoulos, A. P., & Tremoli, E. (1994). Fatty acids and lipids: Biological aspects. *World Review of Nutrition and Dietetics, 75*, 1–197.
Hamazaki, T., & Okuyama, H. (2001). Fatty acids and lipids: New findings. *World Review of Nutrition and Dietetics, 88*, 1–260.
Harris, W. S. (1997). n-3 fatty acids and serum lipoproteins: human studies. *American Journal of Clinical Nutrition, 65*(5), 1645S–1654S.
Harris, W. S. (2004). Fish oil supplementation: evidence for health benefits. *Cleveland Clinic Journal of Medicine, 71*(3), 208–221.
Harris, W. S., Ginsberg, H. N., Arunakul, N., Shachter, N. S., Windsor, S. L., Adams, M., & Osmundsen, K. (1997). Safety and efficacy of Omacor in severe hypertriglyceridemia. *Journal of Cardiovascular Risk, 4*(5–6), 385–391.
Keogh, J. (2003). Discovering nutrition. *Nutrition & Dietetics, 60*(3), 217–218.
Kroetz, D. L., & Zeldin, D. C. (2002). Cytochrome P450 pathways of arachidonic acid metabolism. *Current Opinion in Lipidology, 13*(3), 273–283.
Lagarde, M., Spector, A. A., Galli, C., Hamazaki, T., & Knapp, H. R. (1999). Fatty acids and lipids from cell biology to human disease. *Lipids, 34*(Suppl.), S1–S350.
Landmesser, U., Spiekermann, S., Dikalov, S., Tatge, H., Wilke, R., Kohler, C., & Drexler, H. (2002). Vascular oxidative stress and endothelial dysfunction in patients with chronic heart failure: role of xanthine-oxidase and extracellular superoxide dismutase. *Circulation, 106*(24), 3073–3078.
Ledger, H. P. (1968). Body composition as a basis for a comparative study of some East African mammals. *Symposium of the Zoological Society of London, 21*, 289–310.
Lewis, R. A., Austen, K. F., & Soberman, R. J. (1990). Leukotrienes and other products of the 5-lipoxygenase pathway: biochemistry and relation to pathobiology in human diseases. *New England Journal of Medicine, 323*(10), 645–655.
Moghadasian, M. H. (2008). Advances in dietary enrichment with n-3 fatty acids. *Critical Reviews in Food Science and Nutrition, 48*(5), 402–410.
Monnink, S. H., van Haelst, P. L., van Boven, A. J., Stroes, E. S., Tio, R. A., Plokker, T. W., & van Gilst, W. H. (2002). Endothelial dysfunction in patients with coronary artery disease:

a comparison of three frequently reported tests. *Journal of Investigative Medicine, 50*(1), 19–24.
Moyad, M. A. (2002). Complementary therapies for reducing the risk of osteoporosis in patients receiving luteinizing hormone-releasing hormone treatment/orchiectomy for prostate cancer: a review and assessment of the need for more research. *Urology, 59*(4), 34–40.
Moyad, M. A. (2005). An introduction to dietary/supplemental omega-3 fatty acids for general health and prevention: part II. *Urologic Oncology: Seminars and Original Investigations, 23*(1), 36–48.
Panza, J. A., Quyyumi, A. A., Brush Jr, J. E., & Epstein, S. E. (1990). Abnormal endothelium-dependent vascular relaxation in patients with essential hypertension. *New England Journal of Medicine, 323*(1), 22–27.
Park, J. B., Charbonneau, F., & Schiffrin, E. L. (2001). Correlation of endothelial function in large and small arteries in human essential hypertension. *Journal of Hypertension, 19*(3), 415–420.
Rizzoni, D., Porteri, E., Guelfi, D., Muiesan, M. L., Valentini, U., Cimino, A., & Rosei, E. A. (2001). Structural alterations in subcutaneous small arteries of normotensive and hypertensive patients with non–insulin-dependent diabetes mellitus. *Circulation, 103*(9), 1238–1244.
Ross, R. (1999). Atherosclerosis—an inflammatory disease. *New England Journal of Medicine, 340*(2), 115–126.
Saini, R. K., & Keum, Y. S. (2018). Omega-3 and omega-6 polyunsaturated fatty acids: Dietary sources, metabolism, and significance–A review. *Life Sciences, 203*, 255–267.
Salem Jr, N., Simopoulos, A. P., Galli, C., Lagarde, M., & Knapp, H. R. (1996). Fatty acids and lipids from cell biology to human disease. *Lipids, 31*(Suppl.), S1–S326.
Schiffrin, E. L., Park, J. B., Intengan, H. D., & Touyz, R. M. (2000). Correction of arterial structure and endothelial dysfunction in human essential hypertension by the angiotensin receptor antagonist losartan. *Circulation, 101*(14), 1653–1659.
Schofield, I., Malik, R., Izzard, A., Austin, C., & Heagerty, A. (2002). Vascular structural and functional changes in type 2 diabetes mellitus: evidence for the roles of abnormal myogenic responsiveness and dyslipidemia. *Circulation, 106*(24), 3037–3043.
Simopoulos, A. P. (1991). Omega-3 fatty acids in health and disease and in growth and development. *American Journal of Clinical Nutrition, 54*, 438–463.
Simopoulos, A. P. (1997). W-3 fatty acids in the prevention–management of cardiovascular disease. *Canadian Journal of Physiology and Pharmacology, 75*, 234–239.
Simopoulos, A. P. (2002). Omega-3 fatty acids in wild plants, nuts and seeds. *Asia Pacific Journal of Clinical Nutrition, 11*, S163–S173.
Simopoulos, A. P., Kifer, R. R., & Martin, R. E. (Eds.). (1986). *Health Effects of Polyunsaturated Fatty Acids in Seafoods*. Orlando, FL: Academic Press.
Simopoulos, A. P., Kifer, R. R., Martin, R. E., & Barlow, S. M. (1991). Health effects of Ω3 polyunsaturated fatty acids in seafoods. *World Review of Nutrition and Dietetics, 66*, 1–592.
Sprecher, H. (2000). Metabolism of highly unsaturated n-3 and n-6 fatty acids. *Biochimica et Biophysica Acta, 1486*(2–3), 219–231.
Stenvinkel, P. (2001). Endothelial dysfunction and inflammation—is there a link? *Nephrology, Dialysis, Transplantation, 16*(10), 1968–1971.

Stevenson, R. E., Allen, W. P., Pai, G. S., Best, R., Seaver, L. H., Dean, J., & Thompson, S. (2000). Decline in prevalence of neural tube defects in a high-risk region of the United States. *Pediatrics, 106*(4), 677–683.

Taddei, S., Virdis, A., Mattei, P., Ghiadoni, L., Sudano, I., & Salvetti, A. (1996). Defective L-arginine–nitric oxide pathway in offspring of essential hypertensive patients. *Circulation, 94*(6), 1298–1303.

Thambyrajah, J., Landray, M. J., McGlynn, F. J., Jones, H. J., Wheeler, D. C., & Townend, J. N. (2000). Abnormalities of endothelial function in patients with predialysis renal failure. *Heart, 83*(2), 205–209.

Tilley, S. L., Coffman, T. M., & Koller, B. H. (2001). Mixed messages: modulation of inflammation and immune responses by prostaglandins and thromboxanes. *Journal of Clinical Investigation, 108*(1), 15–23.

Wei Wo, C. K., & Draper, H. H. (1975). Vitamin E status of Alaskan Eskimos. *American Journal of Clinical Nutrition, 28*(8), 808–813.

White, B. (2009). Dietary fatty acids. *American Family Physician, 80*(4), 345–350.

CHAPTER 17

MARINE-DERIVED NATURAL FLAVONOIDS AND THEIR BIOLOGICAL ACTIVITIES

AARTI TIWARI,[1] VIMAL KUMAR YADAV,[1] SANDEEP KUMAR SINGH,[1] AJAY KUMAR SHUKLA,[1] and MANISH KUMAR[2]

[1]*Institute of Pharmacy, Dr. Ram Manohar Lohia Avadh University, Ayodhya, Uttar Pradesh, India*

[2]*Department of Pharmacy, Madhav University, Pindwara, Rajasthan, India*

ABSTRACT

Because oceans cover more than 70% of the Earth's surface, marine species provide an abundant and limitless supply of structurally varied bioactive chemicals. Due to the various biological environments in which they live, these species have acquired unique characteristics and bioactive substances that are, in most cases, unmatched by their terrestrial equivalents. Due to an increasing interest in their promising biological/pharmacological properties, marine flavonoids have been widely investigated in recent decades. Flavones and flavonols, which are typically isolated from marine plants, are the most prevalent groups of marine flavonoids. While most flavonoids are hydroxylated and methoxylated, certain marine flavonoids have an uncommon substitution pattern, specifically the presence of sulfate, chlorine, and amino groups, which is not typical in terrestrial organisms. This chapter provides information about the biological activity of marine-derived natural flavonoids.

Antioxidants as Nutraceuticals. Nayan A. Gujarathi, Raj K. Keservani, Rajesh K. Kesharwani, Bhushan R. Rane, Yogeeta Sameer Goyal (Eds.)

17.1 INTRODUCTION

Biologists and chemists from all around the globe are researching marine-natural flavonoids and developing novel products. Marine natural sources have flavonoids, used as bioactive natural compounds with the potential to act as nutritional supplements (Keservani & Sharma, 2014), medicines, cosmetics, agrochemicals, molecular probes, and enzymes. Marine flavonoids are potential bio-chemicals. It is a completely unexplored resource (Martins et al., 2019), and has low molecular weight secondary metabolites. Marine flavonoids are present in both terrestrial and marine plants. Recent research has found that marine flavonoids offer a wide range of biologically beneficial properties, and as a result, these natural compounds have gotten a lot of attention (Fernando et al., 2022). The isolation of marine flavonoids, particularly flavones (68 compounds) and flavonols has increased dramatically during the last 50 years (23 compounds). Despite the range and structural complexity of marine flavonoids, only a few families, including the *Hydrocharitaceae*, *Zosteraceae*, *Rhodomelaceae*, *Juncaceae*, and *Tamaricaceae*, have been isolated (Erdman et al., 2007). The key sources of flavonoids (51%) are seagrasses and halophytes (28%). Nonetheless, these natural flavonoid compounds have been isolated from a variety of marine sources such as mangroves, algae, mollusks, fungi, corals, and bacteria (El-Bondkly et al., 2021).

17.2 FLAVONOIDS

17.2.1 FLAVONES

The extraction of four flavone C-glycosides from the green alga *Nitella hookeri* is the first report on marine flavones (*Characeae*). These flavones are vicenin and lucenin and are reported by Markham and Porter (Markham & Porter, 1969). Despite this, there was insufficient material to do thorough characterization using NMR investigations. The bulk of marine flavones, including 33 glycosides and 31 aglycones, include hydroxyl and methoxy groups, making these the most prevalent substituents in this family of marine chemicals (Xiao, 2017). The flavones like Polyhydroxylated, with three and four hydroxyl groups at positions 5, 3′, 4′, 5, 7, 4′, and 5, 7, 3′, 4′ being particularly prevalent (Cook & Samman, 1996; Musialik et al., 2009; Martins et al., 2019). Marine sources have also yielded flavones with 5 and 6 hydroxyl groups. It's worth noting that flavones containing hydroxyl and methoxy groups at less frequent locations, such as C-6 and C-8, are also found. The bulk of methylated flavones is O-methylated, while C-methylation is uncommon (Buckingham & Munasinghe, 2015; Andersen & Markham, 2005; Gu et al., 2022). There are just two C-methylated marine flavones that are both on the B ring. Nearly 70% of flavones are mono-O-methylated, with this group appearing more commonly in positions 7 and 3′. Furthermore, 20% of the flavones are di-O-methylated, whereas the remaining 10% are tri-O-methylated. The bulk of the 33 flavone glycosides are O-glycosides, with only four being C-glycosides. About two-thirds of the 29 flavonoids O-glycosides are 7-O-glucosides. Five 4′-O-glucosides, two 7-O-xylosides, and one 3′-O-glucoside make up the rest (Martins et al., 2019; Buckingham & Munasinghe, 2015).

17.2.2 FLAVONOLES

Flavonols are the second most common kind of flavonoids found in the ocean. The bulk of flavonols, including 14 flavonolosides and 9 aglycones, are polyhydroxylated. Trihydroxylated at positions 5, 7, 4′, and tetrahydroxylated at positions 5, 7, 3′, more than two-thirds of these compounds are trihydroxylated. Most flavonols have trisubstituted hydroxyl and methoxy groups at 5, 7, 4′, and tetrasubstituted hydroxyl and methoxy groups at 5, 7, 3′, 4′. The occurrence of substitution patterns not usually encountered in the terrestrial environment, such as methyl and sulfate groups, as well as a chlorine atom at C-3′ (compound 86), has been recorded (Cook & Samman, 1996; Musialik et al., 2009; Martins et al., 2019).

17.2.3 OTHER FLAVANOIDS

Flavonoids (Keservani & Sharma, 2014) from other classes, such as flavanones, flavan-3-ols, isoflavones, and dihydrochalcones, have also been identified from the sea. Actinoflavoside and thalassodendrone are two flavonoids that have a unique substitution pattern that is not seen in the terrestrial environment. Actinoflavoside is a flavanone that has an aminodeoxy sugar moiety at C-7 and was found in *Streptomyces* sp. Thalassodendrone is a dihydrochalcone with a 6′-O-rhamnosyl-(1”‘ 6”)-glucopyranosyl substituent group isolated from Thalassodendrinciliatum. Only 27 of the 93 flavonoids isolated from marine sources have been reported in the marine environment, highlighting the relevance of this habitat in the finding of flavonoids with a distinct structure (Cook & Samman, 1996; Musialik et al., 2009; Martins et al., 2019).

17.3 BIOLOGICAL ACTIVITY OF MARINE-DERIVED NATURAL FLAVONOIDS

Because of their unusual substitution pattern and interesting biological actions, some marine flavonoids have piqued the interest of scientists. Several flavonoids have been found to have antifouling and anti-feedant properties in addition to pharmacological (antioxidant, antimicrobial, antitumor, anticoagulant, and anti-diabetic) properties, demonstrating their potential as lead compounds in the pharmaceutical and chemical industries. Some marine flavonoids, such as apigenin (Salehi et al., 2019), luteolin (López-Lázaro et al., 2009), quercetin (Razavi et al., 2009), kaempferol (Calderon-Montano et al., 2011), catechin (González-Paramás et al., 2019), and their glycosides, are widely distributed in the plant world, have been isolated from terrestrial sources, and are regularly found in food and medicinal herbs (Sharma et al., 2020; Rane et al., 2020a, b, c). Apigenin, luteolin, quercetin, kaempferol, and catechin, for example, have been shown to have neuroprotective (Keservani et al., 2016b), anti-inflammatory, antioxidant, and anticancer action in various studies, indicating that they could be used as nutraceuticals (Keservani et al., 2010a, b, 2020; Yashin et al., 2017; Asif & Khodadadi, 2013.). Aside from these functions, apigenin, luteolin, quercetin, and kaempferol have been shown to have positive effects on the cardiovascular system (Keservani et al., 2016a), type-2 diabetes, and the prevention and treatment of liver illnesses. Flavonoids found in nature, such as kaempferol, luteolin, quercetin, and catechin, have been shown to be effective against a wide spectrum of bacteria and viruses (Boeing et al., 2021; Perez-Vizcaino & Duarte, 2010; Dubey et al., 2021).

17.3.1 ANTICOAGULANT ACTIVITY

The thrombin enzyme is responsible for the creation of fibrin clots, the conversion of fibrinogen into fibrin, and the activation of other substrates in the final coagulation cascade (factors V, VIII, XI, and XIII) (Norris, 2003). Thrombin can also facilitate additional clotting events and improve coagulation and peeling efficiency, making its direct blockage an effective anticoagulant approach. The identification of quercetin-3-O-arabinoside and quercetin-3-O-rhamnoside as strong inhibitors of human thrombin activity was based on a bioassay-guided chemical fractionation of the extract of white mangrove (*Laguncularia racemosa*) (Martins et al., 2019). The ability of these compounds to interact with thrombin was discovered by high-performance liquid chromatography (HPLC) examinations of thrombin samples treated with them (Wang et al., 2008). In reality, natural thrombin was eluted at 28.1 minutes under identical chromatographic conditions; Thrombin treated with flavonoids 84 and 85 was eluted at 25.2 and 23.8 minutes, respectively, indicating that both of these flavonoids reduced thrombin hydrophobicity. Enzymatic tests were used to confirm the efficiency of these flavonoids in inhibiting thrombin (Correia-da-Silva et al., 2011).

17.3.2 ANTIDIABETIC ACTIVITY

Several *in vitro* and *in vivo* investigations have shown that dietary flavonoids improve glucose homeostasis via a variety of mechanisms, including a reduction in carbohydrate digestion due to α-glucosidase inhibition. Despite this, only two marine flavonoids have been shown to have this action. Ma et al. investigated the *in vitro* α-glucosidase inhibitory activity of aspergivone A and B, which were isolated from the fungus *Aspergillus candidus* cultured from the gorgonian coral *Anthogorgia ochracea* collected from the South China Sea, using deoxynojirimycin (IC_{50} = 42.40 g/mL), acarbose (IC_{50} = 457 g/mL). Both flavonoids showed some inhibitory action, with compound 87 having an IC_{50} of 244 g/mL and compound 86 having just 30% inhibition at 100 g/mL (Munhoz & Frode, 2018; Babu et al., 2013).

17.3.3 ANTIOXIDANT ACTIVITY

Flavonoids have been shown to be scavengers of numerous oxidizing species, including reactive oxygen species (ROS) such as superoxide anion, hydroxyl, and peroxyl radicals, as well as singlet oxygen quenchers. However, studies of marine flavonoids' antioxidant activity have been confined to scavenging effects against diphenyl-picrylhydrazyl (DPPH) and 2,2′-azino-bis[3-ethylbenzothiazoline-6-sulfonate] (ABTS) radicals, as well as electron spin resonance spectroscopy. When compared to the positive control (IC_{50} = 18.0 g mL^{1}), butylated hydroxytoluene, Feng et al. found that apigenin and 5,3′,4′-trihydroxy-7-methoxyflavone (19), isolated from the aerial parts of the mangrove plant *Avicennia marina*, had moderate DPPH scavenging activity (IC_{50} = 52.0 and 37.0 g mL^1, respectively). Using the ABTS radical cation decolorization assay, Behery et al. assessed the antioxidant activity of apigenin, luteolin, chrysoeriol, hydnocarpin, and luteolin-7-O-D-glucoside, all isolated from the halophyte *Juncus acutus* L. The number of free phenolic groups in a compound's molecule was discovered to be a factor in its antioxidant effectiveness, according to the findings. In fact, whereas luteolin had the maximum scavenging activity (90.7% at 1 mg/mL), apigenin, chrysoeriol, hydnocarpin, and luteolin-7-O-D-glucoside had relatively moderate scavenging activity (68–75% at 1 mg/mL). Hydroxyl radicals were produced in a cell-free environment and analyzed by electron spin resonance spectroscopy to assess the scavenging action of isorhamnetin-3-O-D-glucoside and quercetin-3-O-D-glucoside, both obtained from *Salicornia herbacea.* When compared to the control group, both drugs showed good radical scavenging capacity (80 and 94% inhibitory actions, respectively, at 10 M concentrations) (100% inhibitory activity). The overall findings for marine flavonoids with antioxidant activity are consistent with the findings for other flavonoids with similar structures. In fact, it's been suggested that the amount and position of hydroxyl groups in the flavone scaffold affect their scavenging capacity, with the presence of catechol groups promoting this activity (Amic et al., 2007; Behery et al., 2013).

17.3.4 ANTICANCER ACTIVITY

The anticancer action of marine flavonoids, as well as flavonoids from other parts of the world, has been well-researched and reviewed. Nonetheless, information on the anticancer potential of flavonoids found only in the marine environment is limited. Penimethavone was tested *in vitro* against cervical (HeLa), human laryngeal epithelial (Hep-2), rhabdomyosarcoma (RD), and non-small cell lung cancer (A549) cell lines by Hou et al. Penimethavone cytotoxicity was shown to be selective and moderate in HeLa (IC_{50} = 8.41 g mL^1) and RD (IC_{50} = 8.18 g mL^1) cells. MMPs (matrix metalloproteinases), especially MMP-9 and MMP-2, are key enzymes in extracellular matrix degradation and play a role in a variety of diseases, including cancer. In a human fibrosarcoma cell line, Kong et al. extracted quercetin-3-O-D-glucoside and isorhamnetin-3-O-D-glucoside from *Salicornia herbacea* and investigated their inhibitory effects on MMP-9 and MMP-2 (HT1080). When compared to phorbol 12-myristate 13-acetate, both flavonols reduced MMP-9 and MMP-2 expression and activity by roughly 60% at 10 M (PMA).

The promoter activity of AP-1 was investigated by transfecting HT1080 cells with AP-1 binding sites including luciferase constructs to confirm that these flavonoid glycosides exert their inhibitory effects by interfering with AP-1 transcription factor binding. The reporter activity was increased by up to 2-fold in the PMA-stimulated group but was inhibited by treatment with these flavonoid glycosides. As a result, the inhibitory action of these flavonoid glycosides on MMP-9 and MMP-2 could be explained by the transcription factor AP-1 down-regulating those genes. However, there was no significant change in AP-1 luciferase activity between these two flavonoid glycosides in a comparative study. As a result, these findings suggested that flavonol glycosides could be used as chemopreventive drugs (Mao et al., 2018; George et al., 2017).

17.4 OTHER BIOLOGICAL ACTIVITIES

The highest part of the earth is covered by marine sources, approximately 70%. It offers good sources of natural bioactive molecules. Researchers can easily collect and isolate the bioactive molecules. Commonly, flavones and flavonols containing bioactive molecules are found in marine sources. These flavonoids have potential therapeutic activities. They may be a good alternative drug for the treatment of critical diseases like cancer, etc. (Beatriz et al., 2019). Hozzein et al. investigated and found that marine flavonoids have potential therapeutic roles. These flavonoids are used for the treatment and management of various diseases. Marine flavonoids have been found to have the following activities: antimicrobial, antioxidant, anti-inflammatory, anticancer, and anti-diabetic activities. However, a challenging task is isolating and characterizing flavonoids from natural sources. Therefore, there is a need to discover more economical and develop suitable methods for the isolation of marine flavonoids (Hozzein et al., 2021). Algae are the oldest and biggest sources of polyphenols. These polyphenols show intriguing structural diversity. Among the algal polyphenols, phlorotannins are mainly found in brown seaweeds and contain enormous value as potent modulators of biochemical processes linked to untreatable diseases. These types of phlorotannins have potential therapeutic properties such as anticancer, immunomodulatory, antidiabetic, antioxidant, anti-inflammatory, angiotensin-I-converting enzyme (ACE-I), butyrylcholinesterase (BChE), and acetylcholinesterase (AChE), etc. (Priyan et al., 2021; Roleda et al., 2018, 2019). The common bioactive molecules and their marine sources are shown in Table 17.1.

TABLE 17.1 List of Common Bioactive Molecules and Their Marine Sources

Sl. No.	Name of Marine Sources	Bioactive Molecules	References
1	*Himanthalia elongate*	Myricetin quercetin and Kaempferol	Rajauria et al. (2018).
2	*Tetraselmis suecica* and *Nannochloropsis gaditana*	flavonol glycoside rhamnosyl hexosyl-methyl-quercetin (quercetin 3-O-neohesperidosid)	Haoujar et al. (2019)
3	*S. muticum, Sargassum vulgare, Hypnea spinella, U. pinnatifida, Chondrus crispus, and Halopytis incurvus, S. spongiosa, Scenedesmus, Phaeodactylum tricornutum* and *P. purpureum*	Daidzin, genistein, sissotrin, formononetin, and biochanin A	Lee et al. (2006); Liu et al. (2009).
4	*Nitella hookeri*	Lucenin-I, Orientin, Isoorientin, Vicenin-1, Vitexin, Isovitexin	Haoujar et al. (2019)
5	*Sargassum pallidum*	Flavone	Liu et al. (2009)
6	*T. suecica* and *N. gaditana*	Apigenin-7-O-rutinoside	Lee et al. (2006); Haoujar et al. (2019)
7	*Osmundea pinnatifida*	Scutellarein 4-methyl ether	Sabina et al. (2009)
8.	*H. pluvialis*	Dihydroquercetin Dihydrokaempherol	Lee et al. (2013); Lopes et al. (2016); Fernando et al. (2020)

The above common natural sources of bioactive molecules possess many therapeutic activities. These bioactive molecules have been obtained from various natural sources, but not all natural sources are available in all seasons. Therefore, marine natural algae have become a good alternative for obtaining bioactive molecules. The most common bioactive molecules are Myricetin, Quercetin, Kaempferol, Apigenin, Genistein, etc. These bioactive molecules have potential activities against various diseases such as anti-aging, anti-inflammatory activity, immunomodulatory activity, cardioprotective, antimicrobial activity, anti-parasitic activity, etc. These polyphenolic molecules have the ability to inhibit the germination of pathogenic spores in plants and combat fungal infections in humans (Salas et al., 2011).

The most common natural bioactive molecules such as Quercetin, Kaempferol, Rutin, and many other phenolic and flavonoids have been found in various activities present in marine algae. It means that these activities are present in natural marine sources in the form of flavonoids. Therefore, more research work is needed to obtain suitable bioactive molecules for the treatment of diseases. These common flavonoids and their mechanism of action are shown in Table 17.2.

TABLE 17.2 List of Common Bioactive Molecules and Mechanisms of Biological Activities

Sl. No.	Biological Activity	Mechanism	References
1.	Anti-aging property	Flavonoids remove the superoxide, peroxyl radicals, and reveal antiaging properties	Cerqueira et al. (2003); Portinho et al. (2012).
2.	Anti-inflammatory activity	Campferol-3-O-methyl is a flavonoid that inhibits the formation of nitric oxide and prostaglandin E2. It is blocking the activity of enzymes cyclooxygenase and 5-lipoxygenase.	Soares et al. (2015); Behling et al. (2004); Soares et al. (2015); Moutinho et al. (2018)
3.	Antioxidant effect, besides anticancer and protective actions on the cardiovascular, renal, and hepatic systems	Quercetin and catechin block the cyclooxygenase-2 (COX-2) and lipoxygenase enzymes of arachidonic acid metabolism	Behling et al. (2004); Soares et al. (2015)
4.	Immunomodulatory activity	Flavonoids stimulate immune response. The definite mechanism is unknown	Fischer et al. (2008)
5.	Cardioprotective effects	Quercetin and its glycosides prevent LDL (Low-density lipid). It also prevents oxidative modification. Therefore, it can be used in the treatment of heart failure and arrhythmia. Polyphenolic compounds are positive regulation of sodium-potassium pump (Naþ/KþATPase)	Asher et al. (2012); Zhao et al. (2010)
6.	An antimicrobial activity like antiviral, antifungal	Polyphenols and flavonoids have antimicrobial inhibitory activity. Kaempferol and Quercetin bind to viral envelope proteins and interfere with activities of virus binding and penetration into the cell, as well as DNA synthesis, due to interference in viral DNA polymerase, respectively.	Oliveira et al. (2013); Calderon-Montano et al. (2011); Brum (2006); Winter et al. (1989)
7.	Antiparasitic activity	Antimicrobial and anti-inflammatory action of quercetin in the treatment of trypanosomiasis	Tasdemir et al. (2006)

17.5 FUTURE PERSPECTIVES

Industrial biotechnology is used for the production of active components which are used as supportive materials for the development of foodstuffs, cosmetics, and green fuel. This technology is old but still very popular. In modern times, the demands of people have increased towards naturally derived products. The suitability of natural therapeutics and meeting the demands of people can be achieved by using metabolic engineering. The metabolic engineering technology is not very old. These technologies use algae to produce biochemical compounds from natural sources. These algae are used to produce various other biomolecules such as vitamins, enzymes, lipids, recombinant proteins, pigments, alcohols, amino acids, etc. These algae are the richest sources of antioxidant compounds, which are also used for the treatment and management of various diseases like cancer. The biosynthesis mechanism is a key factor for the development of bioactive compounds from this method. The antioxidant compounds such as polyphenolics and flavonoids are identified and confirmed in their purest form by using stereo, regiospecificity, and iron-catalyzed biomimetic oxidative cross-coupling of these reactions. These reactions are used for the development of suitable modifications that offer prenylated, acylated, glycosylated phloroglucinols, halogenated, and the development of novel derivative products. These modified polyphenolic and flavonoid compounds have more desirable bioactive effects than their precursors. On the other hand, in-depth studies related to research should be carried out to establish the cheap, patient acceptability of developed natural products in all parameters.

17.6 CONCLUSION

The study of the marine environment is expanding because it has one of the world's largest biological resources, containing a diverse range of creatures with distinct biological systems and traits that are key sources of bioactive natural compounds. This chapter provided an overview of the most important classes of marine flavonoids, with flavones and flavonols being the most representative. Flavones and flavonols are primarily extracted from plants such as seagrasses, halophytes, and mangroves, with the *Hydrocharitaceae* family having a high incidence. The presence of sugar moieties is frequent in marine flavonoids, which makes them extremely polar. Marine flavonoids attract scientists' attention due to their pharmacological action. Although various research on the biological potential of these marine natural products has been published, the biological potential of the majority of the flavonoids isolated entirely from the marine environment has yet to be fully studied. As a result, future exploitation of these marine natural compounds is predicted to aid Medicinal Chemistry in the development of novel medications with novel modes of action.

KEYWORDS

- **acetylcholinesterase**
- **butyrylcholinesterase**
- **flavonoids**
- **reactive oxygen species**
- **rhabdomyosarcoma**
- **streptomyces**

REFERENCES

Amic, D., Davidovic-Amic, D., Beslo, D., Rastija, V., Lucic, B., & Trinajstic, N. (2007). SAR and QSAR of the antioxidant activity of flavonoids. *Current Medicinal Chemistry, 14*(7), 827–845.

Andersen, O. M., & Markham, K. R. (2005). *Flavonoids: Chemistry, Biochemistry and Applications* (1st eds). CRC Press. Pp. 1256. https://doi.org/10.1201/9781420039443.

Asher, G. N., Vieira, A. J., Weaver, M. A., Dominik, R., Caughey, M., & Hinderliter, A. I. (2012). Effect of hawthorn standardized extract on flow mediated dilation in prehypertensive and mildly hypertensive adults: A randomized, controlled cross-over trial. *BMC Complementary and Alternative Medicine, 12*, 1–7.

Asif, M., & Khodadadi, E. (2013). Medicinal uses and chemistry of flavonoid contents of some common edible tropical plants. *Archives of Advances in Biosciences, 4*(3), 1–20.

Babu, P. V. A., Liu, D., & Gilbert, E. R. (2013). Recent advances in understanding the anti-diabetic actions of dietary flavonoids. *The Journal of Nutritional Biochemistry, 24*(11), 1777–1789.

Beatriz T. Martins, Marta Correia da Silva, Madalena Pinto, Honorina Cidade, & Anake Kijjoa. (2019). Marine natural flavonoids: Chemistry and biological activities. *Natural Product Research, 33*(22), 3260–3272. https://doi.org/10.1080/14786419.2018.1532001.

Behery, F. A., Naeem, Z. E. M., Maatooq, G. T., Amer, M. M., & Ahmed, A. F. (2013). A novel antioxidant phenanthrenoid dimer from *Juncus acutus* L. *Natural Product Research, 27*(2), 155–163.

Behling, E. B., Sendão, M. C., Francescato, H. D. C., Antunes, L. M. G., & Bianchi, M. D. L. P. (2004). Flavonoid Quercetin: Aspectos Gerais E. *Aliment Nutr Brazilian J Food Nutr, 15*, 285–292.

Boeing, T., Tafarelo Moreno, K. G., Gasparotto Junior, A., Mota da Silva, L., & de Souza, P. (2021). Phytochemistry and pharmacology of the genus *Equisetum* (*Equisetaceae*): A narrative review of the species with therapeutic potential for kidney diseases. *Evidence-based Complementary and Alternative Medicine*, 2021, pp. 1–17.

Brum, L. P. (2006). Atividade antiviral dos compostos fenólicos (ácidos ferúlico e transcinâmico) edos flavonoides (quercetina e kaempherol) sobre os herpesvirus bovino 1, herpesvirus bovino 5 e vírus da cinomose canina [thesis, Federal University of Viçosa] https://www.locus.ufv.br/bitstream/123456789/336/1/texto%20completo.pdf.

Buckingham, J., & Munasinghe, V. R. N. (2015). *Dictionary of Flavonoids with CD-ROM.* (1st ed.). CRC Press. Pp. 1199. https://doi.org/10.1201/b18170.

Calderon-Montano, J. M., Burgos-Moron, E., Perez-Guerrero, C., & Lopez-Lazaro, M. (2011). A review on the dietary flavonoid Kaempferol. *Mini Reviews in Medicinal Chemistry, 11*(4), 298–344.

Cerqueira, F., Cordeiro-Da-Silva, A., Araujo, N., Cidade, H., Kijjoa, A., & Nascimento, M. S. J. (2003). Inhibition of lymphocyte proliferation by prenylated flavones: Artelastin as a potent inhibitor. *Life Sciences, 73*, 2321–2334.

Cook, N. C., & Samman, S. (1996). Flavonoids chemistry, metabolism, cardioprotective effects, and dietary sources. *The Journal of Nutritional Biochemistry, 7*(2), 66–76.

Correia-da-Silva, M., Sousa, E., Duarte, B., Marques, F., Cunha-Ribeiro, L. M., & Pinto, M. M. (2011). Dual anticoagulant/antiplatelet persulfated small molecules. *European Journal of Medicinal Chemistry, 46*(6), 2347–2358).

Dewick, P. M. (2002). Medicinal Natural Products: A Biosynthetic Approach. New York, NY: John Wiley & Sons. 552 pages. ISBN: 978–0-470–74168–9.

Dixon, R. A., & Pasinetti, G. M. (2010). Flavonoids and isoflavonoids: From plant biology to agriculture and neuroscience. *Plant Physiology, 154*(2), 453–457.

Dubey, R. S., Verma, N. K., Shukla, A. K., Naidu, M. A. (2021). Diabetes mellitus-a report on antidiabetic medicinal plants and their potent bioactive molecules. *Journal of Medicinal Pharmaceutical & Allied Sciences, 10*(3), 2949–2960.

El-Bondkly, E. A. M., El-Bondkly, A. A. M., & El-Bondkly, A. A. M. (2021). Marine endophytic fungal metabolites: A whole new world of pharmaceutical therapy exploration. *Heliyon, 7*(3), e06362.

Erdman Jr, J. W., Balentine, D., Arab, L., Beecher, G., Dwyer, J. T., Folts, J., & Messina, M. (2007). Flavonoids and heart health: Proceedings of the ILSI North America flavonoids workshop, May 31–June 1, 2005, Washington, DC. *The Journal of Nutrition, 137*(3), 718S–737S.

Fernando, I. P. S., Lee, W., & Ahn, G. (2022). Marine algal flavonoids and phlorotannins; an intriguing frontier of biofunctional secondary metabolites. *Critical Reviews in Biotechnology, 42*(1), 23–45.

Fernando, I. P. S., Ryu, B., Ahn, G., et al. (2020). Therapeutic potential of algal natural products against metabolic syndrome: A review of recent developments. *Trends in Food Science & Technology, 97*, 286–299.

Fischer, G., H€ubner, S. O., Vargas, G. D., & Vidor, T. (2008). Imunomodulação pela própolis. *Arquivos do Instituto Biológico, 75*, 247–253.

George, V. C., Dellaire, G., & Rupasinghe, H. P. V. (2017). Plant flavonoids in cancer chemoprevention: Role in genome stability. *Journal of Nutritional Biochemistry, 45, 1–14.*

González-Paramás, A. M., Ayuda-Durán, B., Martínez, S., González-Manzano, S., & Santos-Buelga, C. (2019). The mechanisms behind the biological activity of flavonoids. *Current Medicinal Chemistry, 26*(39), 6976–6990.

Gu, X., Hao, D., & Xiao, P. (2022). Research progress of Chinese herbal medicine compounds and their bioactivities: Fruitful 2020. *Chinese Herbal Medicines*, *14*(2), 171–186.

Haoujar, I., Cacciola, F., Abrini, J., et al. (2019). The contribution of carotenoids, phenolic compounds, and flavonoids to the antioxidative properties of marine microalgae isolated from Mediterranean Morocco. *Molecules, 24*(22), 4037.

Hozzein, W. N., Mohany, M., Alhawsawi, S. M. M., Zaky, M. Y., Al-Rejaie, S. S., & Alkhalifah, D. H. M. (2021). Flavonoids from marine-derived Actinobacteria as anticancer drugs. *Current Pharmaceutical Design, 27*(4), 505–512.

Ilekuttige Priyan Shanura Fernando, WonWoo Lee, & Ginnae Ahn. (2021). Marine algal flavonoids and phlorotannins; An intriguing frontier of biofunctional secondary metabolites. *Critical Reviews in Biotechnology, 42*(1), 23–45.

Keservani, R. K., & Sharma, A. K. (2014). Flavonoids: Emerging trends and potential health benefits. *Journal of Chinese Pharmaceutical Sciences, 23*(12), 815.

Keservani, R. K., Sharma, A. K., & Kesharwani, R. K. (Eds.). (2020). Nutraceuticals and Dietary Supplements: Applications in Health Improvement and Disease Management, Apple Academic Press, CRC Press. Pp. 1–344. ISBN: 9781771888738.

Keservani, R. K., Sharma, A. K., Kesharwani, R. K., Vyas, N., Raghuvanshi, R., & Jain, S. (2010). Nutraceutical and functional food as future food: A review. *Der Pharmacia Lettre, 2*(1), 106–116.

Lee, S. -H., & Jeon, Y. -J. (2013). Anti-diabetic effects of brown algae derived phlorotannins, marine polyphenols through diverse mechanisms. *Fitoterapia, 86*, 129–136.

Lee, Y. J., Adlercreutzl, H., & Kwon, H. (2006). Quantitative analysis of isoflavones and lignans in sea vegetables consumed in Korea using isotope dilution gas chromatography-mass spectrometry. *Food Science and Biotechnology, 15*, 102–103.

Liu, X., Wang, C-Y., Shao, C-L., et al. (2009). Chemical constituents from *Sargassum pallidum* (Turn.) C. Agardh. *Biochemical Systematics and Ecology, 37*(2), 127–129.

Lopes, G., Andrade, P., & Valent~ao, P. (2016). Phlorotannins: Towards new pharmacological interventions for diabetes mellitus type 2. *Molecules, 22*(1), 56.

López-Lázaro, M. (2009). Distribution and biological activities of the flavonoid luteolin. *Mini Reviews in Medicinal Chemistry, 9*(1), 31–59.

Ma, J., Zhang, X-L., Wang, Y., Zheng, J-Y., Wang, C-Y., & Shao, C-L. (2017). Aspergivones A and B, two new flavones isolated from a gorgonian-derived *Aspergillus candidus* fungus. *Natural Product Research, 32*(1), 32–36.

Mao, X. Y., Jin, M. Z., Chen, J. F., Zhou, H. H., & Jin, W. L. (2018). Live or let die: Neuroprotective and anti-cancer effects of nutraceutical antioxidants. *Pharmacology & Therapeutics, 183*, 137–151.

Markham, K. R., & Porter, L. J. (1969). Flavonoids in the green algae (*Chlorophyta*). *Phytochemistry, 8*(9), 1777–1781.

Martins, B. T., Correia da Silva, M., Pinto, M., Cidade, H., & Kijjoa, A. (2019). Marine natural flavonoids: Chemistry and biological activities. *Natural Product Research, 33*(22), 3260–3272.

Mércia Marques Jucá, Francisco Mauricio Sales Cysne Filho, Jamily Cunha de Almeida, Dara da Silva Mesquita, Jéssica Rodrigues de Moraes Barriga, Kátia Cilene Ferreira Dias, Talita Matias Barbosa, Luna Costa Vasconcelos, Luzia Kalyne Almeida Moreira Leal, José Eduardo Ribeiro, & Silvânia Maria Mendes Vasconcelos. (2018). Flavonoids: Biological activities and therapeutic potential. *Natural Product Research, 34*(5), 692–705.

Moutinho, M. S. S., Aragão, S., Carmo, D., Casaca, F., Silva, S., Ribeiro, J., Sousa, H., Pires, I., & Queiroga, F. (2018). Curcumin and rutin down-regulate cyclooxygenase-2 and reduce tumor-associated inflammation in HPV16-transgenic mice. *Anticancer Research, 38*, 1461–1466.

Munhoz, A., & Frode, T. S. (2018). Isolated compounds from natural products with potential antidiabetic activity-A systematic review. *Current Diabetes Reviews, 14*(1), 36–106.

Musialik, M., Kuzmicz, R., Pawłowski, T. S., & Litwinienko, G. (2009). Acidity of hydroxyl groups: An overlooked influence on antiradical properties of flavonoids. *The Journal of Organic Chemistry, 74*(7), 2699–2709.

Norris, L. A. (2003). Blood coagulation. *Best Practice & Research Clinical Obstetrics & Gynaecology, 17*(3), 369–383.

Oliveira, K. A. de M., Oliveira, G. V. de, Batalini, C., Rosalem, J. A., & Ribeiro, L. S. (2013). Atividade antimicrobiana e quantificação de Flavonoides e Fenóis totais em diferentes extratos de Própolis. *Seminários em Ciências Biológicas e da Saúde, 33*, 211–222.

Onofrejova, L., Vašíčková, J., Klejdus, B., et al. (2010). Bioactive phenols in algae: The application of pressurized liquid and solid-phase extraction techniques. *Journal of Pharmaceutical and Biomedical Analysis, 51*(2), 464–470.

Perez-Vizcaino, F., & Duarte, J. (2010). Flavanols and cardiovascular disease. *Molecular Aspects of Medicine, 31*(6), 478–494.

Portinho, J. A., Zimmermann, L. M., Bruck, M. R., et al. (2012). Beneficial effects of aci. *International Journal of Nutrology, 5*, 15–20.

Priyan, I., Shanura Fernando, Lee, W. W., & Ahn, G. (2021). Marine algal flavonoids and phlorotannins; an intriguing frontier of bifunctional secondary metabolites. *Critical Reviews in Biotechnology, 42*(1), 1–24.

Rajauria, G. (2018). Optimization and validation of reverse phase HPLC method for qualitative and quantitative assessment of polyphenols in seaweed. *Journal of Pharmaceutical and Biomedical Analysis, 148*, 230–237.

Rane, B. R., Bharath, M. S., Patil, R. R., Keservani, R. K., & Jain, A. S. (2020b). Novel Approaches in Nutraceuticals. In R. K. Kesharwani, R. K. Keservani, A. K. Sharma (Eds.), *Enhancing the Therapeutic Efficacy of Herbal Formulations through Novel Drug Delivery Systems* (pp. 241–266). IGI Global International Publisher.

Rane, B. R., Patil, A. S., Keservani, R. K., & Jain, A. S. (2020a). Novel Approaches in Herbal Formulation. In R. K. Kesharwani, R. K. Keservani, A. K. Sharma (Eds.), *Enhancing the Therapeutic Efficacy of Herbal Formulations through Novel Drug Delivery Systems* (pp. 43–68). IGI Global International Publisher.

Rane, B. R., Tadavi, S. A., & Keservani, R. K. (2020c). Naturopathy. In A. K. Sharma, R. K. Keservani, S. P. Gautam (Eds.), *Herbal Product Development* (pp. 321–347). CRC Press, Taylor & Francis Group.

Razavi, S. M., Zahri, S., Zarrini, G., Nazemiyeh, H., & Mohammadi, S. (2009). Biological activity of quercetin-3-O-glucoside, a known plant flavonoid. *Russian Journal of Bioorganic Chemistry, 35*(3), 376–378.

Roleda, M. Y., Marfaing, H., Desnica, N., et al. (2019). Variations in polyphenol and heavy metal contents of wild-harvested and cultivated seaweed bulk biomass: Health risk assessment and implication for food applications. *Food Control, 95*, 121–134.

Roleda, M. Y., Skjermo, J., Marfaing, H., et al. (2018). Iodine content in bulk biomass of wild-harvested and cultivated edible seaweeds: Inherent variations determine species-specific daily allowable consumption. *Food Chemistry, 254*, 333–339.

Sabina, H., & Aliya, R. (2009). Seaweed as a new source of flavone, scutellarein 4-methyl-ether. *Pakistan Journal of Botany, 41*(4), 1927–1930.

Salehi, B., Venditti, A., Sharifi-Rad, M., Kręgiel, D., Sharifi-Rad, J., Durazzo, A., & Antolak, H. (2019). The therapeutic potential of apigenin. *International Journal of Molecular Sciences, 20*(6), 1305.

Sharma, A. K., Keservani, R. K., & Gautam, S. P. (2020). Herbal Product Development. (1st ed.). Apple Academic Press. CRC Press, Taylor & Francis Group. Pp. 376. https://doi.org/10.1201/9781003003182.

Soares, D. J., Moura Neto, L. G., Damaceno, M. N., Souza, P. A., Braga, R. C., & Brasil, I. M. (2015). Atividade anti-inflamatória de produtos de origem vegetal. *Saúde em Revista, 15*, 33–45.

Tasdemir, D., Kaiser, M., Brun, R., Yardley, V., Schmidt, T. J., & Tosun, F. (2006). Antitrypanosomal and antileishmanial activities of flavonoids and their analogues: In vitro, in vivo, structure-activity relationship, and quantitative structure-activity relationship studies. *Antimicrobial Agents and Chemotherapy, 50*, 1352–1364.

Ververidis, F., Trantas, E., Douglas, C., et al. (2007). Biotechnology of flavonoids and other phenylpropanoid-derived natural products. Part I: Chemical diversity, impacts on plant biology and human health. *Biotechnology Journal, 2*(10), 1214–1234.

Wang, J., Huang, Z. G., Cao, H., Wang, Y. T., Hui, P., Hoo, C., & Li, S. P. (2008). Screening of anti-platelet aggregation agents from *Panax not ginseng* using human platelet extraction and HPLC–DAD–ESI-MS/MS. *Journal of Separation Science, 55*, 1173–1180.

Winter, J., Moore, L. H., Dowell, V. R., & Bokkenheuser, V. D. (1989). C-ring cleavage of flavonoids by human intestinal bacteria. *Applied and Environmental Microbiology, 55*, 1203–1208.

Xiao, J. (2017). Dietary flavonoid aglycones and their glycosides: Which show better biological significance? *Critical Reviews in Food Science and Nutrition, 57*(9), 1874–1905.

Yashin, A., Yashin, Y., Xia, X., & Nemzer, B. (2017). Antioxidant activity of spices and their impact on human health: A review. *Antioxidants, 6*(3), 70.

Zhao, G., Gao, H., Qiu, J., Lu, W., & Wei, X. (2010). The molecular mechanism of protective effects of grape seed proanthocyanidin extract on reperfusion arrhythmias in rats in vivo. *Biological and Pharmaceutical Bulletin, 33*, 759–767.

Zuiter, A. S. (2014). Proanthocyanidin: Chemistry and biology: From phenolic compounds to proanthocyanidins. In *Reference Module in Chemistry, Molecular Sciences and Chemical Engineering*, pp. 1–5. Elsevier.

INDEX

A

Absorption, 10, 15, 54, 55, 59–61, 131, 140, 155, 170, 172, 207, 208, 249, 285, 286
Acetate, 60, 157, 206, 316
Acetic acid, 58
Acetylcholinesterase (AChE), 317, 321
Active
  biological effects, 201
  components, 79, 177, 320
  food components, 3
  ingredients, 41, 270
Acute
  coronary events & syndromes, 34, 128
  rheumatic fever (ARF), 31, 181, 192
  viral nasopharyngitis, 79
Acyclic carotenoid, 142
Acyl-CoA: cholesterol acyltransferase (ACAT), 208
Acylglycerols, 298
Adenine monophosphate (AMP), 243
Adhesion molecules, 154, 271, 299
Adipocytes, 206
Adipogenesis, 243, 246
Adipokine, 208, 281
Adiponectin, 154
Adipose tissue, 77, 154, 187
Adrenal glands, 141
Adulteration, 185
Aerva lanata, 234, 237, 247
Aged garlic extract (AGE), 70–72, 74–77, 79, 80, 187, 245, 283, 284
Aging, 10, 17, 29, 32, 36, 41, 89, 184, 186, 191
  population, 10, 32, 191
Agro-climatic conditions, 97, 236
Alanine aminotransferase (ALT), 204
Albumin, 171, 225
Alcohol, 28, 31, 56, 93, 178, 247, 298
  abuse, 28, 320
  consumption, 56
  misuse, 178
Aldosterone secretion, 280
Algae, 312, 317, 318, 320
Alk(en)ylresorcinols (ARs), 239
Alkali extractions, 55
Alkaloids, 10, 93, 95, 98, 158, 241, 246
Alkylresorcinols (ARs), 239, 240, 253
All-cause death, 77, 186
Allergic responses, 79, 211
Allicin, 11, 38, 41, 72, 170, 244, 267, 283
Alliin, 11, 72, 244, 283
Alliinase enzyme, 11, 72, 244
Allium
  cepa, 234, 237, 245
  sativum, 187, 234, 237, 244, 253
Alpha
  glucosidase inhibition, 247
  linolenic acid (ALA), 6, 18, 298, 301
  tocopherol, 108, 109
Aluminum (Al), 93
American diet, 5, 140
Amino
  acids, 10, 93, 95, 96, 184, 247, 270, 320
  groups, 311
Aminodeoxy sugar, 313
Aminotransferase, 211
Anaerobic conditions, 58
Analgesic, 241–243
Angina pectoris, 41, 124, 180, 277, 282
Angiogenesis, 207, 227, 303
Angiotensin, 12, 129, 132, 171, 203, 209, 227–229, 245, 271, 273, 280, 284, 317
  converting enzyme (ACE), 129, 132, 203, 209, 227–229, 245, 273, 284
    inhibitor (ACE-I), 228, 273, 284
  I-converting enzyme (ACE-I), 317
  receptor blockers, 228
Animal
  models, 55, 191, 207, 210, 272, 278, 288, 305
  origin, 108, 298
Anthocyanidins, 221

Anthocyanin, 6, 169, 223, 245, 275
Antiaging, 86, 210, 318, 319
property, 319
Antiangiogenic activity, 207
Anti-atherogenic, 189, 210
action, 189
Anti-atherosclerotic, 129, 145, 188, 203, 208, 241, 242, 277
effect, 188, 242, 246
molecule, 203
Antibiotic
activities, 88
effects, 92
Anticancer, 96, 97, 123, 141, 152, 184, 223, 241, 242, 314, 316, 317, 319
drug combinations, 184
properties, 123, 141
Anticarcinogenic, 54, 96, 278
effect, 96
properties, 242, 278
Anticatatonic activities, 249
Anticoagulant, 33, 314
Anti-collagen antibodies, 31
Antidiabetic, 11, 54, 97, 152, 240, 242, 247–249, 252, 277, 314, 317
activity, 247, 248
effects, 11
Antidiarrheal, 86, 92
activities, 92
Antiestrogenic activity, 10
Anti-feedant properties, 314
Antifibrinolytic activity, 245
Antifungal, 86, 92, 248, 319
Anti-hair fall, 97
Anti-hyperlipidemic properties, 244
Antihypertensive, 12, 39, 41, 72–74, 129, 145, 207, 241, 244, 245, 269–272, 277, 284, 286
effect, 12, 39, 73, 207, 241, 271, 272, 277, 286
mechanism, 129
medications, 74, 129
properties, 245
therapy, 72
Anti-infective properties, 38
Anti-inflammatory, 6, 8, 11, 13, 14, 17, 18, 38, 39, 41, 86, 89, 92, 95, 97, 123, 128, 130, 131, 139, 145, 155, 158, 169, 188, 189, 201, 206, 207, 234, 236, 238–243, 246, 248–250, 252, 270, 271, 281, 284, 287, 297, 314, 317–319
activity, 14, 155, 243, 248, 318
effect, 6, 17, 128, 281
foods, 250
potential, 155, 248
properties, 13, 18, 38, 86, 89, 123, 131, 191, 207, 238, 248, 271, 287
qualities, 189
Antilipidemic effect, 204
Antimicrobial, 97, 158, 201, 206, 250, 269, 270, 314, 317–319
activity, 250, 318, 319
Antioxidant, 3, 5–8, 10, 11, 13–18, 27, 38, 39, 41, 51, 69, 71, 72, 85, 86, 89, 93, 95, 97, 103, 108–112, 121, 122, 124, 126, 127, 129–131, 139–141, 144–147, 151, 154, 156, 158, 159, 167–171, 173, 177, 186, 188, 190, 192, 201, 203–207, 221, 223, 233–236, 238–240, 242, 243, 245–253, 267, 270, 271, 273, 275, 277–279, 282–284, 287, 297, 311, 314–317, 319, 320
action, 141
activity, 13, 14, 38, 109, 129, 240, 243, 247, 271, 273, 275, 315, 316
characteristics, 186
compounds, 8, 10, 156, 251, 320
defense
mechanisms, 279
system, 203
deficiency, 279
effect, 144, 204, 283, 316, 319
enzyme, 170, 203, 205
activity, 11, 207, 243, 246
impact, 129
intake, 126
metabolism, 111
phytochemicals, 245
phytonutrients, 171
polyphenols, 7
potential, 11, 122
property, 5, 6, 11, 13, 15, 39, 103, 110, 124, 127, 144, 159, 245, 248, 249, 271
reduction, 111
rich tomato-based juice, 126
status, 71

supplementation, 18
vitamins, 103, 108, 111, 112
Antioxidative, 39, 189, 205
properties, 189
Anti-parasitic, 318
activity, 319
Antiplatelet, 145, 187, 244, 245, 283
activity, 283
aggregation, 245
effects, 187
Anti-proliferative, 39, 145, 206
Anti-sleep disorders, 168
Antithrombotic, 6, 188–190, 297, 303
Antitumor, 11, 183, 201, 240, 248, 249, 269, 314
activities, 249
pathways, 183
properties, 201
Antiviral, 96, 97, 201, 223, 319
activity, 97
agent, 97
properties, 96, 97
Anti-worm properties, 241
Aorta, 36, 38, 77, 129, 191, 202
Aortic
aneurysm, 38
atherosclerosis, 9
stenosis, 32, 36
Apigenin, 86, 89, 314–316, 318
7-O-rutinoside, 318
Apis mellifera, 209
Apitherapy, 201, 204, 210
Apolipoprotein profile, 7
Apoptosis, 127, 139, 145, 206, 227, 284, 303
Apoptotic markers, 206
Aqueous garlic extract, 72, 245
Arabinoxylans, 239
Arachidonic acid, 156, 247, 273, 319
metabolism, 247, 319
Arginine, 7, 93, 247
Armolipid plus, 277
Arrhythmia, 36, 127, 203, 319
Arterial
blood pressure, 223
compliance, 280
coronary diseases, 300
elastic properties, 144
function, 8
hypertension, 127–129
stiffness, 145, 276
wall, 57, 143, 183, 299
Artery
dilation, 9
rigidity, 286
Arthritis, 4, 28, 30, 152, 298–300
Asafetida, 249, 252
Ascorbate, 111
Ascorbic acid, 109, 171, 205, 279, 280
Aspartate aminotransferase (AST), 204
Aspergillus candidus, 315
Astaxanthin, 10, 277
Asthma, 3, 18, 130, 169, 248
Asymmetric dimethylarginine (ADMA), 203, 208, 279
Asymptomatic, 33, 76
adults, 76
Atheroma, 34
Atheromatous constriction, 34
Atheroprotective benefits, 191
Atherosclerosis, 6, 11, 12, 38, 39, 41, 52, 70, 77, 80, 110, 123, 124, 128, 129, 131, 140, 143, 156, 180, 182, 188, 190, 192, 202, 206–209, 211, 235, 238, 240, 245, 246, 252, 268, 271, 274, 281, 282
progression, 77, 206
Atherosclerotic
conditions, 6, 14
coronary artery, 181
lesions, 11, 191, 274
plaque, 52, 127, 128, 131, 179, 203, 206
Atherothrombotic events, 15
Athletes, 185, 244
Atrial
fibrillation (AF), 37, 129, 182
flutter, 37
septal defect, 36
Autoantibodies, 31
Autoimmune
disorders, 152
reaction, 31
Autophagy, 207
Avial, 249, 251, 252
Avicennia marina, 315
Ayurveda, 233, 236–238, 244
Ayurvedic
medicine, 69, 80
treatments, 237

B

B complex vitamins, 71, 251
Babylonian, 236
Bacterial cell walls, 58
Bacteriostatic properties, 159, 204
Bacteroides, 58
Barley, 55, 60, 222, 236
Baroreflexes, 225
Baseline blood pressure, 73, 276
Bee
 bread, 201
 pollen, 201, 204, 208, 209
 products, 201, 204, 210, 211
 venom, 201
Benzoxazinoids (BXs), 239, 253
Berberine, 277
Bergamot essential oil (BEO), 159
Berry, 6, 157, 169, 222, 275
 fruits, 169
Beta
 blockers, 110
 carotene, 12–14, 109, 126, 140, 144, 250, 251
 glycinin, 8
 sitosterol oleate, 286
Beverage, 9, 16, 85, 98, 122, 169, 222, 274, 275, 287
Bifidobacterium, 58, 172
 longum, 58
Bile, 40, 54, 58–61, 170, 209, 210, 271, 272, 285, 286
 acid, 40, 58–61, 170, 272
  binding, 209, 210
  capacity, 210
 salt
  deconjugase activity, 58
  hydrolase (BSH), 54
  micelles, 285
Biliary
 cholesterol, 155, 286
 micelles, 286
Bilirubin, 171, 271
Biliverdin reductase (BVR), 271
Binding capacity, 59, 171
Bioactive, 3, 5, 7–14, 18, 72, 121, 125, 127, 129, 131, 142, 155, 179, 205, 209, 235, 239, 243, 244, 246, 268–271, 283, 285, 306, 311, 312, 317–320
 chemicals, 125, 235, 311
 component, 3, 5, 7–12, 18, 72, 155, 244
 compounds, 5, 7, 9, 12, 14, 18, 131, 243, 244, 246, 283, 320
 constituents, 269, 270
 dietary elements, 129
 food
  components, 127
  elements, 121
 molecules, 317–319
 natural compounds, 312, 320
 peptides, 269–271
 phytochemicals, 239
 potentials, 285
 substances, 311
 supermolecule mediators, 306
Bioassay-guided chemical fractionation, 315
Biochemical
 compounds, 320
 markers, 204
 processes, 317
Biochemistry, 27, 103, 167, 177, 201, 221, 297
Biodiversity, 236
 species, 236
Biological
 activity, 154, 158, 201, 204, 240, 269, 311, 319
 effects, 221, 236
 environments, 311
 potential, 321
 properties, 201
 resources, 320
 systems, 127, 183, 320
Biomarkers, 78, 79
Biomolecules, 320
Biophytum sensitivum, 234, 237, 247, 248
Biopolymers, 270
Biosynthesis, 241, 320
 mechanism, 320
Black
 chickpeas, 250
 grape, 169
 tea, 9, 13, 85, 86, 89, 92, 275
Bleeding, 79, 187, 190, 207
 time, 190
Blood
 antioxidant levels, 144
 cholesterol, 18, 58, 60, 86, 206, 210, 240, 241
  concentrations, 60, 240

levels, 18, 58, 60
lowering, 241
circulation, 36, 38, 203
clot, 33, 37, 108, 129, 143, 179, 180
clotting, 33, 108
factors, 108
flow, 16, 31, 34, 52, 77, 179, 180, 182, 190, 305
irregularities, 190
glucose, 246
lipid, 8, 38, 57, 189, 209
concentrations, 304
levels, 285
profiles, 40
phospholipids, 186
plasma triglyceride levels, 304
pressure (BP), 3, 4, 6, 8–13, 16–18, 38, 39, 41, 57, 73, 74, 122, 129–131, 171, 177, 187, 189, 202, 205, 225, 227, 228, 238, 239, 244, 245, 247, 251, 267, 269, 272, 273, 275–281, 284, 286, 287
decrease, 279
lowering mechanisms, 239
outcomes, 73
reduction, 73, 122, 228
regulation, 272, 280
rheology, 40, 41
sugar
concentrations, 242
control, 274
vessel, 31, 122, 179, 180, 182, 245, 299, 306
disorders, 30, 123
function, 189
health, 187
narrowing, 180
Blueberries, 221, 275
Blue-green algae (BGA), 269, 270, 289
Body
aches, 85
build, 56
fat, 11, 209, 242
percentages, 242
mass index, 11
odor, 78
weight, 12, 17, 209, 242, 251
Bone, 38, 103
disorders, 30
metabolism, 109
mineral density, 13
mineralization, 39, 123
Boost energy, 85
Botanical products, 184
Bovine thrombin, 205
Bran, 60, 222, 238–240, 251
fractions, 240
husk, 238
layers, 239
Breast cancer, 13, 123, 170
Broken wheat, 234, 237, 239
Brown seaweeds, 317
Buttermilk, 250–252
Butylated hydroxytoluene (BHT), 315
Butyric acid, 58
Butyrylcholinesterase (BChE), 317, 321

C

Cacao beans, 221
Cafestol, 8
Caffeic acid, 11, 86, 89, 169
Caffeine, 8, 9, 89, 93, 95, 96
Calcium, 17, 39, 41, 71, 93, 108, 127, 171, 172, 185, 187, 247, 250–252, 277, 281, 284, 298
absorption, 39
management, 127
metabolism, 108
mobilization, 187
oxalate urolithiasis, 247
phosphate homeostasis, 171, 281
Camellia sinensis, 86, 87, 93, 95, 98, 188
Cancer, 3–5, 10, 12, 13, 17, 18, 28, 30, 54, 71, 96, 109, 139, 144, 152, 157, 168, 183, 184, 186, 202, 238, 239, 268, 298–300, 303, 316, 317, 320
cells, 303
patients, 10, 54
prevention, 96, 109
therapy, 183
treatment, 184
Capsules, 29, 74, 184
Carbohydrates, 10, 17, 55, 58, 93, 96, 251, 252, 283
Carbon atom, 185, 186, 298
Carboxylic acid composition, 305
Cardamom, 88, 89

Cardiac
  arrhythmia, 36, 181, 182, 205
  birth abnormality, 36
  channel mutation, 36
  disease, 34, 42, 76, 243
  dysfunction, 183
  effects, 124, 284
  health, 177, 234, 237
  hypertrophy, 41, 128
  injury, 206
  muscle hyperplasia, 33
  output, 32, 33, 40, 178, 179, 225
  remodeling, 127
  valves, 31
Cardio protective effect, 96
Cardiogenic shock, 181
Cardiomax brand garlic oil, 73
Cardiometabolic
  disorders, 9
  risk factors, 235
Cardiomyocytes, 39, 183
Cardiopathy risk, 55
Cardio-protection, 223
Cardio-protective
  actions, 228
  agent, 177, 204
  characteristics, 187
  effect, 7, 8, 42, 223, 245, 247, 252, 273, 319
  foods, 236
  mechanisms, 211
  nature, 227
  potential, 234, 252
  properties, 131
  role, 11
Cardiospermum halicacabum, 234, 237, 247, 248
Cardiotonic effects, 244
Cardiovascular, 3, 4, 6–10, 12–14, 17, 18, 27, 28, 30, 37–39, 41, 42, 51, 52, 54, 59, 69–71, 76, 78–80, 85, 86, 97, 103, 108, 109, 112, 121–132, 139, 140, 143–145, 147, 151, 152, 157, 158, 162, 167, 171, 172, 177–181, 183, 184, 186–192, 201, 203, 205, 209, 211, 223, 225, 228, 233–236, 238–240, 243, 245, 246, 252, 253, 267–269, 271–273, 275, 277, 279–282, 285, 289, 298, 299, 314, 319
  benefits, 85
  conditions, 41
  disease (CVD), 3, 4, 6, 7, 9, 10, 12, 13, 18, 27, 28, 30, 38, 39, 41, 42, 51, 52, 54, 59, 69–71, 76, 78–80, 97, 122–128, 130–132, 139, 140, 143–145, 147, 152, 157, 158, 162, 177–181, 183, 184, 187–189, 191, 192, 201, 205, 209, 223, 233–236, 238, 239, 243, 245, 246, 252, 253, 267, 268, 271, 272, 275, 280, 285, 289, 298, 299
    mortality, 145, 188
    prevention, 42, 79, 132
    risk factors, 41, 76, 191
  disorders, 28, 121, 122, 129
  event, 103, 108, 112, 124, 167, 171, 172, 191, 223, 225, 228, 279, 282
  health, 122, 131, 145, 187, 277
  mortality, 9, 109, 189
  prevention, 269
  problems, 37, 121, 129
  protective effects, 281
  reserve, 184
  risk, 8, 17, 27, 129, 183, 184, 191, 253, 267, 277
    factors, 129, 183, 184, 191, 253, 267
  system, 14, 39, 80, 122, 128, 130, 205, 211, 279, 314
Carditis, 181
Carminative effects, 242
Carnosine, 159
Carotene, 58, 109, 124, 126, 140, 143, 145, 147, 282
  rich diet, 145
Carotenoid, 5, 10, 12–14, 18, 40, 95, 103, 108, 122, 124–127, 131, 139–143, 146, 147, 171, 239, 269, 270, 282, 283
  pigment, 122, 127
  synthesis, 142
Cashew nuts, 250
Catalase, 203, 243
Catecholamine, 33, 207, 243
  levels, 33
Cell
  death, 183, 207
  membrane, 11, 40, 108, 188, 304
    phospholipids, 304
  migration, 35, 207
  walls, 59

Cellular function, 40
Cellulose, 55, 93
Central nervous system, 249
Cereals, 16, 29, 122, 168, 221, 237, 274
Cerebral blood flow (CBF), 31
Cerebrovascular, 7, 31, 179, 182, 235
  disease, 179, 182, 235
  illness, 31
Ceruloplasmin, 171
C-glycosides, 312, 313
Chalcones, 221
Chavicine, 246
Chemical
  inhibitors, 159
  makeup, 211
  nature, 152
  preservatives, 159
Chemokine, 111
Chemopreventive, 243, 317
  drugs, 317
Chemotherapy, 184
Chest
  discomfort, 35
  pain, 180
Chlorine, 311, 313
  atom, 313
Chlorogenic acid, 86, 89, 169
Chlorophyll, 95, 96
Chloroplast, 141
  membrane, 300
Chocolate, 9, 10, 13, 18, 38, 275, 276
  flavonoids, 38
Cholesterol, 4–9, 11, 12, 14, 15, 17, 38–41, 51–54, 57–62, 70, 75, 88, 92, 111, 127–129, 143, 144, 155, 157, 168, 179, 180, 187, 205, 206, 210, 238, 240–242, 244–246, 269, 274, 285–287, 304
  absorption, 15, 58, 210, 241, 242, 269, 285–287
  accumulation, 129
  assimilation, 58, 286
  binding, 58
  biosynthesis, 187
  control, 168
  deposition, 57
  elimination, 285
  esters, 285
  imbalance, 54
  level, 4, 6, 8, 11, 12, 17, 38, 51, 52, 54, 57, 59, 75, 92, 155, 240, 245, 274, 304
  lowering, 7, 14, 241, 285
    activity, 241
    effect, 14
    properties, 285
  metabolism, 180, 238, 244, 286, 287
  metabolites, 40
  production, 127
  reduction, 53, 58, 61
  synthesis, 129, 157
  transport, 206
  uptake, 246
Cholesteryl esters (CEs), 298
Cholic acid, 58
Chordae tendineae (CT), 31
Chronic
  cardiovascular conditions, 268
  diseases, 3, 17, 18, 30, 202, 239
  heart failure, 190
  illness, 3, 5, 9, 204
  inflammation, 144
  inflammatory
    disease, 238
    disorders, 30
  non-communicable diseases, 279
  obstructive pulmonary disease, 234
  poor diet, 233
  renal failure, 299
Chrysin, 205–207
Cigarette
  smoking, 52, 56, 61, 180
  use, 178
Cinnamon, 169, 170
Citrus
  bergamot, 154
  fruits, 6, 159, 221
Clinical
  evidence, 160, 189, 210
  implications, 132, 174
  manifestations, 35
  measure, 78
  prognosticators, 80
  research, 42
  significance, 32
  studies, 42, 171, 190, 191, 239, 244
  trial, 14–16, 18, 38, 70, 71, 74, 79, 109, 112, 122, 123, 155, 168, 210, 269, 273, 284
Clostridium, 58

Clove, 72, 88, 89, 169
Coagulation, 70, 79, 108, 182, 299, 314
  cascade, 314
  factors, 70, 182
  malfunction, 79
Cocoa, 9, 13, 38, 41, 168, 275–277
  flavanols, 276
Coconut
  kernel protein (CKP), 247
  milk, 234, 237, 247, 250
  oil, 249, 250
Cocos nucifera L., 247
Coenzyme Q (CoQ), 41, 177, 188
Collagen, 109, 207
  synthesis, 109
Colon cancer, 172
Complementary medicines, 73, 185
Computed tomography (CT), 76, 80
Congenital
  abnormalities, 35
  cardiac disease, 35
  heart
    disease, 35, 52, 179, 235
    disorders, 178
Conjugated dienes (CD), 126, 132
Connective tissue, 37, 38
  disorder, 37
Consumption, 5, 6, 8, 10, 13, 17, 39, 40, 54, 60, 86, 122, 124, 130, 131, 151, 186, 187, 189, 204, 209, 223, 238–240, 244, 246, 253, 272, 275–278, 280, 282, 287, 297, 300, 301
Conventional
  drugs, 11, 160
  milling, 238
Corals, 312
Coriander, 170, 249, 252
Coronary arteries
Coronary
  artery, 52, 76, 77, 157, 244
  atherosclerosis, 144
  blood supply, 181
  calcium (CAC), 69, 80, 187
  disease (CAD), 33, 34, 76, 80, 123, 139, 144, 156, 162, 180, 186, 189, 268, 278, 281, 289, 299
  heart disease (CHD), 14, 51, 52, 56, 60, 61, 77, 109, 128, 129, 140, 146, 147, 169, 171, 179, 180, 186, 190, 235, 239, 240, 278, 297
  insufficiency, 124, 282
  occlusion, 181
  spasm, 180
  syndromes, 181
  thrombosis, 180, 181
Cosmetics, 169, 209, 312, 320
COVID-19, 53, 97, 202
C-phycocyanin, 40, 272, 273
Creatine kinase MB (CK-MB), 204
Culinary aromatic plants, 242
Cultural heritage, 236
Cumin, 234, 237, 242, 252
  seeds, 234, 237, 242
Cuminum cyminum, 234, 237, 242
Curculigo orchioides, 234, 237, 247, 248
Curcumin, 38, 39, 41, 154, 158
Curry leaves, 249, 250, 252
Cyanobacterium, 40, 269, 270
Cyclooxygenase (COX), 11, 211, 223, 243, 246, 248, 273, 305, 319
  2 (COX-2), 243, 248, 273, 305, 319
Cymbopogon, 86, 90, 92
  citratus, 86, 90
Cynodon dactylon, 234, 237, 247, 248
Cysteine, 72, 158, 283
Cytokine, 77, 154, 157, 186
  production, 33
Cytosolic calcium, 225
Cytotoxic, 159, 183, 223
  effect, 159
Cytotoxicity, 316

D

Dairy products, 16, 54, 104, 108, 172
Dark chocolate, 5, 9, 10, 276
Dasapushpam, 234, 237, 252
D-dimer testing, 33
De novo lipogenesis (DNL), 208
Decameric peptide, 272
Deep
  loam soil, 93
  vein thrombosis, 178, 179, 182
  venous thrombosis (DVT), 33, 34
Dehydroepiandrosterone sulfate (DHEA-S), 209, 210
Delta tocotrienols, 154, 157

Desaturation, 298, 302
method, 302
Detoxification, 85, 240, 251
Diabetes, 4, 18, 28, 30, 32, 34, 41, 54–57, 128, 129, 144, 157, 168, 183, 184, 202, 206, 208, 225, 238, 239, 241, 245, 252, 267, 268, 279, 300
induced cardiovascular disorders, 241
mellitus, 28, 34, 184, 202, 239, 267, 279
Diabetic
cardiac myopathy, 241
group, 284
nephropathy, 41
patients, 75, 243
women, 239
Diagnosis, 28, 33, 37, 38
Diallyl
disulfide (DADS), 12, 72, 283
sulfide (DAS), 283
trisulfide (DATS), 72, 283
Diastolic
blood pressure, 70, 187, 273, 276, 277, 279
function, 273, 282
Dietary
antioxidants, 58, 140, 171
approaches, 16, 42, 59, 167
assessment methods, 190
changes, 223, 268
cholesterol intake, 286
components, 17, 18, 58
constituents, 184
consumption, 278
deficiency, 104
factors, 4, 27
fat uptake, 179
fiber, 12, 51, 54, 55, 57, 60, 62, 139, 158, 168, 170, 173, 238–240, 249, 251, 252
flavonoids, 315
functional components, 287
habits, 4, 159
ingredient, 184
intake, 159, 278, 279
items, 179
lycopene, 122, 123, 131, 142
management, 167
modifications, 238, 268
patterns, 3, 5, 15, 178
phytochemicals, 234, 253
polyphenols, 223
protein, 209, 210
recommendations, 61
reference intake (DRI), 170, 173
sources, 108, 141
strategies, 18, 42
Supplement Health and Education Act (DSHEA), 179, 184, 185, 202
to stop hypertension (DASH), 16, 167
treatments, 27
variables, 70
whole grains, 8
Digestion, 55, 85, 141, 169, 250–252, 315
Digestive
enzymes, 170, 285
juice acids, 59
problems, 242
process, 252
system, 171, 238
tract, 15
Diode array detector, 222
Diphenyl-picrylhydrazyl (DPPH), 315
Disability-adjusted life years (DALYs), 4, 31, 143
Docosahexaenoic acid (DHA), 6, 7, 18, 185, 186, 189, 297, 298, 300–303, 305, 306
Double
blind, 73–77, 124, 223, 280, 282
bond, 142, 186, 285, 298
Dyslipidemia, 27, 41, 78, 152, 154, 157, 159, 160, 162, 179, 184, 235, 267
Dysphagia, 78
Dysplastic syndrome, 182
Dyspnea, 32

E

Eclipta prostata, 237, 247, 248
Edema, 31–33, 248
Eicosapentaenoic acid (EPA), 6, 18, 185, 189, 246, 298, 301
Electrocardiogram parameters, 203
Electron
spin resonance spectroscopy, 315, 316
transport chain, 188
Emilia sonchifolia, 234, 237, 247, 248
Endosperm, 238, 239
Endothelial
apoptosis, 110

cells, 9, 13, 39, 110, 183, 202, 207, 226, 227, 271, 299
damage, 33, 129
dysfunction, 6, 14, 39, 124, 144, 151, 155, 156, 189, 207–209, 228, 235, 268, 282, 297, 299, 304, 306
effects, 145
function, 15, 40, 124, 131, 202, 209, 272, 277–280, 282, 283, 286, 299, 302, 305
injury, 179
nitric oxide synthase, 156, 202, 203, 227
oxidative stress, 239
protective, 188
vasodilator function, 209
Endothelium, 31, 33, 110, 122, 123, 129, 183, 187, 189, 203, 207, 245, 272, 281, 299, 302
dependent vasorelaxation, 187, 207, 272
Epicardial adipose tissue (EAT), 77, 281
Epicatechin (EC), 9, 93–95, 188, 245, 275
3-gallate (ECG), 9, 93, 275
gallate, 95, 188
Epidemiological
data, 131
evidence, 12, 143
research, 70
studies, 4, 9, 14, 18, 61, 122, 128, 129, 131, 279, 299
Epidural hematoma (EDH), 79
Epigallocatechin (EGC), 9, 86, 93–96, 98, 155, 188, 275
gallate (EGCG), 9, 86, 93, 95, 96, 98, 188, 155, 275
Epidemiological
evidence, 12
studies, 128
Epigenetics, 172
Estradiol (E2), 210
Ethanolic extract, 206
European
population, 123
societies of hypertension and cardiology, 77
Union (EU), 34
Evolvulus alsinoides, 234, 237, 247, 249

F

Fabaceae family, 241
Fat soluble vitamins, 108
Fatty
acid (FAs), 6, 7, 10, 156, 172, 189, 190, 206, 210, 239, 240, 270, 297–301, 304–306
content, 301, 303
exposure, 305
fish, 301
streak, 223
Fenugreek seeds, 241
Fermentation, 170
Fermented
red ginseng, 187
soy, 154
Fever, 88, 92, 169, 179, 181
Fiber, 56, 168, 170
Fire-fighter aged garlic extract research, 77
Fish oil, 6, 177, 186
supplements, 6, 186
Flavanols, 95
Flaviola health study, 276
Flavone, 311, 318, 320
Flavonoids, 9, 13, 18, 38, 85, 86, 89, 98, 140, 167, 169, 206–208, 221, 223, 239, 241, 245, 246, 251, 267, 275, 278, 279, 287, 311–321
Flavonols, 313
Flax seed, 10, 154, 156
Foam cell formation, 111
Folic acid, 7, 17, 76, 158, 242, 251, 277, 298
Food
and Drug Administration (FDA), 7
groups, 56
supplements, 161
Fragile red blood cells, 108
Framingham
heart offspring study, 124, 282
risk, 76, 78
factors, 76
Frank-starling mechanism, 33
Free radicals, 183
Fruits and vegetables, 5, 104
Functional
fiber, 170
food, 3–7, 11, 18, 29, 42, 235, 245, 267
Fusobacterium, 58

G

Gallate, 95
Gallocatechin, 94
Garlic, 11, 38, 70–73, 78–80, 159, 177, 187, 234, 283
  formulations, 71, 74, 79, 284
  groups, 74
  ingestion, 283
  supplementation, 70
Gas chromatography (GC), 222, 229
Gastrointestinal
  intolerances, 78
  tract (GIT), 54, 155, 172
Gender, 31
Genetics, 3, 31, 121
Genistein, 318
GID-spirulina, 272
Ginger, 11, 86, 88, 242, 243, 250
  derived terpenes, 242
  pickle, 250
Gingerenone-A, 243
Ginseng, 177, 186
Glutamic
  oxaloacetic transaminase (GOT), 209
  pyruvic transaminase (GPT), 209
Glutathione
  peroxidase (GPx), 170, 203, 227
  reductase (GRx), 170, 203, 207, 211
  s-transferase (GST), 203, 207, 211
Google, 69
Grain, 56
Grape, 169
  seeds, 275
Green
  leafy vegetables, 108
  tea, 9, 85, 86, 88, 89, 92, 93, 95–97, 154, 155, 159, 168, 177, 188, 275, 277
Guava, 56

H

Haptoglobin 2–2 genotype, 111
Harappa, 236
Health
  benefits, 3, 5, 6, 10–14, 29, 30, 54, 86, 89, 97, 122, 125, 151–153, 155, 204, 206, 245, 248, 269
  characters, 89
  systems, 29
Healthier tea, 88, 89
Healthy
  eating habits, 184
  lifestyle, 62
Heart, 32, 34, 76, 109, 121, 122, 152, 178, 181
  attack, 178, 181
  disease, 77, 121, 122
  disorders, 152
  failure with preserved ejection fraction (HFpEF), 32
Hemorrhagic stroke, 31
Herbal drugs, 235
High
  blood
    lipid levels, 128, 143
    pressure, 268, 279
  density
    lipids (HDL), 52
    lipoprotein (HDL), 9, 56, 273, 274, 304
  fructose diets, 205
  performance liquid chromatography (HPLC), 315
Himanthalia elongate, 318
Histidine, 160
Honeybee, 201
Hormones, 77
Human
  beings, 297
  clinical trials, 69
  trials, 98, 278
  umbilical vein
    endothelial cells (HUVECs), 207
    phospholipase C (HUVECs), 206
Hydrocharitaceae, 312, 320
  family, 320
Hydroquinone, 86, 89
Hydroxybenzoic derivatives, 169
Hydroxyl radicals, 316
Hypercholesterolemia, 32, 34, 69, 74, 80, 128, 180, 183, 208, 238, 274
Hyperlipidemia, 52
Hypertension, 4, 10, 16, 27, 31, 32, 34, 38, 39, 41, 52, 56, 60, 61, 69–74, 80, 108, 122–124, 127–129, 131, 139, 157, 167, 168, 172, 173, 180, 182, 184, 186, 187, 189, 191, 207, 208, 221, 223, 225, 228, 229, 238, 240, 252, 269, 272, 273, 276, 284, 287, 289, 299

Hypertensive patients, 73, 74, 77, 245, 272, 299
Hypnea spinella, 318

I

Immunomodulatory, 97, 319
  activity, 319
In vitro, 126, 127, 140
Industrial biotechnology, 320
Inflammation, 6, 8, 9, 15, 16, 39, 52, 77, 121, 123, 128, 143, 144, 152, 170, 172, 179, 191, 202, 205, 207, 208, 227, 235, 269, 272, 273, 287, 299, 303–306
Insoluble fiber, 55
Insulin sensitization, 247
Interferon-gamma (IFN-γ), 243
Interleukin-6 (IL-6), 155, 243, 248, 271, 272
Intimal damage, 34
Ipomoea obscura, 234, 237, 247, 249
Iron, 6, 185
Ischemic, 4, 7, 17, 31, 36, 110, 128, 180, 182, 188, 189, 202, 235, 278
  heart disease, 4, 143, 203
  stroke, 31
Isoflavones, 13, 221
Isomerization, 142
Isoorientin, 318
  2′O rhamnoside, 86, 89
Isovitexin, 318

J

Jaggery, 250, 252
Japanese
  garlic preparation, 74
  knotweed, 275
Jaundice, 242, 248
Juncaceae, 312
Junctional connectivity, 145
Juncus acutus L., 316
Junk food, 4
  consumption, 28

K

Kaempferol, 86, 89, 95, 160, 207, 245, 314, 318, 319
  glucoside, 245
Karkkidaka kanji, 234, 236–239, 247, 252
Karuka, 234, 237, 247
Kayyonni, 234, 237, 247
Kerala, 4, 233–237, 249–252
  sadhya, 234, 236, 249–252
Kidney
  disease, 202, 208
  disorders, 157
  function markers, 209
  oxidized glutathione, 186
Krebs cycle activity, 157
Kwai garlic powder (KB GP), 73–75, 187
Kyolic brand aged garlic extract (KB AGE), 73–78, 80
  formulation, 76

L

Lactic acid bacteria (LAB), 54
Lactobacillus, 58, 172
Lactococcus lactis subsp. biovar, 59
L-arginine, 7, 72, 76, 207
Left ventricular (LV), 32, 124, 225, 273, 282
  ejection fraction (LVEF), 32
Legumes, 5, 7, 16, 55, 169, 221, 240, 274
Lemongrass, 86, 88, 89, 92
Lentils, 56
Leukocyte adherence, 33
L-gulonolactone oxidase, 109
Lignans, 10, 13, 156, 169, 221–223, 239, 246, 275
Lignin, 55, 96, 170
Lipid, 8, 11, 29, 34, 52, 60, 61, 71, 93, 96, 127, 143, 155, 157, 183, 203, 206, 208, 225, 252, 267, 273, 300, 320
  peroxidation, 103, 108, 111, 126, 128, 188, 205, 246, 269
  profile, 6–8, 12, 13, 40, 130, 154, 155, 225, 238, 248, 277
Lipoxins (LXs), 304
Lipoxygenase (LOX), 11, 183, 305, 319, 248
  activity, 248
Liver, 104, 108, 209
Low-density
  lipid (LDL), 7–16, 39–41, 52, 55, 57–59, 61, 70, 78, 110, 112, 126–129, 140, 143–145, 154, 155, 157, 161, 169, 172, 183, 188–190, 203, 205, 206, 208, 210, 239, 240, 242, 244–246, 248, 273, 275, 277, 285, 286, 304, 305, 319
    breakdown, 127

concentration, 242
elimination, 127
levels, 8, 155, 244
protein oxidation, 190
lipoprotein (LDL), 3, 5, 17, 55, 140, 147, 156, 162, 179, 183, 187, 188, 203, 211, 228, 241, 246, 253, 274
cholesterol (LDL-C) receptors, 5, 7, 8, 10, 12, 14, 16, 17, 39–41, 52, 58, 59, 61, 78, 127–129, 143, 145, 179, 188, 208, 210, 239, 244, 246, 248, 273, 285, 286, 305
oxidation, 8, 9, 12, 13, 15, 57, 110, 126, 129, 154, 161, 169, 188, 240, 245, 275
receptor, 127, 155
L-tryptophan-rich, 241
Lucenin, 318
Luteolin, 86, 89, 206, 314, 316
Lycopene, 13, 14, 41, 121–132, 139–147, 171, 267, 282, 283, 287

M

Macrophage scavenger receptors, 111
Major royal jelly proteins (MRJP 1–9), 209, 210
Malnutrition, 152, 251
Marfan syndrome (MFS), 37, 38
Marine
flavonoids, 312, 317, 320
sources, 312, 318
Matcha, 89, 95
Medicinal
chemistry, 321
plants, 234, 237
value, 88, 89
Mediterranean diets, 16, 167
Meta-analysis, 8, 14, 73–75, 77, 78, 145, 188, 244, 276–278, 284
Metabolic health, 86
Metabolism, 8, 13, 15, 54–56, 59–61, 70, 108, 109, 123, 131, 132, 145, 157, 180, 203, 204, 208–210, 238, 240, 243, 244, 247, 284, 286, 287, 300, 305, 319
Metal binding proteins, 171
Metalloproteinases (MMPs), 157, 207, 227, 316
Methyl allyl trisulfide (MATS), 283
Mitogen-activated protein kinase (MAPK), 243
Monocytes, 111
Monounsaturated fats (MUFAs), 7, 154, 156, 298
Mortality, 3, 9, 17, 18, 31, 35, 52, 55, 60, 74, 76, 79, 109, 111, 131, 140, 143, 145, 156, 178, 181, 188, 189, 202, 225, 238, 239, 252
Mung bean, 234, 240
protein, 240
Mushrooms, 10, 104
Mutagens, 111
Myocardial infarction, 6, 8, 9, 34, 74, 76, 111, 123, 124, 127, 171, 181, 203–205, 277, 281, 282, 284
Myricetin, 160, 318

N

N acetyl cysteine (NAC), 80, 154, 157, 158, 171
Nannochloropsis gaditana, 318
Nano-formulations, 144
Nanotechnology, 132
Natural
medicinal value, 98
sources, 268
Necrosis, 36
Niacin, 154, 159
Niemann-pick C1 Like 1 (NPC1L1), 285
Nitella hookeri, 312, 318
Nitric oxide (NO), 9, 11, 15, 38, 110, 111, 127, 129, 156, 172, 183, 187, 189, 203, 205, 207–209, 211, 227, 229, 239, 243, 245, 248, 272, 273, 278–280, 299, 319
bioavailability, 208, 239
generation, 129
synthase (NOS), 207, 208, 248
Njavara
grains, 238
rice, 237, 238
bran oil, 238
NOD- like receptor family (NLRP), 243
Non-communicable disease (NCD), 4, 28, 233, 279
Nuclear factor-kappa B (NF-kB), 112, 206, 211, 272, 243, 247

Nutraceutical, 3, 4, 27–30, 38, 41, 42, 51, 69, 85, 103, 121, 122, 139, 140, 142, 151, 152, 154, 156, 160, 162, 167, 168, 172, 173, 177, 201, 202, 204, 221, 233, 236, 239, 245, 249, 267, 268, 287, 289, 297, 311, 314
  compound, 142
Nutrient-rich foods, 267
Nutritional, 267, 287
  aspects, 267
  supplements, 287
Nuts, 3, 5, 7, 16–18, 104, 156, 250, 267, 286, 298

O

Oats, 56
Ocimum sanctum, 86, 90, 98
O-glucosides, 313
Omega 3 fatty acid (Ω3FAs), 6, 7, 17, 39, 41, 140, 154–156, 177, 189, 190, 297–305
Omega-6 fatty acid, 300
Onion stalk extract, 246
Online platform, 112, 173, 229
Oolong tea, 86
Orientin, 318
Oryza sativa, 234, 237, 253
Osmundea pinnatifida, 318
Oxidative
  damage, 182
  stress reduction, 7
  vulnerability, 7
Oxidized LDL (oxLDL), 6, 39, 41, 156, 203, 206–209, 242
  mediated apoptosis, 206

P

Panax, 186
Panchakarma, 237
Pantetheine, 159
Pantethine, 154, 157
Patent ductus arteriosus (PDA), 36
P-coumaric acid, 245
Peaches, 56
Peas, 56
Pedaliaceae, 156
Penimethavone, 316
Pepper, 246
Peptostreptococcus, 58
Peripheral
  arterial disease (PAD), 123, 179, 182
  vascular disease (PVD), 171, 182, 281
pH range, 93
Pharmacological agents, 52
Phenolic compounds, 5–7, 10, 13, 86, 89, 124, 143, 158, 211, 240, 242, 275, 278, 282
Phosphorus, 6
Phycocyanin, 270
Phycocyanobilin, 271
Physical
  exams, 35
  inactivity, 235
Physiological antioxidants, 171
Phytochemicals, 12
Phytoestrogens, 13
Phytosterol, 5, 7, 8, 12, 39, 154, 155, 267, 285–287, 289
  ingestion, 286
Piper nigrum, 234, 237, 246
Piperine, 246, 247
Plant
  derived flavonoids, 13
  stanol, 14, 39
  sterols, 14, 15, 39
Plantation, 87
Plaque stability, 77
Platelet aggregation, 187
Pleiotropic effects, 228
Polyhydroxylated, 312
Polyphenol, 7, 9, 10, 13, 15, 17, 93, 96, 97, 140, 168, 173, 179, 202, 206, 208, 221–223, 225, 227–229, 250, 267, 270, 274–277, 279, 287, 289, 317, 319
  subtypes, 221
Polyphenolic
  compound, 319
  constituents, 86
Polyunsaturated fatty acid (PUFA), 7, 16, 168, 172, 173, 185, 192, 298, 300, 302–306
Pomegranate, 154, 158
  juice, 154
Portfolio diet, 17
Post-menopausal women, 7, 11, 13

Potassium, 6, 93
Prebiotics, 13, 139, 168, 172, 173, 202
Probiotics, 51–55, 58–62, 139, 140, 167, 168, 171–173
Propolis, 206, 207, 211
Protein, 96, 203
Protopanaxadiol (PPD), 186
Pulmonary stenosis, 36
Pulse, 56
  wave velocity (PWV), 69, 70, 77, 78, 80, 276, 277

Q

Quality, 73, 74, 130, 167, 168, 185, 233
Quercetin, 41, 86, 89, 95, 207, 245, 246, 314–316, 318, 319
  glucosides, 245
Quotation, 85

R

Randomized controlled trials, 190, 276–278
Raw cocoa powder, 10
Reactive oxygen species (ROS), 6, 14, 39, 70, 80, 127, 128, 132, 140, 143, 147, 152, 159, 183, 186, 190, 192, 203, 205–209, 211, 227, 228, 239, 243, 275, 279, 289, 315, 321
  generation, 127, 205, 208
  levels, 239, 275
  production, 205, 207, 209
  regulating enzymes, 186
Recommended
  dietary allowances, 108
  dose, 154
Red ginseng extract (RGE), 187
Redox reactions, 109, 111
Reduced dilatation, 299
Renin-angiotensin system, 241
Retinol, 108, 111
Rhabdomyosarcoma (RD), 316, 321
Rheumatic heart disease (RHD), 31, 32, 56, 178, 179, 181, 192
Rhizome, 88, 92
Rhodomelaceae, 312
Rice, 56, 237, 251, 252
  bran, 56
Rickets, 108
Risk
  assessment, 77
  factor, 61
Rotterdam study, 144
Royal jelly (RJ), 201, 204, 209–211

S

Saffron, 41, 169
Salicornia herbacea, 316
S-allyl cysteine (SAC), 72, 245
  sulfoxide, 72, 245
S-allylmercaptocysteine (SAM), 72
Sardar Bhagwan Singh University, 51, 151, 297
Sargassum
  pallidum, 318
  vulgare, 318
Saturated fatty acids FAs, 298
Scutellarein, 318
Sesame, 154, 156
Sesame, 156
Short-chain fatty acid (SCFA), 58, 60, 239
Signal transducer, and activators of transcription (STAT), 243
Signaling molecule, 111, 157, 284
S-methylcysteine, 246
Smooth muscle
  cell, 34
    proliferation, 111
  relaxant, 97
Soluble fiber, 7, 8, 55, 59–61
Soy, 155, 278
  isoflavones, 278
  proteins, 5, 8
Spices, 168, 169, 246
Spirulina, 40, 41, 267–274, 287–289
  maxima, 40, 273, 274
  platensis, 272, 274
Spontaneously hypertensive rats (SHRs), 241, 271
Stilbenes, 222, 223
Streptococcal bacteria, 179, 181
Streptomyces, 313
Stroke, 4, 9, 28, 31, 37, 38, 40, 72, 74, 110, 111, 123, 124, 129, 171, 180, 182, 186, 188, 189, 202, 234, 240, 277, 281, 282
Sung dynasty, 85
Superoxide dismutase (SOD), 124, 170, 203, 211, 227, 243, 283

Supplement, 42, 72, 79, 88, 109, 111, 131, 154, 178, 184, 185, 189, 209
Supraventricular tachycardia (SVT), 37
Systemic arterial hypertension (SAH), 273, 289

T

T lymphocytes, 31, 129
Tamaricaceae, 312
Taxifolin, 221
Testosterone (T), 210
Tetraselmis suecica, 318
Theaceae, 86
Theaflavins (TF), 86, 95, 98, 275
Theobroma cacao, 275
Therapeutic
  potential, 226
  value, 98, 152
Thrombin, 314, 315
Thrombosis, 33
Thromboxanes (TX), 172, 303, 304
Thrombus propagation, 34
Tolerance, 74, 189, 243
Toll-like receptor (TLR), 243
Tomato
  based products, 122, 132, 139, 140, 142
  fruit, 142
  products, 123
  supplementation, 124
Topical preparations, 86
Total cholesterol (TC), 6, 8, 10–12, 15, 16, 39, 40, 70, 74, 75, 80, 157, 203, 205, 208, 210, 239–241, 244, 269, 274, 277, 304
  levels, 304
Traditional
  food, 233, 236
  knowledge, 236
Transglutaminase (TG), 39, 129, 155, 157, 205, 206, 210, 244
Triacylglycerol (TAG), 52, 59
Triglyceride (TG), 7, 11, 12, 39, 41, 52, 70, 128, 132, 143, 154, 156, 162, 172, 190, 202, 203, 239–241, 244, 246, 304, 305
  levels (TG), 190, 203, 239, 304
Trigonella foenum-graceum, 234, 237, 241
Triticum aestivum L., 234, 237, 238
Tulsi, 86, 88, 92
Tumor necrosis factor (TNF), 155, 162, 206, 243, 248, 272
  alpha (TNF-α), 206, 243, 248, 272
Turmeric, 38, 40, 88, 89, 169, 170, 249, 250, 252
  curcumin, 41

U

Ubiquinol, 111
United States, 32, 52, 53, 123, 184, 185
Unsaturated fatty acids, 7, 10, 156, 158
Uric acid, 243
Urinary tract infections (UTI), 158
US Department of Agriculture (USDA), 300
Uzhinja, 234, 237, 247

V

Valvular
  activity, 13
  cell adhesion
    molecule (VCAM), 157, 223
    protein 1 (VCAM-1), 31
  heart disease (VHD), 32
  smooth muscle, 6, 14, 39, 41, 110, 225, 245, 281
  system, 16, 31, 178
Vasoconstriction, 12, 127, 190, 225, 245
Vasorelaxation, 9, 187, 207, 272
Vegetarian diet, 17
Ventricular
  fibrillation (VF), 37, 205
  tachycardia (VT), 37
Veratrum grandiflorum, 157
Vernonia cinerea, 234, 237, 247, 249
Very low-density lipoprotein (VLDL), 241, 304
Vigna radiata, 234, 237, 240
Virchow triad, 33
Viscous fibers, 17
Vitamin, 5, 6, 29, 40, 58, 71, 93, 95, 103–105, 108, 110–112, 124, 130, 140, 143, 158, 167, 179, 184, 191, 206, 234, 236, 250–252, 267, 270, 279, 282, 298, 320
  A, 108, 109
  B3, 154
  C, 39, 41, 96, 109, 110, 154, 159, 171, 177, 190
    level, 190
  D, 39, 41, 171, 281
    receptor (VDR), 39

E, 6, 14, 39, 41, 110, 111, 177, 190, 191
forms, 111
supplements, 111
Vitexin, 318

W

Walnuts, 7
Watermelon, 142
Water-soluble fiber, 55, 60
Western countries, 86, 300
Wheat, 56, 108, 238, 239
bran (WB), 56, 239, 240
foods, 238
White
adipose tissue, 243
tea, 89
Whole grains, 8
World Health Organization (WHO), 4, 28, 31, 32, 34, 52, 123, 178, 201, 202, 234, 253, 268, 289
Wound infections, 158

X

Xanthine, 183, 227, 243, 247
oxidase, 183, 227, 243, 247
enzyme activity, 247
Xenobiotics, 169

Y

Yeast, 171
Yellow plantains, 250
Yogurt, 172
Younger population, 4

Z

Zinc, 17, 71, 185, 251, 252
Zingerone, 243
Zingiber officinale, 86, 98, 234, 237
Zoology, 233
Zosteraceae, 312